D0912990

Trauma and Emergency Radiology

Editor

STEPHAN W. ANDERSON

RADIOLOGIC CLINICS OF NORTH AMERICA

www.radiologic.theclinics.com

Consulting Editor
FRANK H. MILLER

July 2019 • Volume 57 • Number 4

ELSEVIER

1600 John F. Kennedy Boulevard • Suite 1800 • Philadelphia, Pennsylvania, 19103-2899

http://www.theclinics.com

RADIOLOGIC CLINICS OF NORTH AMERICA Volume 57, Number 4
July 2019 ISSN 0033-8389, ISBN 13: 978-0-323-67833-9

Editor: John Vassallo (j.vassallo@elsevier.com)
Developmental Editor: Donald Mumford

Radiologic Clinics of North America (ISSN 0033-8389) is published bimonthly by Elsevier Inc., 360 Park Avenue South, New York, NY 10010-1710. Months of issue are January, March, May, July, September, and November. Periodicals postage paid at New York, NY and additional mailing offices. Subscription prices are USD 508 per year for US individuals, USD 933 per year for US institutions, USD 100 per year for US students and residents, USD 594 per year for Canadian individuals, USD 1193 per year for Canadian institutions, USD 683 per year for international individuals, USD 1193 per year for international institutions, and USD 315 per year for Canadian and international students/residents. To receive student and resident rate, orders must be accompanied by name of affiliated institution, date of term and the signature of program/residency coordinatior on institution letterhead. Orders will be billed at individual rate until proof of status is received. Foreign air speed delivery is included in all *Clinics* subscription prices. All prices are subject to change without notice. **POSTMASTER:** Send address changes to *Radiologic Clinics of North America*, Elsevier Health Sciences Division, Subscription Customer Service, 3251 Riverport Lane, Maryland Heights, MO63043. **Customer Service: Telephone: 1-800-654-2452** (U.S. and Canada); **1-314-447-8871** (outside U.S. and Canada). **Fax: 1-314-447-8029. E-mail: journalscustomerservice-usa@elsevier.com (for print support); journalsonlinesupport-usa@elsevier.com (for online support).**

Reprints. For copies of 100 or more of articles in this publication, please contact the Commercial Reprints Department, Elsevier Inc., 360 Park Avenue South, New York, New York 10010-1710. Tel.: +1-212-633-3874; Fax: +1-212-633-3820; E-mail: reprints@elsevier.com.

Radiologic Clinics of North America also published in Greek Paschalidis Medical Publications, Athens, Greece.

Radiologic Clinics of North America is covered in *MEDLINE/PubMed (Index Medicus), EMBASE/Excerpta Medica, Current Contents/Life Sciences, Current Contents/Clinical Medicine, RSNA Index to Imaging Literature, BIOSIS, Science Citation Index,* and *ISI/BIOMED.*

Printed in the United States of America.

Contributors

CONSULTING EDITOR

FRANK H. MILLER, MD, FACR
Lee F. Rogers MD Professor of Medical
Education, Chief, Body Imaging Section and
Fellowship Program, Medical Director, MRI,
Department of Radiology, Northwestern
Memorial Hospital, Northwestern University
Feinberg School of Medicine, Chicago, Illinois,
USA

EDITOR

STEPHAN W. ANDERSON, MD
Professor, Department of Radiology, Boston
University Medical Campus, Boston,
Massachusetts, USA

AUTHORS

ZOHAIB Y. AHMAD, MD
Resident Physician, Department of
Radiology, Boston University Medical
Center, Boston, Massachusetts,
USA

ARMONDE A. BAGHDANIAN, MD
Assistant Professor, Department of Radiology,
University of San Francisco, San Francisco,
California, USA

ARTHUR H. BAGHDANIAN, MD
Assistant Professor, Department of Radiology,
University of San Francisco, San Francisco,
California, USA

ALEXANDER B. BAXTER, MD
NYU Langone Health/Bellevue Hospital, New
York, New York, USA

NICHOLAS M. BECKMANN, MD
Department of Diagnostic and Interventional
Imaging, McGovern Medical School,
The University of Texas Health Science
Center at Houston, Houston, Texas,
USA

MARK P. BERNSTEIN, MD
NYU Langone Health/Bellevue Hospital, New
York, New York, USA

SARAH BIXBY, MD
Associate Professor, Department of
Radiology, Boston Children's Hospital,
Boston, Massachusetts, USA

NAGA R. CHINAPUVVULA, MD
Department of Diagnostic and Interventional
Imaging, McGovern Medical School,
The University of Texas Health Science
Center at Houston, Houston, Texas,
USA

MARIZA O. CLEMENT, MD, MSE
Assistant Professor, Department of
Radiology, Boston Medical Center, Boston
University, Boston, Massachusetts,
USA

MATTHEW DIAMOND, MD
Resident, Department of Radiology, Boston
Medical Center, Boston, Massachusetts,
USA

DAVID DREIZIN, MD
Assistant Professor, Department of Diagnostic
Radiology and Nuclear Medicine, R Adams
Cowley Shock Trauma Center, University of
Maryland School of Medicine, Baltimore,
Maryland, USA

MICHAEL P. GEORGE, MD, MFA
Instructor, Department of Radiology, Boston
Children's Hospital, Boston, Massachusetts,
USA

SHAHMIR KAMALIAN, MD
Instructor, Department of Radiology, Director
of the Emergency Radiology CT, Division of
Emergency Radiology, Massachusetts General
Hospital, Harvard Medical School, Boston,
Massachusetts, USA

GENE KIM, MD
Radiology Resident, Department of Radiology,
Boston Medical Center, Boston University
School of Medicine, Boston, Massachusetts,
USA

CHRISTINA A. LeBEDIS, MD
Associate Professor, Department of Radiology,
Boston Medical Center, Boston,
Massachusetts, USA

JOHN LEE, MD
Resident, Department of Radiology, Boston
Medical Center, Boston, Massachusetts, USA

MICHAEL H. LEV, MD, FAHA, FACR
Professor, Department of Radiology, Chief,
Division of Emergency Radiology,
Massachusetts General Hospital, Harvard
Medical School, Boston, Massachusetts, USA

NICOLAS MURRAY, MD, FRCPC
Emergency and Trauma Radiology, Vancouver
General Hospital, Vancouver, Canada

JASON W. NASCONE, MD
Associate Professor, Department of
Orthopaedics, University of Maryland School
of Medicine, R Adams Cowley Shock Trauma
Center, Baltimore, Maryland, USA

HRISTINA NATCHEVA, MD
Assistant Professor, Department of Radiology,
Boston Medical Center, Boston University
School of Medicine, Boston, Massachusetts,
USA

SAVVAS NICOLAOU, MD, FRCPC
Professor of Radiology, Emergency and
Trauma Radiology, Vancouver General
Hospital, Vancouver, Canada

SADIA R. QAMAR, MBBS
Emergency and Trauma Radiology, Vancouver
General Hospital, Vancouver, Canada

LATIFA SANHAJI, MD
Department of Diagnostic and Interventional
Imaging, McGovern Medical School, The
University of Texas Health Science Center at
Houston, Houston, Texas, USA

CLINT W. SLIKER, MD
Associate Professor, Department of Diagnostic
Radiology and Nuclear Medicine, Division of
Emergency and Trauma Imaging, University of
Maryland Medical Center, Baltimore,
Maryland, USA

JENNIFER W. UYEDA, MD
Assistant Professor, Department of Radiology,
Brigham and Women's Hospital, Boston,
Massachusetts, USA

O. CLARK WEST, MD
Department of Diagnostic and Interventional
Imaging, McGovern Medical School, The
University of Texas Health Science Center at
Houston, Houston, Texas, USA

YUHAO WU, MD
Faculty of Medicine, University of British
Columbia, Emergency and Trauma Radiology,
Vancouver General Hospital, Vancouver,
Canada

MATTHEW G. YOUNG, DO
NYU Langone Health/Bellevue Hospital,
New York, New York, USA

Contents

Damage control surgery is a staged surgical procedure in a patient who has suffered penetrating or blunt abdominal traumatic injury with severe metabolic derangements. Multidetector computed tomography scanning is a vital tool for patient management in the damage control patient, providing many uses, including assessing the extent of traumatic injury, evaluating areas that were not surgically explored, evaluating for injuries that were missed during the initial surgery, and assessing the stability of surgical repair. Understanding the postsurgical multidetector computed tomography appearance of these patients can aid the radiologist in protocol optimization and provide immediate accurate diagnoses.

Imaging evaluation of small bowel obstruction (SBO) is essential for determining the appropriate clinical treatment for a patient. The current recommendations for the evaluation of SBO, including protocols, are reviewed. A method for evaluating SBO including the criteria for diagnosis, finding the transition point, determining the cause, and identifying the presence of ischemia is discussed.

Acute abdominopelvic pain, a common symptom in emergency department patients, is challenging given the spectrum of differential diagnoses encompassing multiple organ systems, ranging from benign self-limiting to life-threatening and emergent. Diagnostic imaging is critical given its high accuracy and management guidance. A contrast-enhanced computed tomography (CT) scan is preferred given its widespread availability and speed of acquisition. MR imaging may be appropriate, usually performed for specific indications with tailored protocols. It is accurate for diagnosis and may be an alternative to CT. This article discusses the advantages and disadvantages, protocols, and appearances of MR imaging of common diagnoses.

Stroke is the clinical syndrome of acute onset of neurologic deficit caused by ischemia or hemorrhage. Neuroimaging has a crucial role in differentiating ischemic from hemorrhagic stroke. Advanced neuroimaging has become essential in the management of patients with acute ischemic stroke mainly because of improved awareness of the imaging findings and their role in patient selection for novel treatment options as highlighted in recent clinical trials, including "late window"

(8–24 hours post ictus!) intra-arterial thrombectomy. This article focuses on the role of neuroimaging in the management of patients with acute ischemic stroke.

Conventional imaging in the acute setting of brain trauma, relevant pathophysiology of injury, and advanced imaging techniques that may provide value in understanding the immediate management and long-term sequela of traumatic brain injury are reviewed. Key imaging findings that can guide clinical management related to such injuries as concussions, hematomas, dissections, dural atrioventricular fistula, and diffuse axonal injury are discussed. The role and accuracy of computed tomography, dual-energy computed tomography, computed tomography angiography, and magnetic resonance angiography in the acute setting are evaluated. In addition, caveats related to imaging the elderly and pediatric population are addressed.

The neck visceral space is a complex region housing several vital structures. Diagnostic imaging plays an important role in the evaluation of neck visceral injuries. Many injuries are initially missed by both clinicians and radiologists because of their infrequency and the high likelihood of other more obvious injuries. Understanding which diagnostic modality to apply at given point in the work-up; recognizing relevant clinical signs, symptoms, and injury mechanisms; and knowing pertinent direct and indirect imaging findings of injury allow radiologists to either directly render the correct diagnosis or choose the most appropriate tool for doing so.

Every year in North America, approximately 3 million patients are evaluated for spinal injury. Of blunt trauma patients presenting to the emergency department, 3% to 4% will have a cervical spine injury, and up to 18% will suffer a thoracolumbar spine injury. Failure to identify an unstable spine injury can lead to devastating outcomes.

Cardiovascular injuries represent the second most common cause of death among trauma victims in the United States. Motor vehicle collisions account for more than 80% of all blunt thoracic trauma. Given the nonspecific nature and variable severity of presenting symptoms, such as chest pain and shortness of breath, as well as confounding and overlapping clinical presentations in the setting of additional injuries, diagnosis of cardiovascular injuries can be challenging. This article reviews the clinical entities of acute aortic syndrome and pulmonary embolism, their imaging findings, and diagnostic challenges.

Cardiac trauma carries high mortality rates and should be considered in all patients presenting with chest trauma. These patients can have a wide range of clinical presentations, from being asymptomatic to being in hemodynamic collapse. Currently, multidetector computed tomography is the gold-standard diagnostic imaging modality for all patients with abnormal electrocardiogram and/or Troponin I levels following chest trauma. In this article, we discuss pathophysiology of cardiac trauma, review the role of medical imaging, and present the spectrum of abnormal findings in traumatic cardiac injuries.

Shoulder girdle trauma is one of the most common injuries encountered in emergency centers. These injuries can be easily overlooked due to the complex osteology of the shoulder. Although radiographs are usually sufficient for assessing traumatic shoulder injuries, cross-sectional imaging is sometimes indicated to assess portions of the shoulder not well visualized by radiographs. In this article, the authors review the spectrum of shoulder girdle injuries: sternoclavicular dislocations, clavicle fractures, acromioclavicular separations, shoulder dislocations, scapula fractures, and scapulothoracic dissociation. They also discuss the presentation, imaging evaluation, and classification of these injuries with emphasis on pitfalls in imaging diagnosis and indications for computed tomography/magnetic resonance.

Acetabular fractures are encountered by radiologists in a wide spectrum of practice settings. The radiologist's value in the acute and long-term management of acetabular fractures is augmented by familiarity with systematic computed tomography–based algorithms that streamline and simplify Judet-Letournel fracture typing, together with an appreciation of the role of imaging in initial triage, operative decision making, postoperative assessment, prognostication, and evaluation of complications. The steep increase in incidence of acetabular fractures in the elderly over the past several decades places special emphasis on familiarity with geriatric fracture patterns.

Missed fractures are common in pediatric trauma patients. Pediatric bone differs from adult bone in its composition and response to injury, leading to fracture patterns that may be subtle, radiographically unfamiliar, and challenging to distinguish from normal variation. Familiarity with the unique fracture types of the pediatric skeleton and site-specific injury patterns is critical, because prompt diagnosis can significantly alter clinical management and outcome. This article examines the unique features of pediatric bone contributing to missed fractures, the incidence of missed fractures, common injury types of the pediatric skeleton, and frequently missed site-specific fracture patterns, highlighting problem-solving techniques for challenging cases.

RADIOLOGIC CLINICS OF NORTH AMERICA

FORTHCOMING ISSUES

September 2019
Imaging of the Upper Limb
Giuseppe Guglielmi and Alberto Bazzocchi,
Editors

November 2019
Neuroradiology
Jacqueline A. Bello and Shira E. Slasky, *Editors*

January 2020
**Imaging the ICU Patient or Hospitalized
Patient**
Travis Henry and Vincent Mellnick, *Editors*

RECENT ISSUES

May 2019
Ultrasound
Jason M. Wagner, *Editor*

March 2019
Topics in Spine Imaging
Lubdha M. Shah, *Editor*

January 2019
Cardiac CT Imaging
Suhny Abbara and Prabhakar Rajiah, *Editors*

RELATED SERIES

Magnetic Resonance Imaging Clinics
Neuroimaging Clinics
PET Clinics

THE CLINICS ARE AVAILABLE ONLINE!
Access your subscription at:
www.theclinics.com

PROGRAM OBJECTIVE

The objective of the *Radiologic Clinics of North America* is to keep practicing radiologists and radiology residents up to date with current clinical practice in radiology by providing timely articles reviewing the state of the art in patient care.

TARGET AUDIENCE

Practicing radiologists, radiology residents, and other healthcare professionals who provide patient care utilizing radiologic findings.

LEARNING OBJECTIVES

Upon completion of this activity, participants will be able to:
1. Review the role of medical imaging in traumatic cardiac injury, traumatic brain injury, and spine trauma.
2. Discuss the role of neuroimaging in the management of patients with acute ischemic stroke
3. Recognize advantages and disadvantage of MR imaging in evaluating acute abdominopelvic pain in the emergency setting.

ACCREDITATION

The Elsevier Office of Continuing Medical Education (EOCME) is accredited by the Accreditation Council for Continuing Medical Education (ACCME) to provide continuing medical education for physicians.

The EOCME designates this enduring material for a maximum of 15 *AMA PRA Category 1 Credit*(s)™. Physicians should claim only the credit commensurate with the extent of their participation in the activity.

All other healthcare professionals requesting continuing education credit for this enduring material will be issued a certificate of participation.

DISCLOSURE OF CONFLICTS OF INTEREST

The EOCME assesses conflict of interest with its instructors, faculty, planners, and other individuals who are in a position to control the content of CME activities. All relevant conflicts of interest that are identified are thoroughly vetted by EOCME for fair balance, scientific objectivity, and patient care recommendations. EOCME is committed to providing its learners with CME activities that promote improvements or quality in healthcare and not a specific proprietary business or a commercial interest.

The planning committee, staff, authors and editors listed below have identified no financial relationships or relationships to products or devices they or their spouse/life partner have with commercial interest related to the content of this CME activity:
Zohaib Y. Ahmad, MD; Stephan W. Anderson, MD; Armonde A. Baghdanian, MD; Arthur H. Baghdanian, MD; Alexander B. Baxter, MD; Nicholas M. Beckmann, MD; Mark P. Bernstein, MD; Sarah Bixby, MD; Naga R. Chinapuvvula, MD; Mariza O. Clement, MD, MSE; Matthew Diamond, MD; David Dreizin, MD; Michael P. George, MD, MFA; Shahmir Kamalian, MD; Alison Kemp; Gene Kim, MD; Pradeep Kuttysankaran; Christina A. LeBedis, MD; John Lee, MD; Frank H. Miller, MD, FACR; Nicolas Murray, MD, FRCPC; Jason W. Nascone, MD; Hristina Natcheva, MD; Savvas Nicolaou, MD, FRCPC; Sadia R. Qamar, MBBS; Latifa Sanhaji, MD; Clint W. Sliker, MD; Jennifer W. Uyeda, MD; John Vassallo; O. Clark West, MD; Yuhao Wu, MD; Matthew G. Young, DO.

The planning committee, staff, authors and editors listed below have identified financial relationships or relationships to products or devices they or their spouse/life partner have with commercial interest related to the content of this CME activity:
Michael H. Lev, MD, FAHA, FACR: is a consultant/advisor for General Electric Company and Takeda Pharmaceutical Company Limited.

UNAPPROVED/OFF-LABEL USE DISCLOSURE

The EOCME requires CME faculty to disclose to the participants:
1. When products or procedures being discussed are off-label, unlabelled, experimental, and/or investigational (not US Food and Drug Administration [FDA] approved); and
2. Any limitations on the information presented, such as data that are preliminary or that represent ongoing research, interim analyses, and/or unsupported opinions. Faculty may discuss information about pharmaceutical agents that is outside of FDA-approved labelling. This information is intended solely for CME and is not intended to promote off-label use of these medications. If you have any questions, contact the medical affairs department of the manufacturer for the most recent prescribing information.

TO ENROLL

To enroll in the *Radiologic Clinics of North America* Continuing Medical Education program, call customer service at 1-800-654-2452 or sign up online at http://www.theclinics.com/home/cme. The CME program is available to subscribers for an additional annual fee of USD 327.60.

METHOD OF PARTICIPATION

In order to claim credit, participants must complete the following:

1. Complete enrolment as indicated above.
2. Read the activity.
3. Complete the CME Test and Evaluation. Participants must achieve a score of 70% on the test. All CME Tests and Evaluations must be completed online.

CME INQUIRIES/SPECIAL NEEDS

For all CME inquiries or special needs, please contact elsevierCME@elsevier.com.

Preface
Trauma and Emergency Radiology

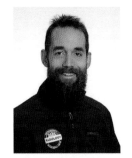

Stephan W. Anderson, MD
Editor

I sincerely hope that the reader will enjoy this issue of *Radiologic Clinics of North America*, dedicated to the ongoing evolution of trauma and emergency imaging. This issue offers an in-depth, multifaceted review of a number of topics of critical importance to trauma and emergency imaging. Given the breadth of the field of trauma and emergency imaging, this issue is truly a head-to-toe endeavor, from stroke and brain trauma imaging to easily missed fractures of the pediatric foot and ankle. Furthermore, this field is inherently multimodal in nature, from radiographic examinations to cutting-edge MR imaging. While far from exhaustive, our objective was to represent evolving applications of imaging, such as the article focused on damage control laparotomy, common, critically important applications such as stroke and bowel imaging, as well as those facets of our field in which known challenges and pitfalls occur, such as easily missed pediatric extremity fractures.

My sincere thanks to all of the contributing authors; their tremendous dedication to this project is deeply appreciated, and its success is a direct result of their efforts. We were fortunate to be able to draw upon a deeply experienced team of experts in their respective areas of trauma and emergency imaging. I would also like to express my gratitude to the staff at Elsevier for all of their assistance throughout the development and completion of this issue. We hope you find this issue to be a helpful resource in the interpretation of trauma and emergency imaging examinations.

Stephan W. Anderson, MD
Department of Radiology
Boston University Medical Campus
FGH Building, 3rd Floor
820 Harrison Avenue
Boston, MA 02218, USA

E-mail address:
sande@bu.edu

Radiol Clin N Am 57 (2019) xi
https://doi.org/10.1016/j.rcl.2019.03.001
0033-8389/19/© 2019 Published by Elsevier Inc.

Multidetector Computed Tomography Imaging of Damage Control Surgery Patients

Zohaib Y. Ahmad, MD[a], Arthur H. Baghdanian, MD[b],
Armonde A. Baghdanian, MD[b],*

KEYWORDS

- Damage control • MDCT • Abdominal trauma • Penetrating abdominal injury
- Blunt abdominal injury

KEY POINTS

- Damage control surgery is a staged surgical management for trauma patients with severe metabolic derangements.
- Multidetector computed tomography scanning is used to assess for the extent of trauma, missed surgical injury, injury in surgically unexplored areas, or surgical repair stability.
- Understanding the common postsurgical appearance of damage control patients can aid the radiologist in protocol optimization and accurate diagnosis.

INTRODUCTION

Patients undergoing damage control surgery (DCS) are being increasingly evaluated with multidetector computed tomography (MDCT) imaging as a tool to help direct medical and surgical management. DCS consists of multiple staged laparotomies implemented in patients with abdominopelvic trauma who are at risk for a deadly hemorrhagic coagulopathy if they undergo conventional surgery, a process that has been described by some surgeons as the "bloody vicious cycle."[1] In this setting, the first stage is an abbreviated laparotomy consisting of intraabdominal packing for hemostasis and potential repair of life-threatening intraabdominal organ injury. The patient is then rushed to the intensive care unit (ICU) for attention to the metabolic derangements of coagulopathy, hypothermia, and acidosis, and it is later that definitive surgical repair is completed. MDCT can be critical either immediately after the first staged laparotomy or sometime before the second laparotomy in determination of the full extent of the traumatic abdominopelvic injury or injuries missed during the initial laparotomy.[1,2]

The prior use of multistage laparotomies during the world wars involved treating hepatic trauma patient in the field by using nonsterile packing. However, these attempts were not very successful because patients frequently succumbed to sepsis despite adequate hemostasis and subsequent full surgical treatment of their injuries.[3,4] A resurgence of interest arose in the staged laparotomy process after the work of Drs Stone and Burch showed increased survival in patients with severe hepatic trauma that had never before been achieved.[3] Over the following 2 decades, damage control has increasingly been used as the standard of care.

There has been an increase in DCS cases and associated imaging owing to an increase in the incidence of traumatic injuries throughout the

Disclosure Statement: None.
[a] Department of Radiology, Boston University Medical Center, 820 Harrison Avenue, FGH Building, 4th Floor, Boston, MA 02115, USA; [b] Department of Radiology, University of San Francisco, 505 Parnassus Avenue, Room M392, Box 0628, San Francisco, CA 94143, USA
* Corresponding author.
E-mail address: Armonde.baghdanian@ucsf.edu

Radiol Clin N Am 57 (2019) 671–687
https://doi.org/10.1016/j.rcl.2019.02.003
0033-8389/19/© 2019 Elsevier Inc. All rights reserved.

radiologic.theclinics.com

United States. The National Center for Injury Prevention and Control, a subdivision of the Centers for Disease Control and Prevention, counts a total of 201,410 nonfatal injuries in 2015 to 2016 owing to firearms, an increase from 141,242 nonfatal injuries in 2005 to 2006.[5] An epidemiologic study on traumatic injuries within the United States describes an increasingly older, severely injured population with multiple comorbidities, noting an increase of traumatic discharges of those aged 45 to 64.[6] Although lower extremity injury is most common in both unintentional and assault nonfatal firearm injuries, lower trunk (abdominal) injuries consisted of 19% of assault nonfatal firearm injuries.[7] Furthermore, from 1999 to 2012, the rates of nonfatal firearm assaults increased by 52%.[7] Further studies showed not only a 31.7% increase in firearm injures between 2006 and 2012, but also an increase in severity in injuries within this population.[8] With such an increase, there has been a correlative increase in DCS cases, making a radiologist's knowledge of the imaging appearance and potential imaging and surgical pitfalls critical to the management of these patients.

METABOLIC DERANGEMENTS AND THE PATIENT UNDERGOING DAMAGE CONTROL SURGERY

The need for DCS stems from the need to quickly address the metabolic derangements that occur in the setting of severe abdominopelvic trauma. Such trauma leads to intraabdominal hemorrhage, creating a shock state that leads to progressive heat loss, lactic acidosis, and coagulation dysfunction, further exacerbated by large-scale blood transfusions.[9–11] Hypothermia has also been shown to affect intrinsic and extrinsic coagulation factors, further exacerbating the coagulopathy.[12] This state leads to what is known in surgical circles as the bloody vicious cycle, which results in uncontrollable intraoperative hemorrhage. These patients are also at risk for ventricular arrhythmias. This situation historically has led to an increase in mortality with a conventional surgical approach.[13,14] Furthermore, longer times of the initial staged surgery has lead to an increase in morbidity and mortality including longer ICU stays and multiorgan dysfunction.[9,15]

Therefore, identifying the damage control patient involves a multitude of factors. Asensio and colleagues[16] describes exsanguinating as a syndrome in patients who have experienced abdominopelvic trauma, with certain factors mandating DCS based on patient mortality: a pH of less than or equal to 7.2 and a body temperature of less than or equal to 34°C in patients who have had more than 5000 mL in blood loss (**Table 1**).

Table 1	
Metabolic derangements as indication for damage control	
Metabolic Derangement	**Factor for Indication**
Coagulation dysfunction	Not used for indication
Lactic acidosis	pH of ≤7.2
Hypothermia	Body temperature of ≤34°C

From Asensio JA, Mcduffie L, Roldán G, et al. Reliable variables in the exsanguinated patient which indicate damage control and predict outcome. 2002. Available at: https://www.americanjournalofsurgery.com/article/S0002-9610(01)00809-1/pdf. Accessed November 4, 2018; with permission.

SURGICAL TECHNIQUE

DCS has 3 main universal stages, the first of which involves initial surgical exploration for the stabilization of acutely lethal injuries. The patient is then immediately transported to the ICU for reversal of metabolic derangements and coagulopathy. Once the metabolic derangements have been addressed, the now more stable patient is then returned to the operating room for definitive surgical treatment.[1,2]

A midline incision is performed. Any hemoperitoneum is evacuated, and the abdomen is packed to prevent further hemorrhage. The source of hemorrhage, if found, is controlled by direct measures, such as sutures, clips, ligatures, or electrocautery. Furthermore, packing should attempt to approximate the disrupted tissue planes, to provide adequate hemostasis. This involves placing packing material above and below the liver; other areas of surgical packing include the splenic fossa (**Fig. 1**A) and the paracolic gutters (**Figs. 2**C and **3**C).[17–19] The small bowel is examined from the ligament of Treitz to the cecum to identify areas of injury. In some cases, the retroperitoneum is explored to assess for involvement.[17] Often, if there is no concern for retroperitoneal or renal injury, the retroperitoneum is left unexplored. This is important to note by radiologists because areas that are surgically unexplored are at risk of having undiscovered injuries that can lead to rapid patient decompensation.

There are certain maneuvers used to access the retroperitoneum, including the Mattox and Kocher maneuvers. The Mattox maneuver involves mobilizing the left-sided colon as well as rotating the spleen, left kidney, and pancreatic tail to assess the periaortic tissue and lumbar veins. The classic Kocher maneuver involves creating an incision at the points of peritoneal reflection of the duodenum to assess the duodenum and pancreatic head as

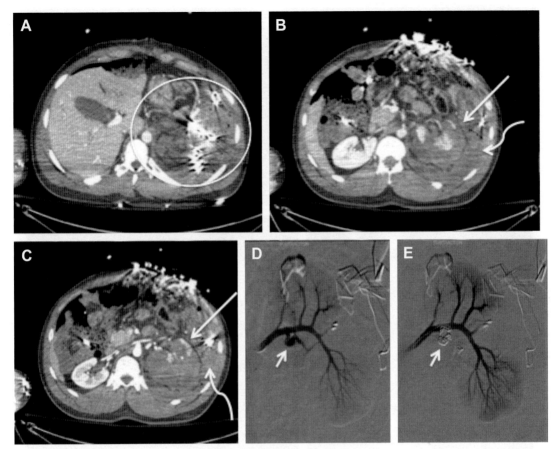

Fig. 1. A 33-year-old man who was run over by a truck. Axial MDCT IV contrast portal venous phase images show that the patient underwent an (*A*) emergent splenectomy with multiple surgical packing material placed within the splenic fossa (*circle*). (*B, C*) A fractured left kidney (*long arrows*) with associated retroperitoneal hematoma (*curved arrows*). A towel clip covering of the open abdomen was placed. The patient was taken to the angiography suite where (*D*) multiple pseudoaneurysms (*short arrows*) were seen and were embolized (*E*).

well as the aorta, inferior vena cava, and the right side of the lesser sac. The extended Kocher maneuver adds on by mobilizing the right colon to assess the right kidney and the retrohepatic inferior vena cava. The Catell-Braasch maneuver excises the attachment of the small bowel mesentery to the posterior peritoneum to allow for the further evaluation of the retroperitoneal duodenum and the right-sided retroperitoneal structures.[19–21] It is important for the radiologist to know what maneuvers were performed to understand postsurgical anatomy and to pay close attention to areas that were surgically unexplored.

Once there is hematologic control, the patient's abdomen is left open with a vacuum dressing, and the patient is sent immediately to the ICU for reversal of the patient's metabolic derangements. Hemodynamic optimization measures include red blood cells and other blood product transfusions, rewarming, and reversal of the patient's coagulopathy.

Once the patient is stable enough for repeat surgery, the patient is returned to the operating room to remove the intraabdominal packing and undergo definitive surgical management of the traumatic injuries and final closure of the abdomen.[1,17,19,21]

MULTIDETECTOR COMPUTED TOMOGRAPHY SCANNING IN THE DAMAGE CONTROL SETTING

Given the increase in DCS over the past 2 decades, more of these critically injured patients are undergoing MDCT after the initial surgery making it an essential tool in helping guide patient management.

INDICATIONS

There is a paucity of studies within the literature on the use of MDCT in the setting of DCS. However,

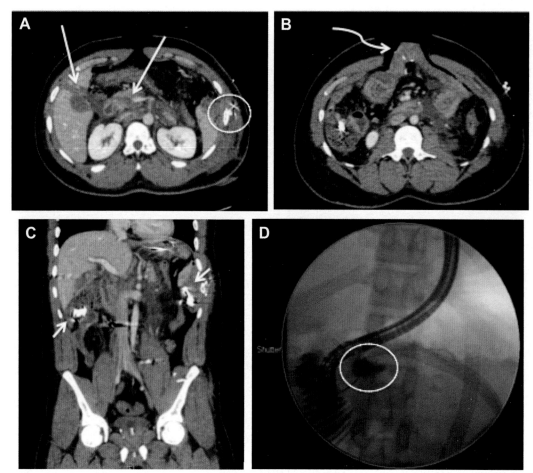

Fig. 2. A 27-year-old-man status post gunshot wound to the flank. Axial MDCT intravenous contrast portal venous phase images show (*A*) the transverse trajectory of the bullet resulting in a liver laceration and pancreatic head laceration (*long arrows*) with bullet fragments in the left abdominal subcutaneous tissues and an associated rib fracture (*circle*). (*B*) Note the proximal small bowel resection and open abdomen (*curved arrow*). Coronal images (*C*) show packing in the right and left hemiabdomen (*short arrows*) that can mimic bowel loops or fecal matter. Endoscopic retrograde cholangiopancreatography (*D*) was completed to assess the pancreatic duct, noting injury of the duct at the pancreatic head with a contrast leak (*circle*).

given the accessibility and speed of CT imaging, many patients are obtaining imaging immediately after the initial laparotomy before transport to the ICU.

MDCT can either be obtained in the immediate initial postoperative setting or later after admission to the ICU, but before the second staged laparotomy (**Fig. 4**). Reasons for MDCT include (1) evaluation for traumatic injury in regions of the abdomen and pelvis that were not surgically explored, (2) evaluation for traumatic injuries that may have been missed during the initial surgery, (3) evaluation of effective surgical repair, and (4) evaluation for foreign bodies that may have been missed during the initial surgery.[19]

In patients with persistent clinical instability despite resuscitative measures in the ICU, such as unstable vital signs, continued transfusion/

vasopressor requirements, or worsening coagulopathy, MDCT may be obtained to assess for uncontrolled acute abdominal/pelvic injury. MDCT may also be used to assess for failure of surgical repairs or injuries that may have been missed at the first laparotomy. In addition, MDCT can provide a roadmap for the surgeons to use when they reoperate on the patient as the next step in damage control (see **Fig. 4**).[19] Understanding these reasons can aid the radiologist in properly protocoling and assessing these MDCT studies for the question at hand.

PROTOCOL

Understanding the mechanism of injury to the chest, abdomen, and pelvis sustained from a traumatic injury aids in designing the technique and protocol

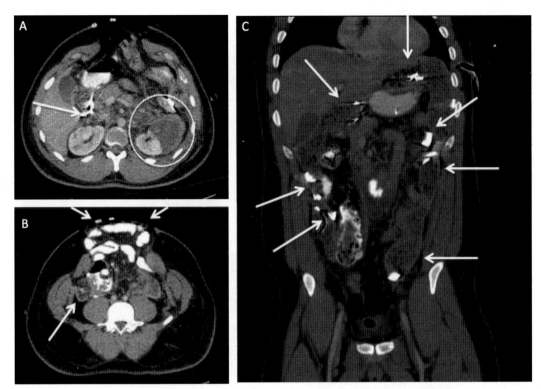

Fig. 3. A 32-year-old man status post gun shot wound to the abdomen. Axial (*A, B*) MDCT intravenous and oral contrast portal venous phase images demonstrate a grade intravenous left renal laceration (*circle*) and contrast filled bowel herniating through the open abdomen (*short arrows*). Coronal image (*C*) demonstrates packing underneath the liver, in the right-sided peritoneal lesser sac, and the bilateral paracolic gutters (*long arrows*).

of MDCT. The assessment of traumatic intraabdominal injuries in patients undergoing DCS is best evaluated with multiphase contrast enhanced imaging with arterial, portal venous, and also delayed phase imaging being obtained when necessary (**Box 1**).[22]

The use of noncontrast imaging can be considered, given that many of these patients may have multiple, highly dense foreign bodies internally, depending on the mechanism of injury, that can create suboptimal scans from a beam hardening artifact. Imaging before the administration of contrast may aid in the identification of these foreign bodies or even bone fragments that may mimic contrast extravasation on the postcontrast phase imaging.[19]

Arterial phase imaging is commonly used in the setting of pelvic fractures to assess for arterial or solid organ injury within the pelvis. Furthermore, arterial phase imaging can help to identify traumatic vascular injuries such as arterial lacerations, dissections, pseudoaneurysms, and traumatic vascular occlusions. Arterial phase imaging also helps to diagnose posttraumatic vascular malformations such as pseudoaneurysms and arteriovenous fistulas (see **Fig. 1**; **Fig. 5**).[19,23]

Enteric contrast can be considered in certain settings, such as in penetrating trauma with

patients at risk for a small or large bowel injury. Furthermore, enteric contrast can assess the surgical success or failure of a recent anastomosis.[19] The use of enteric contrast has been shown to not be necessary in the setting of blunt trauma. However, in patients undergoing DCS, secondary signs of bowel injury such as free air, bowel wall thickening, and hyperenhancement from shock bowel, as well as mesenteric stranding and hematomas, are already present as a consequence of the initial laparotomy. Therefore, the use of enteric contrast may be crucial to help diagnose a bowel injury (**Fig. 6**).[24–26]

IMAGING OF THE POSTOPERATIVE ABDOMEN
Postoperative Appearance

Postoperatively, the abdominal incision site is kept open to limit the risk of abdominal compartment syndrome, and the visceral edema from fluid resuscitation and reperfusion make it difficult to close the skin (see **Figs. 2** and **5**; **Figs. 7–11**).[18] This open abdomen is also conducive for expedited entry for the second staged laparotomy. Commonly, a wound vacuum dressing is placed, with surgical towels protecting any herniated loops

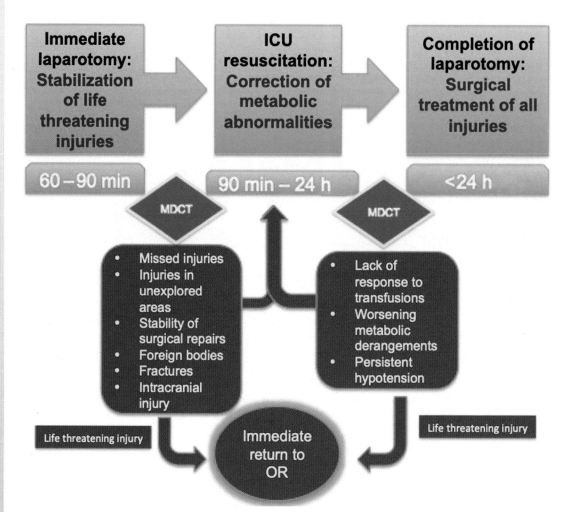

Fig. 4. Timing of MDCT during DCS. OR, operating room. (*From* Baghdanian AA, Baghdanian AH, Khalid M, et al. Damage control surgery: use of diagnostic CT after life-saving laparotomy. Emerg Radiol 2016;23(5):483–95; with permission.)

of edematous bowel. This strategy also decreases the risk of skin and tissue necrosis.[18,19]

Packing in the damage control setting is usually done with laparotomy pads. As described, packing has been used to control intraabdominal hemorrhage while the injury is repaired surgically or the patient's metabolic derangements are controlled. In this setting, packing is inserted at areas of injury and throughout the abdomen in the 4 quadrants.[18,19] Laparotomy pads are visible on radiography and MDCT, because they contain a radiopaque band attached to a gauze pad (see **Figs. 2** and **3**). The pads are made of polymers that prevent tissue necrosis and also contain hemostatic agents.[18,19] The radiopaque band is readily visible on MDCT and, with this knowledge, the adjacent gauze can be identified. Because the gauze pad absorbs surrounding bodily fluids, it can appear as an abscess, hematoma, or feculent material (see **Fig. 8**).[19] Also, compression of the pad on adjacent structures should be assessed because overpacking can increase the intraabdominal pressure and cause compression of the inferior vena cava.[17,19]

Given the nature of trauma and the subsequent surgery, foreign bodies are commonly discovered within the abdomen, which have to be completely reported on the imaging study. This practice helps the surgeon to know if there is a risk for further injury or potential infection. In the setting of gunshot wounds, the knowledge of an entry site and either an exit site or a retained bullet will help in identifying the trajectory (see **Fig. 2**).[19,27,28] Besides causing beam-hardening artifact, foreign bodies can have a variety of appearances, whether it is due to the number or the method of fragmentation of the bullet. The location of the foreign body should be described

Box 1
Clinical usefulness of different MDCT techniques

- Noncontrast
  - Foreign bodies
  - Bone fragments
  - Fractures
- Intravenous arterial and portal venous phase
  - Vascular injury
  - Posttraumatic vascular malformation
  - Abdominal solid organ injury
- Intravenous delayed phase
  - Confirmation of active extravasation
  - Urinary collecting system injury
  - Ureteral injury
- CT cystogram
  - Bladder injury
  - Distal ureteral injury
- Oral contrast
  - Distal esophageal and small bowel injury
- Rectal contrast
  - Rectal and large bowel injury

in detail, including adjacent neurovascular and visceral structures, because there is a risk of soft tissue erosion over time and potential injury if the patient may require MR imaging.[19]

It should be noted that, because this is an abbreviated surgery only to control active injury and minimize the time to intensive care treatment of the metabolic derangements, the surgical findings on MDCT will be reflective of this time-saving process.[17]

Hepatic Injury

Throughout the history of DCS and before, management of hepatic injury has been widely discussed.[3,4,29,30] Traditionally, packing has been used to control hepatic hemorrhage, especially by reapproximating the tissue planes that were injured. Of note, packing material is commonly placed superior and inferior or anterior and posterior to the liver to provide adequate compression for hemostasis (see **Fig. 10**).[29] Balloon catheter tamponade has also been used for hemostasis in injuries that completely traverse the liver. In this technique, a Sengstaken-Blakemore tube with both a gastric and an esophageal balloon is passed through the

injury tract, and the gastric balloon is inflated behind the liver as an anchor. The esophageal balloon is then inflated within the tract to provide hemostasis. This tube is brought through the skin and can be left in place for 48 to 72 hours.[29] To properly assess for liver hemorrhage, a multiphase MDCT should be completed with arterial and portal venous phases to assess for active hemorrhage. An acknowledgment of these areas may lead to hepatectomy or hepatorrhaphy for hemostasis. Persistent hemorrhage may also be treated with angiographic embolization (see **Fig. 8**).[31] Posttraumatic parenchymal vascular injuries, such as arteriovenous fistulas and pseudoaneurysms, may be seen given the hypervascularity of the liver.[31,32] In addition, hepatic infarcts may be seen after treatment and from traumatic devascularization, which is exacerbated by the shock physiologic state (see **Fig. 8**). For the radiologist, it is important to understand the methods for liver hemostasis as well as the sequelae of liver parenchymal and vascular injury.

Splenic Injury

Both penetrating and blunt traumas can result in splenic injury and hemorrhage. In this setting, total splenectomy is completed in the damage control setting because a repair or subtotal resection is not time conducive. After splenectomy, packing is placed in the splenic fossa for postoperative hemostasis (see **Fig. 1**). If no active hemorrhage is identified, multiphase MDCT can be used to assess for active contrast extravasation.[22,33–35] Splenic infarcts or splenic vein thrombosis can be seen owing to profound hypoperfusion state of patients undergoing DCS in physiologic shock.[36]

Upper Gastrointestinal Injury

Given the ligamentous attachment of the stomach, complete perioperative evaluation of the stomach cannot be completed. If an injury is detected during laparotomy, temporary measures are undertaken, such as nonradiopaque sutures for small perforations and contiguous bands of metallic surgical staples for larger injuries. Further surgical management of the stomach, such as gastric bypass, is reserved for the later laparotomy. MDCT evaluation should include evaluation of suture lines for surgical site dehiscence or anastomotic failure that may appear as a hematoma or hemorrhage.[19,21] The distal esophagus should also be evaluated carefully because injury from shear forces at the gastroesophageal junction can be missed easily during the initial laparotomy.[37] The use of enteric

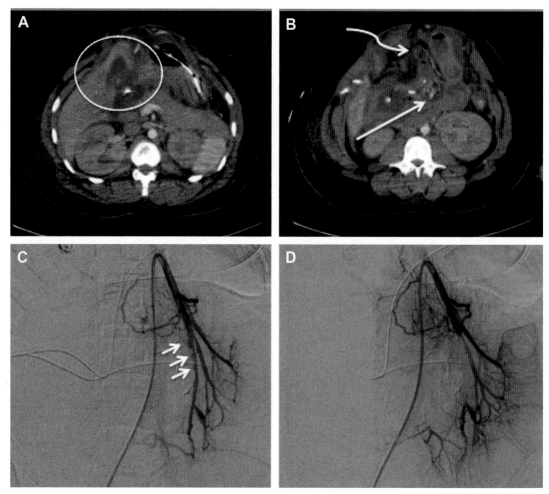

Fig. 5. A 29-year-old woman status post multiple stab wounds to the abdomen. Axial MDCT with intravenous contrast in the late arterial phase (*A, B*) demonstrates a grade II liver laceration (*circle*), multiple loops of herniating bowel (*curved arrow*), and narrowing of the superior mesenteric artery (*long arrow*). The patient was taken to angiography (*C, D*) where multiple pseudoaneurysms of the superior mesenteric artery are visualized (*short arrows*). A stent was successfully placed over the injured superior mesenteric artery segment (*D*).

contrast may be essential to detect subtle injuries when the mechanism of injury or surgical findings raise clinical suspicion. Enteric contrast can greatly aid the radiologist in detecting stomach injury or surgical repair failure because the repair itself is often not visible on MDCT (**Fig. 12**).

These abbreviated techniques are extended to the duodenum and adjacent pancreas because definitive surgical treatments such as duodenal exclusion or pancreaticoduodenectomy have high postoperative morbidity and mortality rates.[38,39] A temporary jejunostomy can be offered for duodenal injuries while the pancreas can be temporarily stabilized with packing and surgical drains.[29] It is possible to do an abbreviated pancreatoduodenectomy with stapling of the pylorus, pancreatic neck, and proximal jejunum, ligation of the common bile duct, and tube placement within the gallbladder.[29] Evaluation on MDCT for proximal bowel injuries can be aided with enteric contrast, especially with an edematous duodenum (see **Fig. 6**). This edema can extend to the pancreas owing to shock, and should not be confused for a direct pancreatic injury.[25] Because the evaluation of the pancreatic duct is limited owing artifacts from packing and edema, endoscopic retrograde cholangiopancreatography or MR imaging/magnetic resonance cholangiopancreatography can be obtained postoperative to evaluate for pancreatic ductal injury (see **Figs. 2** and **11**).[19] For the radiologist, understanding the extent of injury within the pancreas is important for follow-up, especially if there is a concern for a pancreatic ductal injury.

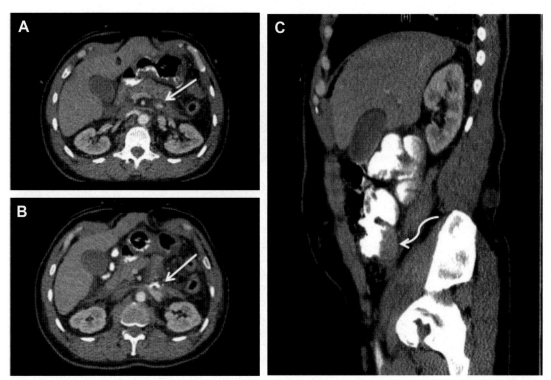

Fig. 6. A 50-year-old man status post stab wound. Oral and rectal contrast agents were administered. Axial MDCT intravenous contrast portal venous phase images (*A*) and (*B*) demonstrate an oral contrast leak from the duodenojejunal junction, consistent with a duodenal injury (*straight arrows*). Without oral contrast, this duodenal injury would not be possible to diagnose on MDCT. Sagittal MDCT images (*C*) demonstrate a cecal hematoma (*curved arrow*) that was easier to visualize with enteric contrast and later needed surgical repair.

Lower Gastrointestinal Injury

During initial laparotomy, the surgeon runs through the small bowel for any injuries and will proceed with any repair of enterotomies or bowel resection. Given the need for an abbreviated surgery, end-ligated noncontinuous loops of bowel after resection will be placed within the abdominal cavity with the anastomosis completed at the later staged laparotomy (see **Fig. 7**; **Fig. 13**).[17] Enterotomies are repaired during the initial laparotomy to limit intestinal spill, thereby decreasing the incidence of sepsis.[1,21] More extensive bowel injuries are ligated or stapled on both sides of the injured segment of bowel.[29] In this setting, the large bowel is not commonly exteriorized with ostomy formation owing to concern for retraction of the transected colon in the setting of abdominal wall edema.[29] With diffuse bowel edema and the increased incidence of complications of an ostomy with an open abdomen, full anastomotic repair is delayed until the later staged laparotomy.[26,40,41] In the shock state, the bowel will be edematous, and on MDCT, it is common to see submucosal enhancement of the bowel (see **Figs. 7** and **9**).[25] To evaluate for bowel injury on MDCT, water-soluble enteric contrast should be administered, especially to see any missed enterotomies or failed anastomoses. It should be noted that, if active hemorrhage is a concern, bowel contrast can mask extravasation

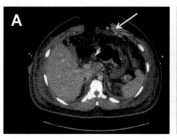

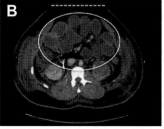

Fig. 7. A 19-year-old man status post gunshot wound to the abdomen. An axial MDCT intravenous contrast portal venous phase image show (*A*) patient had a partial colectomy (*arrow*). (*B*) Note the multiple loops of small bowel remarkable for wall thickening in a patient with shock bowel (*circle*). The patient has an open anterior abdominal wall (*dashed line*).

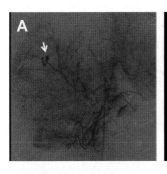
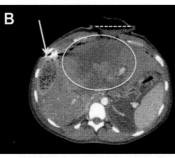

Fig. 8. A 26-year-old women was in a motor vehicle collision. The patient was taken to the angiography suite, where (*A*) active contrast extravasation (*short arrow*) was noted in a distal branch of the right hepatic artery. After embolization, MDCT intravenous contrast portal venous phase imaging shows (*B*) a large geographic area of hypoattenuation (*circle*) in the liver, which represents a laceration with a superimposed infarct. Packing material can be seen lateral to the liver, mimicking fecal matter, hematoma, or an abscess (*long arrow*). The patient has an open abdomen (*dashed line*).

of intravenous contrast into the bowel making it difficult to diagnose intraluminal hemorrhage. If bowel repair is completed, follow-up imaging is advised owing to an increased risk of complications such as fistula and intraabdominal abscess formation.[42] Attention to the proximal jejunum and antimesenteric borders of the left and right colon is warranted; shear force injury to these structures is commonly missed during the initial laparotomy.[37] Differentiating a diffusely edematous bowel that is commonly seen in the damage control setting versus an actual bowel injury is an important distinction for the radiologist to make.

Vascular Injury

Vascular injury is also commonly seen in the form of lacerations, traumatic dissections, and

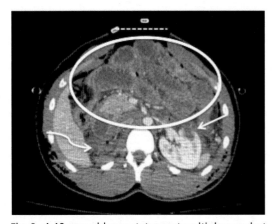

Fig. 9. A 19-year-old man status post multiple gun shot wounds to the abdomen. An axial MDCT intravenous contrast portal venous phase image demonstrates that the patient underwent an emergent right nephrectomy (*curved arrow*). There is a grade 3 left renal laceration (*arrow*). Note that the bowel wall is diffusely thick walled (*circle*) extending into the anterior abdominal surgical defect (*dashed line*), consistent with shock bowel secondary to a low perfusion state. The patient has an open abdomen (*dashed line*).

pseudoaneurysm formation (see **Fig. 11; Fig. 14**). Vessels may be ligated or repaired in the initial laparotomy because they are life-threatening injuries. In addition, patients may present for angiography for the management of cases that are difficult to treat surgically or for which an endovascular approach is more feasible. Arterial injury such as that involving the iliac arteries and the superior mesenteric arteries can be temporarily stented/shunted.[29,43] In difficult to treat cases, amenable vessels that have end-organ collateral flow may also be embolized in the interest of time. Venous injury such as injury to the iliac veins and inferior vena cava must be controlled with direct repair or stenting. Temporary hemostasis of the retrohepatic inferior vena cava can be achieved with packing.[29] A knowledge of the method of treatment of vascular injuries is essential for the radiologist not to miss persistent vessel injury or postsurgical complications such as iatrogenic dissection or posttreatment thrombosis.

Retroperitoneal Injury

Close attention to the retroperitoneum during review of MDCT images is important for patients undergoing DCS, because there may be injuries not known to the clinicians either owing to a lack of surgical exploration or the presence of injuries that are difficult to detect during the initial surgical exploration. During the initial stage of surgery, control of hemorrhage and bowel injury are the primary concerns. The repair of urologic injuries is usually deferred to a later operation in the interest of expediting transport of patients to the ICU. Given the ability for the perirenal fascia to tamponade renal hemorrhage, these areas of the retroperitoneum are often left undisturbed unless there is an expanding hematoma, a pulsatile hematoma, or a hemorrhage outside the fascia. Therefore, evaluation of the retroperitoneum on

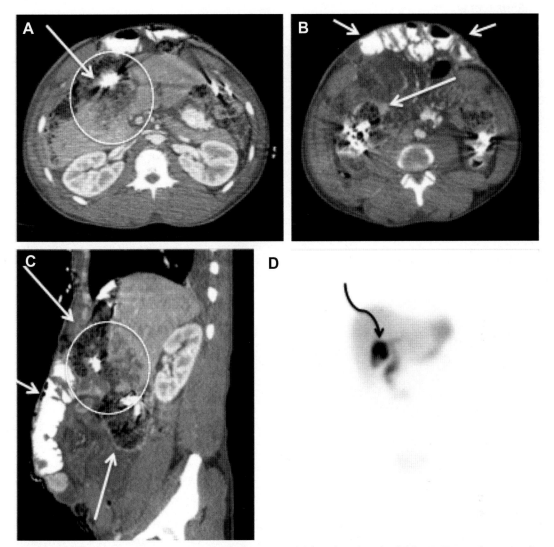

Fig. 10. A 26-year-old man status post gunshot injury. Axial (*A*, *B*) and sagittal (*C*) MDCT portal venous phase intravenous and oral contrast images demonstrate a grade V liver laceration (*circle*) with packing anterior, posterior, and through the point of injury in the liver (*straight long arrows*). The patient underwent a cholecystectomy at the initial laparotomy. There are contrast opacified loops of small bowel herniating through the anterior abdominal surgical defect (*straight short arrows*). Nuclear medicine hepatobiliary iminodiacetic acid scan (*D*) demonstrates leakage of radiotracer at the site of injury (*curved arrow*) consistent with biliary injury.

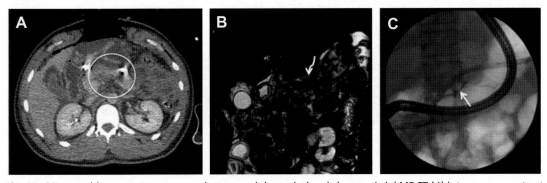

Fig. 11. 29-year-old man status post gun shot wound through the abdomen. Axial MDCT (*A*) intravenous contrast portal venous phase images demonstrate a pancreatic laceration (*circle*). Coronal magnetic resonance cholangiopancreatography T2-weighted fat-suppressed image (*B*) demonstrates attenuation of the mid pancreatic duct (*short curved arrow*). Endoscopic retrograde cholangiopancreatography (*C*) image demonstrates active extravasation of contrast from the pancreatic duct (*short straight arrow*) at the site of laceration.

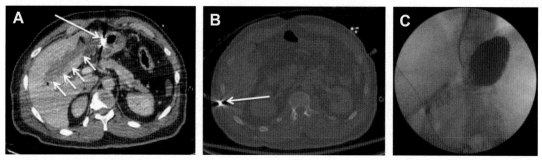

Fig. 12. A 54-year-old man status post gun shot wound to the abdomen. Axial (*A, B*) MDCT intravenous contrast portal image in the venous phase. Upon initial surgery, patient was found to have a grade 4 liver laceration (*short arrows*) and injury to the gastric antrum, which was repaired. Retained radiopaque bullets were identified on MDCT anterior to the gastric wall and within the subcutaneous tissues of the right flank (*long arrows*). An upper gastrointestinal fluoroscopic study (*C*) with water-soluble contrast demonstrates no leakage from the gastric wall repair.

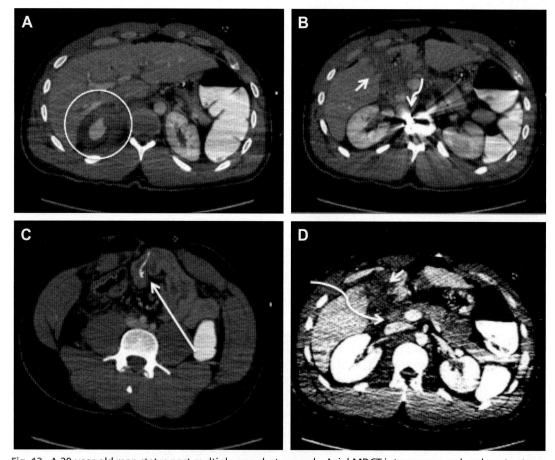

Fig. 13. A 29-year-old man status post multiple gun shot wounds. Axial MDCT intravenous and oral contrast portal venous phase images demonstrate a (*A*) grade 1 right renal laceration with a perirenal hematoma (*circle*) that was not discovered during the initial surgery. The patient also had a (*B, D*) grade 4 liver laceration (*short arrow*) with a bullet fragment adjacent to the spine (*short curved arrow*). Patient had resection of his small and large bowel with (*C*) noncontinuous ligated ends of bowel left in the abdomen for reanastomosis at the next laparotomy (*long arrow*). A focal hyperdensity was noted anterior to the inferior vena cava (*long curved arrow*) (*D*) that given the bullet trajectory was diagnosed as a paracaval hematoma. Further exploration on the second laparotomy demonstrated an injury to the inferior vena cava, which was surgically repaired.

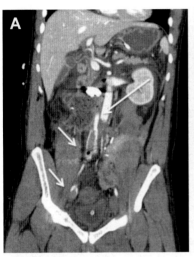 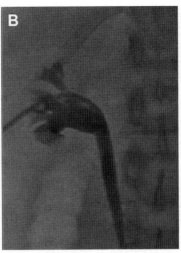 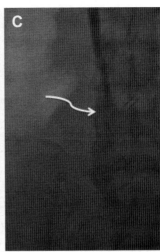

Fig. 14. A 22-year-old man status post gun shot wound. A coronal MDCT with intravenous contrast portal venous phase image (*A*) demonstrates traumatic occlusion within the aorta (*long straight arrow*) and the inferior vena cava extending into the right iliac vein (*short straight arrows*). Owing to concern for a left ureteral injury, a percutaneous nephroureterogram was completed, demonstrating a preserved left renal pelvis (*B*) with sudden cut off of contrast of the left mid ureter (*C*) (*curved arrow*), for which a left percutaneous nephrostomy tube was placed to allow drainage of urine.

MDCT can be valuable (see **Fig. 13**; **Fig. 15**) to exclude the presence of unknown injuries.

If there is concern for high-grade renal injury with hemodynamic instability, the retroperitoneum may be explored surgically. If a high-grade renal injury involving the renal vascular pedicle with an uninjured contralateral kidney is found, a nephrectomy can be performed with the interest of expediting patient transport to the ICU for resuscitation (see **Fig. 9**).[19,44] The use of multiphase imaging is key for complete evaluation of renal parenchymal injury, including active intraparenchymal contrast extravasation and to diagnose traumatic vascular malformations such as arteriovenous fistulas and pseudoaneurysms (see **Fig. 1**).

Urinary extravasation is of a lesser priority than bowel perforation, given that urine in the abdominal cavity has a more delayed onset to sepsis than the presence of fecal matter. Temporary measures such as placement of ureteral stents or urinary diversion with percutaneous nephrostomy drainage can serve as temporizing measures until definitive repair is completed. Furthermore, transurethral catheter placement or suprapubic cystostomy catheter placement can be performed for bladder injuries, given the difficulty of surgical repair in the DCS setting.[44] Delayed contrast imaging is beneficial to assess the renal collecting system and proximal ureters for injury demonstrated on MDCT as contrast leaks, because these injuries are difficult to ascertain during the initial laparotomy (see **Fig. 15**).[19,37] If a bladder injury is suspected, such as with pelvic ring fractures,

retroperitoneal involvement of penetrating trauma, or high-velocity deceleration injuries, a CT cystogram can be performed to assess for injury to the bladder wall. Likewise, if pelvic fractures or blood products in the pelvis are identified on MDCT, a CT cystogram should be performed to evaluate for bladder injury (**Fig. 16**).[19]

USE OF ANGIOGRAPHY IN DAMAGE CONTROL SURGERY

Interventional angiography can have many uses in the damage control setting. Angiography can provide treatment for arterial hemorrhage without disrupting the tissue planes or packing that surgeons have placed during the initial laparotomy. The role of interventional angiography lies in the setting of internal hemorrhage that is not amenable to surgical repair. The patient is taken for angiography either when (1) an arterial injury is identified during the initial laparotomy or (2) the patient becomes hemodynamically unstable while in the ICU and the initial surgery had already addressed the surgically amenable hemorrhages.[23] Although hepatic packing can lead to hemostasis, intrahepatic hemorrhage may not be amenable to surgical repair and may need angiography to identify the source of the bleeding and subsequent embolization (see **Fig. 8**).[45]

Frequent indications for angiography are the identification of an expanding retroperitoneal or pelvic hematoma. As described, the retroperitoneum may not be explored surgically during the initial laparotomy owing to the tamponade effect of the

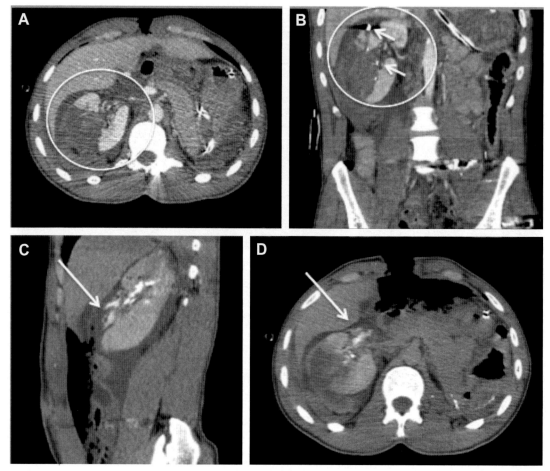

Fig. 15. A 26-year-old man status post gunshot wound. Axial (*A*) and coronal (*B*) MDCT intravenous contrast portal venous phase images demonstrate a grade 4 right kidney laceration (*circle*) with perirenal hematoma and multiple bullet fragments (*short arrows*). The patient also underwent left nephrectomy and splenectomy owing to severe injuries to those organs. The right-sided retroperitoneum was not evaluated during the initial surgery. Sagittal (*C*) and axial (*D*) MDCT intravenous contrast delayed phase images demonstrates proximal right ureteral injury (*long arrows*).

retroperitoneal fascia.[23,44] A pelvic angiogram may also be performed in the setting of pelvic fracture and persistent hemodynamic instability (see **Fig. 1**).[23] Once the patient has reached the ICU and has undergone imaging studies, the identification of complex vascular injuries such as hepatic or splenic arteriovenous fistula formation or pseudoaneurysms may indicate the need for angiography and embolization.[23,45,46]

Furthermore, if the patient becomes hemodynamically unstable in the ICU, interventional angiography can be used as an adjunct or replacement for

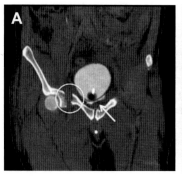
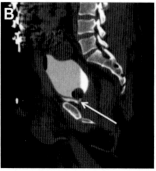

Fig. 16. A 33-year-old man status post motor vehicle accident. Axial and sagittal (*A*, *B*) MDCT cystoscopy images demonstrate a displaced right superior pubic ramus fracture (*circle*). Contrast is seen distending the bladder as well as extraluminal contrast in the retropubic space (*arrows*) from a bladder neck injury.

urgent reexploration, because the initial surgery would have dealt with the hemorrhages that were surgically amenable. This process has been associated with improved outcomes in these patients.[46,47]

SUMMARY

With an increasing incidence of severe traumatic injuries, understanding the usefulness of MDCT in the imaging of patients undergoing DCS can help to guide patient management. MDCT serves as a tool to help detect missed injuries from the initial laparotomy, assess the stability of surgical repairs, or any explore areas not investigated during the initial laparotomy, such as within the retroperitoneum. In addition, MDCT helps as a problem-solving tool when patients are not improving in the ICU despite medical resuscitative measures. A radiologist's knowledge of the indications for DCS and the details of the surgical procedures related to staged laparotomy help to optimize imaging protocols. A radiologist's understanding of the common appearance of patients undergoing DCS with multiple traumatic injuries, the post-staged laparotomy appearance of an open abdomen with surgical packing, and the many findings of a hypoperfused physiology are crucial in providing immediate and accurate diagnoses. MDCT has proved to be a crucial tool in the management of patients undergoing DCS with the radiologist's understanding a key to its success.

REFERENCES

1. Moore EE, Burch JM, Franciose RJ, et al. Staged physiologic restoration and damage control surgery. World J Surg 1998;22(12):1184–90 [discussion: 1190–1]. Available at: http://www.ncbi.nlm.nih.gov/pubmed/9841741. Accessed October 29, 2018.
2. Rotondo MF, Schwab CW, McGonigal MD, et al. "Damage control": an approach for improved survival in exsanguinating penetrating abdominal injury. J Trauma 1993;35(3):375–82 [discussion: 382–3]. Available at: http://www.ncbi.nlm.nih.gov/pubmed/8371295. Accessed October 29, 2018.
3. Waibel BH, Rotondo MMF. Damage control surgery: it's evolution over the last 20 years. Rev Col Bras Cir 2012;39(4):314–21. Available at: http://www.ncbi.nlm.nih.gov/pubmed/22936231. Accessed October 29, 2018.
4. Roberts DJ, Ball CG, Feliciano DV, et al. History of the innovation of damage control for management of trauma patients: 1902-2016. Ann Surg 2017; 265(5):1034–44.
5. WISQARS leading causes of nonfatal injury reports. Available at: https://webappa.cdc.gov/sasweb/ncipc/nfilead.html. Accessed October 29, 2018.
6. DiMaggio C, Ayoung-Chee P, Shinseki M, et al. Traumatic injury in the United States: in-patient epidemiology 2000-2011. Injury 2016;47(7):1393–403.
7. Fowler KA, Dahlberg LL, Haileyesus T, et al. Firearm injuries in the United States. Prev Med (Baltim) 2015; 79:5–14.
8. Kalesan B, Zuo Y, Xuan Z, et al. A multi-decade joinpoint analysis of firearm injury severity. Trauma Surg Acute Care Open 2018;3(1):e000139.
9. Garrison JR, Richardson JD, Hilakos AS, et al. Predicting the need to pack early for severe intra-abdominal hemorrhage. J Trauma 1996;40(6):923–7 [discussion: 927–9]. Available at: http://www.ncbi.nlm.nih.gov/pubmed/8656478. Accessed October 29, 2018.
10. Steinemann S, Shackford SR, Davis JW. Implications of admission hypothermia in trauma patients. J Trauma 1990;30(2):200–2. Available at: http://www.ncbi.nlm.nih.gov/pubmed/2304115. Accessed October 29, 2018.
11. Jurkovich GJ, Greiser WB, Luterman A, et al. Hypothermia in trauma victims: an ominous predictor of survival. J Trauma 1987;27(9):1019–24. Available at: http://www.ncbi.nlm.nih.gov/pubmed/3656464. Accessed October 29, 2018.
12. Gubler KD, Gentilello LM, Hassantash SA, et al. The impact of hypothermia on dilutional coagulopathy. J Trauma 1994;36(6):847–51. Available at: http://www.ncbi.nlm.nih.gov/pubmed/8015007. Accessed November 4, 2018.
13. Stone HH, Strom PR, Mullins RJ. Management of the major coagulopathy with onset during laparotomy. Ann Surg 1983;197(5):532–5. Available at: http://www.ncbi.nlm.nih.gov/pubmed/6847272. Accessed October 29, 2018.
14. Asensio JA, Petrone P, O'Shanahan G, et al. Managing exsanguination: what we know about damage control/bailout is not enough. Proc (Bayl Univ Med Cent) 2003; 16(3):294–6. Available at: http://www.ncbi.nlm.nih.gov/pubmed/16278701. Accessed November 4, 2018.
15. Sharp KW, Locicero RJ. Abdominal packing for surgically uncontrollable hemorrhage. Ann Surg 1992;215(5):467–74 [discussion: 474–5]. Available at: http://www.ncbi.nlm.nih.gov/pubmed/1616383. Accessed October 29, 2018.
16. Asensio JA, Mcduffie L, Roldán G, et al. Reliable variables in the exsanguinated patient which indicate damage control and predict outcome. 2002. Available at: https://www.americanjournalofsurgery.com/article/S0002-9610(01)00809-1/pdf. Accessed November 4, 2018.
17. Bowley DM, Barker P, Boffard KD. Damage control surgery–concepts and practice. J R Army Med Corps 2000;146(3):176–82. Available at: http://www.ncbi.nlm.nih.gov/pubmed/11143684. Accessed October 29, 2018.

18. Shapiro MB, Jenkins DH, Schwab CW, et al. Damage control: collective review. J Trauma 2000;49(5): 969–78. Available at: http://www.ncbi.nlm.nih.gov/pubmed/11086798. Accessed October 29, 2018.

19. Baghdanian AA, Baghdanian AH, Khalid M, et al. Damage control surgery: use of diagnostic CT after life-saving laparotomy. Emerg Radiol 2016;23(5): 483–95.

20. Mattox KL, Moore EE, Feliciano DV. Trauma. New York: McGraw-Hill Medical; 2013.

21. Burch JM, Ortiz VB, Richardson RJ, et al. Abbreviated laparotomy and planned reoperation for critically injured patients. Ann Surg 1992;215(5):476–83 [discussion: 483–4]. Available at: http://www.ncbi.nlm.nih.gov/pubmed/1616384. Accessed October 29, 2018.

22. Uyeda JW, LeBedis CA, Penn DR, et al. Active hemorrhage and vascular injuries in splenic trauma: utility of the arterial phase in multidetector CT. Radiology 2014;270(1):99–106.

23. Hoffer EK, Borsa JJ, Bloch RD, et al. Endovascular techniques in the damage control setting. Radiographics 1999;19(5):1340–8.

24. Stuhlfaut JW, Soto JA, Lucey BC, et al. Blunt abdominal trauma: performance of CT without oral contrast material. Radiology 2004;233(3):689–94.

25. Prasad KR, Kumar A, Gamanagatti S, et al. CT in post-traumatic hypoperfusion complex—a pictorial review. Emerg Radiol 2011;18(2):139–43.

26. Miller PR, Chang MC, Hoth JJ, et al. Colonic resection in the setting of damage control laparotomy: is delayed anastomosis safe? Am Surg 2007; 73(6):606–9 [discussion: 609–10]. Available at: http://www.ncbi.nlm.nih.gov/pubmed/17658099. Accessed October 29, 2018.

27. Richardson JD, Bergamini TM, Spain DA, et al. Operative strategies for management of abdominal aortic gunshot wounds. Surgery 1996;120(4): 667–71. Available at: http://www.ncbi.nlm.nih.gov/pubmed/8862376. Accessed October 29, 2018.

28. Dreizin D, Borja MJ, Danton GH, et al. Penetrating diaphragmatic injury: accuracy of 64-section multidetector CT with trajectography. Radiology 2013; 268(3):729–37.

29. Hirshberg A, Walden R. Damage control for abdominal trauma. Surg Clin North Am 1997;77(4): 813–20. Available at: http://www.ncbi.nlm.nih.gov/pubmed/9291983. Accessed October 29, 2018.

30. Feliciano DV, Pachter HL. Hepatic trauma revisited. Curr Probl Surg 1989;26(7):453–524. Available at: http://www.ncbi.nlm.nih.gov/pubmed/2663381. Accessed October 29, 2018.

31. Sugimoto K, Horiike S, Hirata M, et al. The role of angiography in the assessment of blunt liver injury. Injury 1994;25(5):283–7. Available at: http://www.ncbi.nlm.nih.gov/pubmed/8034343. Accessed October 29, 2018.

32. Ivatury RR, Nallathambi M, Gunduz Y, et al. Liver packing for uncontrolled hemorrhage: a reappraisal. J Trauma 1986;26(8):744–53. Available at: http://www.ncbi.nlm.nih.gov/pubmed/3488414. Accessed October 29, 2018.

33. Atluri S, Richard HM, Shanmuganathan K. Optimizing multidetector CT for visualization of splenic vascular injury. Validation by splenic arteriography in blunt abdominal trauma patients. Emerg Radiol 2011;18(4):307–12.

34. Stuhlfaut JW, Anderson SW, Soto JA. Blunt abdominal trauma: current imaging techniques and CT findings in patients with solid organ, bowel, and mesenteric injury. Semin Ultrasound CT MR 2007; 28(2):115–29. Available at: http://www.ncbi.nlm.nih.gov/pubmed/17432766. Accessed October 29, 2018.

35. Anderson SW, Lucey BC, Rhea JT, et al. 64 MDCT in multiple trauma patients: imaging manifestations and clinical implications of active extravasation. Emerg Radiol 2007;14(3):151–9.

36. Boscak A, Shanmuganathan K. Splenic trauma: what is new? Radiol Clin North Am 2012;50(1): 105–22.

37. Hirshberg A, Wall MJ, Allen MK, et al. Causes and patterns of missed injuries in trauma. Am J Surg 1994;168(4):299–303.

38. Gupta V, Wig JD, Garg H. Trauma pancreaticoduodenectomy for complex pancreaticoduodenal injury. Delayed reconstruction. JOP 2008;9(5):618–23. Available at: http://www.ncbi.nlm.nih.gov/pubmed/18762693. Accessed October 29, 2018.

39. Lopez PP, Benjamin R, Cockburn M, et al. Recent trends in the management of combined pancreatoduodenal injuries. Am Surg 2005;71(10): 847–52. Available at: http://www.ncbi.nlm.nih.gov/pubmed/16468533. Accessed October 29, 2018.

40. Murray JA, Demetriades D, Colson M, et al. Colonic resection in trauma: colostomy versus anastomosis. J Trauma 1999;46(2):250–4. Available at: http://www.ncbi.nlm.nih.gov/pubmed/10029029. Accessed October 29, 2018.

41. Ordoñez CA, Pino LF, Badiel M, et al. Safety of performing a delayed anastomosis during damage control laparotomy in patients with destructive colon injuries. J Trauma 2011;71(6):1512–8.

42. Ott MM, Norris PR, Diaz JJ, et al. Colon anastomosis after damage control laparotomy: recommendations from 174 trauma colectomies. J Trauma 2011;70(3): 595–602.

43. Reilly PM, Rotondo MF, Carpenter JP, et al. Temporary vascular continuity during damage control: intraluminal shunting for proximal superior mesenteric artery injury. J Trauma 1995;39(4):757–60. Available at: http://www.ncbi.nlm.nih.gov/pubmed/7473971. Accessed October 29, 2018.

44. Coburn M. Damage control for urologic injuries. Surg Clin North Am 1997;77(4):821–34. Available at: http://www.ncbi.nlm.nih.gov/pubmed/9291984. Accessed October 29, 2018.

45. Johnson JW, Gracias VH, Gupta R, et al. Hepatic angiography in patients undergoing damage control laparotomy. J Trauma 2002;52(6):1102–6. Available at: http://www.ncbi.nlm.nih.gov/pubmed/12045637. Accessed October 29, 2018.

46. Parr MJ, Alabdi T. Damage control surgery and intensive care. Injury 2004;35(7):712–21.

47. Kushimoto S, Arai M, Aiboshi J, et al. The role of interventional radiology in patients requiring damage control laparotomy. J Trauma 2003;54(1):171–6.

Small Bowel Obstruction and Ischemia

Matthew Diamond, MD, John Lee, MD, Christina A. LeBedis, MD*

KEYWORDS

- Small bowel obstruction • Bowel ischemia • Bowel strangulation
- Computed tomography of bowel obstruction • Closed-loop obstruction

KEY POINTS

- Suspected bowel obstruction is best evaluated using CT of the abdomen and pelvis with IV contrast only.
- Identifying and evaluating the transition point is the key to diagnosing and determining the cause of the obstruction.
- When evaluating the obstruction, it is best to determine if the cause is intrinsic, extrinsic, or intra-luminal, keeping in mind that the most common cause of SBO is intra-abdominal adhesions.
- The presence or absence of a closed-loop obstruction, which increases the likelihood of ischemia and failed nonoperative management, should be mentioned when reading MDCT.
- Reduced bowel wall enhancement and mesenteric edema are the most specific and sensitive, respectively, signs of bowel ischemia, a surgical emergency. Mimics of other signs of ischemia limit their usefulness when identified individually.

INTRODUCTION

Small bowel obstruction (SBO) is a common surgical emergency accounting for 20% of emergency surgical procedures of patients presenting with abdominal pain and approximately 300,000 hospitalizations in the United States annually.[1,2] SBO causes high morbidity with an average hospital stay of 8 days and in-hospital mortality rate of 3% per episode.[3] Following abdominal surgery, the incidence of SBO is up to 9%.[3] It is also a significant cause of hospital readmission following abdominal surgery, with 5.7% of all readmissions following open abdominal and pelvic surgery being directly related to SBO.[4] Although the incidence of SBO has been reduced to 1.4% following laparoscopic abdominal surgery compared with 3.8% following open abdominal surgery, SBO continues to be a significant cause of hospitalization and surgical consultation.[5]

Radiologists play a significant role not only in the diagnosis of SBO but also in the guidance of its management. Increasingly, conservative management has been the dominant method of treatment, with only 18% of patients with SBO requiring surgical treatment.[6] Nonoperative management is the treatment of choice in the absence of signs of strangulation, ischemia, and peritonitis and is effective in 70% to 90% of patients.[3] Although there is a slightly decreased risk of recurrence in patients treated operatively, with a 5-year rate of recurrence of 16% versus 20%, there is a high risk of morbidity for surgical interventions including bowel injury.[3,7] It is the radiologist's job to determine the presence not only of SBO but also signs that require immediate surgical exploration and the possible cause of obstruction.

A feared complication of SBO is a strangulated obstruction, which is SBO with ischemia.[8] Strangulation occurs in approximately 10% of cases

Disclosure Statement: Nothing to disclose.
Department of Radiology, Boston Medical Center, 820 Harrison Avenue, FGH Building 3rd Floor, Boston, MA 02118, USA
* Corresponding author.
E-mail address: Christina.LeBedis@bmc.org

Radiol Clin N Am 57 (2019) 689–703
https://doi.org/10.1016/j.rcl.2019.02.002

of SBO and has a greatly increased mortality risk of 20% to 40%.[9,10] Before the advent of multidetector computed tomography (MDCT), there was great difficulty in determining strangulation based on clinical values and abdominal radiographs alone.[10] Recognizing the presence or absence of strangulated bowel is crucial for determining which patients are likely to fail conservative management.

The typical clinical presentation of SBO includes abdominal pain, vomiting, obstipation, and abdominal distention. Indications of possible strangulation include elevated white blood cell count (>10,000/mm^3), elevated lactate, elevated C-reactive protein (>75 mg/L), and peritoneal signs including rebound tenderness and guarding.[3,10,11] The failure of nonoperative treatment is defined by persistent obstruction for longer than 72 hours, drainage volume from nasogastric suction of greater than 500 mL on the third day, or the presence of peritonitis or ischemia.[10] The water-soluble oral contrast challenge is a new technique used in patients with presumed adhesions producing SBO who fail nasogastric tube decompression after 48 hours. Patients who pass the water-soluble oral contrast challenge have been shown to have lower surgical exploration rates and bowel resection, shorter lengths of stay in hospital, and complication rates similar to those in patients who fail.[12]

DEFINITIONS

- Complete or high-grade obstruction: total luminal occlusion without passage of gas or intestinal contents
- Incomplete, partial, or low-grade obstruction: luminal narrowing allowing passage of some gas or intestinal contents
- Simple obstruction: obstruction with an intact blood supply (no signs of ischemia)
- Strangulating obstruction: obstruction with a compromised blood supply resulting in ischemia
- Closed-loop obstruction: a segment of bowel occluded at 2 adjacent points that isolate the lumen of that segment from the remaining bowel

NORMAL ANATOMY AND IMAGING TECHNIQUE

One of the main anatomic considerations when determining the presence of SBO is differentiating small bowel loops from colon. The small bowel contains mucosal folds extending circumferentially around the bowel known as plicae circulares or valvulae conniventes. The large bowel contains thick haustral folds known as plicae semilunares, which do not extend around the whole circumference of the bowel. Small bowel also tends to be more centrally located.

The intestinal tract secretes up to 8.5 L of fluid a day, most of which is reabsorbed within the intestines.[12] Luminal narrowing and obstruction prevents or reduces the passage of material, causing distention of the proximal loops of bowel. Distention of loops of bowel can result in the compromise of circulation beginning with venous return that increases the risk of gangrene and bowel necrosis.[13] The region of bowel most susceptible to vascular compromise and ischemia is just proximal to the site of the obstruction and the transition point.[13] The transition point is the site of obstruction when the bowel goes from distended to collapsed. Identifying the transition point on imaging greatly aids in the diagnosis of SBO, identifying the cause and determining the severity.[1,8,11,13]

ABDOMINAL RADIOGRAPHY

Although abdominal radiographs are often used for screening of SBO, MDCT has become the main imaging modality for SBO. Abdominal radiography has limited value in initial diagnosis and evaluation of SBO because of its low sensitivity for partial low-grade obstruction, with a false-negative rate of up to 20%, a false-positive rate of 42%, and a diagnostic accuracy rate of 50% to 60% for high-grade SBO.[14] Radiography also offers limited evaluation for strangulation and the cause of the obstruction.[14,15]

Abdominal radiographs can be performed in supine, upright, or decubitus positions. The radiographic signs of SBO are presented in **Box 1**.

Box 1
Radiographic signs of SBO

Gas-filled or fluid-filled small bowel loops greater than 3 cm

Distended stomach

Stretch sign

Gasless abdomen

Greater than 2 air-fluid levels (upright or decubitus)

Differing heights of air-fluid levels in the same loop of bowel (upright or decubitus)

Air-fluid levels longer than 2.5 cm (upright or decubitus)

String-of-beads sign (upright or decubitus)

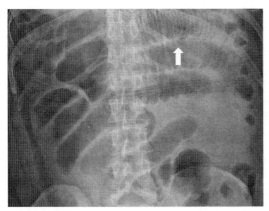

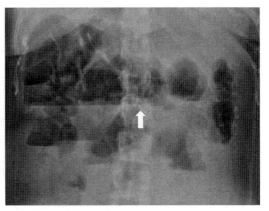

Fig. 1. Supine abdominal radiograph demonstrating a stretch sign (*arrow*).

Fig. 2. Upright abdominal radiograph demonstrating air-fluid levels of different heights with a width great than 2.5 cm (*arrow*).

The signs with the highest sensitivity include more than 2 air-fluid levels, air-fluid levels wider than 2.5 cm, and air-fluid levels of differing heights in the same loop of bowel.[11,14,16,17] Less sensitive signs include a distended stomach, a gasless abdomen, and the stretch and string-of-beads signs. The stretch sign is defined as small bowel gas arrayed as stripes perpendicular to the long axis of the bowel outlining the valvulae conniventes as seen in **Fig. 1**.[11,17] The string-of-beads sign is defined as a series of air-fluid levels measuring less than 1 cm.[17]

Determining severity on radiographs can be difficult. The 2 signs most associated with complete or high-grade obstruction are air-fluid levels of differential heights in the same loop of bowel and air-fluid levels with a width greater than 2.5 cm on upright radiographs, as seen in **Fig. 2**. The presence of both signs showed a positive predictive value of 86% for the presence of complete obstruction.[17]

COMPUTED TOMOGRAPHY
Technique

Although the use of water-soluble positive oral contrast is still widely prevalent, there are multiple drawbacks to using oral contrast with questionable benefits. The current American College of Radiology Appropriateness Criteria recommend evaluating possible high-grade obstruction with an MDCT using intravenous (IV) contrast only unless contraindicated.[15] The use of oral contrast delays care for up to 3 hours, delaying diagnosis and care and decreasing emergency department throughput.[15,18–20] Patients with suspected SBO often have a difficult time ingesting oral contrast because of nausea and vomiting, creating the potential for aspiration of contrast.[18] Oral contrast also increases the radiation dose to the patient when using modern MDCT scanners with automated exposure control.[19–21]

Diagnostic drawbacks of positive oral contrast include obscuring intraluminal causes of bowel obstruction and several signs of bowel ischemia, such as decreased wall enhancement and the presence of intraluminal hemorrhage.[15,22,23] Decreased bowel wall enhancement is the most specific sign of bowel wall ischemia and can be difficult to discern with intraluminal positive contrast, as shown in **Fig. 3**.[22–24] During SBO, normally secreted fluid that has not been reabsorbed

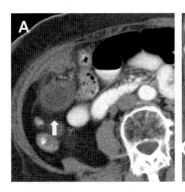

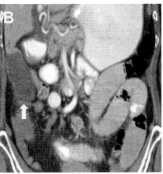

Fig. 3. Axial (*A*) and coronal (*B*) IV contrast-enhanced CT images demonstrating a decreased bowel wall enhancement (*arrows*).

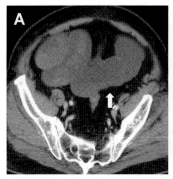 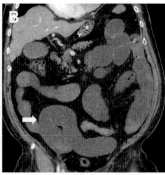

Fig. 4. Axial (*A*) and coronal (*B*) IV contrast-enhanced CT images demonstrating the use of normally secreted fluid that has not been reabsorbed by the bowel as a natural negative contrast in diagnosing bowel obstruction (*arrows*).

by the bowel creates a natural negative contrast in distended loops of bowel that can aid in the diagnosis of intraluminal causes of obstruction, decreased bowel wall enhancement, and intraluminal hemorrhage (**Fig. 4**) instead of obscuring it as does positive oral contrast.

The benefits of using positive oral contrast include the exclusion of high-grade obstruction with the passage of contrast and being able to evaluate for possible resolution of the obstruction using a plain abdominal radiograph.[3,18] On follow-up abdominal radiographs, if contrast material is seen within the colon, either the obstruction has resolved or it is low grade.[3] However, in a large retrospective study involving 1992 patients evaluated with MDCT with IV contrast only for acute abdominal pain, Uyeda and colleagues[20] showed that only 4 patients (0.2%) required repeat CT imaging because of lack of oral contrast.

A typical protocol, summarized in **Table 1**, for MDCT of the abdomen and pelvis for evaluation of suspected acute SBO consists of thin 1.25-mm

axial slice acquisition approximately 70 seconds following the power injection of 100 mL of typically nonionic IV contrast at 3 to 5 mL/s in portal venous phase. The timing of the contrast bolus can be adjusted so that maximum attenuation of the liver is achieved. Additional thick-slice 3.75 mm axial along with 3 to 5 mm coronal and sagittal reformats are created to increase the ability to localize the transition point and assess the cause of the obstruction.[18]

Role of Multidetector Computed Tomography

MDCT plays a critical role in the diagnosis and guidance of treatment of SBO with a reported sensitivity of 90% to 96%, a specificity of 96%, and an accuracy of 95%.[25] When evaluating a suspected obstruction using MDCT several questions need to be answered (**Box 2**).

IMAGING FINDINGS
Diagnostic Criteria

Diagnosing SBO first requires the identification of dilated loops of small bowel, typically 3 cm or greater, with a normal-sized colon less than 6 cm in diameter or 9 cm for the cecum.[11,23,25] Some clinicians use a diameter of 2.5 cm or greater as a cutoff for small bowel dilation, which yields higher sensitivity.[8,11,26,27] A transition point, the point at

Table 1 Typical MDCT protocol for evaluating SBO	
Area of acquisition	Abdomen and pelvis; lung bases to the proximal thighs
IV contrast	100 mL of nonionized iodinated contrast
Injection speed	3–5 mL/s
Oral contrast	None
Phase of acquisition	Portal venous phase: 70 s delay before acquisition
Reconstructions	Thin 1.25-mm and thick 3.75-mm axial slices, 3–5 mm coronal and sagittal reformats

Box 2 Questions to answer for suspected SBO
Is SBO present?
Where is the transition point?
Is there a single transition point or is a closed-loop obstruction present?
What is the cause of the obstruction?
Are there signs of complications such as ischemia, necrosis, or perforation?

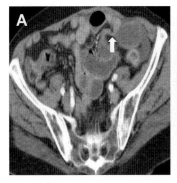
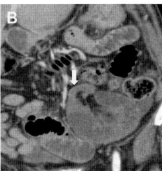

Fig. 5. Axial (*A*) and coronal (*B*) IV contrast-enhanced CT images demonstrating the transition point (*arrows*).

which the bowel transitions from dilated to nondilated loops of bowel, should be identified[8,11,23,25,26] as seen in **Fig. 5**. The presence of dilated loops of small bowel and a transition point within the small bowel are major imaging findings necessary for the diagnosis of SBO. Additional signs of SBO not required for, but can aid in the diagnosis of, SBO include air-fluid levels, collapsed colon, and the small bowel feces sign.[8,11,25,26] SBO diagnostic criteria are summarized in **Table 2**.

Air-fluid levels, collapsed colon, and the small bowel feces sign are unreliable signs of obstruction that may or may not be present.[8,11,28] Air-fluid levels are not specific for obstruction and were seen in 69% of cases of unobstructed cases.[27] Although the colon is more likely to be collapsed, with a greater than 50% difference in the diameter of the proximal dilated small bowel and the colon, in high-grade obstruction it can be of normal size depending on the timing of obstruction.[26]

The small bowel feces sign is the fecalization of material within the small bowel resulting in formation of particulate, partially aerated material as seen in **Fig. 6**. The prevalence of this

sign is low, ranging from 6% to 37%.[26,28] The main utility of the sign is that it most often occurs just proximal to the transition point.[28] Finding the small bowel feces sign can help localize the transition point, which is crucial for diagnosing and assessing the cause of the SBO.

Differential Diagnosis

The list of differential diagnoses is short, consisting of paralytic ileus and large bowel obstruction. Finding the transition point is the key to diagnosing SBO. If a transition point can be located, paralytic ileus is effectively ruled out. If the transition point is within loops of small bowel as opposed to the colon, SBO can be diagnosed and large bowel obstruction excluded.[27] **Table 3** lists the differential diagnosis and key distinguishing diagnostic features between them and SBO.

Severity of the Obstruction

Determining the severity of an obstruction can be difficult on MDCT. Although the passage of positive oral contrast past the point of obstruction effectively rules out high-grade obstruction, oral contrast is not frequently used for reasons previously stated. The presence or absence of multiple signs have been suggested to determine the grade of the obstruction, although having a high-grade obstruction does not always indicate that nonoperative management will fail.[1,25,29,30] What is crucial for the clinical management of the patient is to evaluate the transition point for the presence of a closed-loop obstruction, cause of the obstruction, and signs of ischemia.

Closed-Loop Obstruction

Once the diagnosis of SBO is made, the first step in evaluating the obstruction is to identify whether

Table 2 Diagnostic criteria for SBO	
Major criteria (necessary for diagnosis)	Dilated loops of small bowel ≥3 cm with normal-sized colon (<6 cm)
	Transition point from dilated to nondilated bowel within the small bowel
Minor criteria (not necessary but useful for diagnosis)	Air-fluid levels Collapsed colon Small bowel feces sign

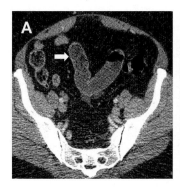
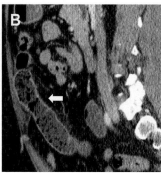

Fig. 6. Axial (*A*) and sagittal (*B*) IV contrast-enhanced CT images demonstrating fecalization of material within the small bowel, known as a small bowel feces sign (*arrows*).

there is a single transition point or a closed-loop obstruction. Closed-loop obstructions occur when a segment of bowel is isolated at 2 or more adjacent points, effectively isolating the segment from the remainder of the bowel.[8,11,18,25] When a closed-loop obstruction is present, gas and material can no longer pass through the lumen of bowel, resulting in the buildup of secreted fluid causing further dilation of bowel and compression of surrounding mesentery, predisposing to the bowel to vascular compromise and ischemia.[18,25] Even without overt signs of ischemia, closed-loop obstruction is considered a precursor to bowel ischemia and therefore, is often considered a surgical emergency.[25]

The CT signs of a closed-loop obstruction depend on the cause and orientation of the loops. The causes of closed-loop obstructions include adhesions, internal and external hernias, and a small bowel volvulus.[25,31] At the site of a closed-loop obstruction, the bowel often gradually tapers to a point causing a beak sign, as seen in **Fig. 7**. When a closed-loop obstruction is caused by a single adhesive band or single site of a hernia, the 2 adjacent transition points often form into beak signs.[1] The dilated fluid-filled segment of bowel in a

closed-loop obstruction can also form a "C" or a "U" configuration based on the orientation of the segment in axial, coronal, and sagittal planes, as seen in **Fig. 8**. The segment will converge on the site of the obstruction.[11,25] The presence of 2 or more beak signs and a "C" or "U" configuration of a dilated loop of bowel is associated with the failure of nonoperative treatment.[1]

A small bowel volvulus with a twisting mesenteric stalk can cause a closed-loop obstruction that appears as a radial distribution of fluid-filled dilated loops of bowel around a single point. This configuration is also known as the spoke-wheel sign and carries an incidence of concurrent bowel ischemia in up to 46% of patients.[31] As seen in **Fig. 9**, the vessels of radially distributed loops of bowel converge on a single central point.

Table 3 Differential diagnosis for SBO	
Differential Diagnosis	Distinguishing Features
Paralytic ileus	Dilated loops of bowel without a transition point
Large bowel obstruction	Transition point within the colon

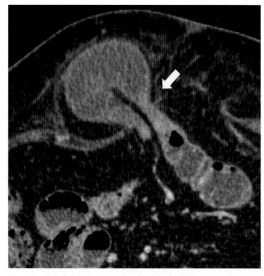

Fig. 7. Axial IV contrast-enhanced CT image demonstrating a beak sign (*arrow*).

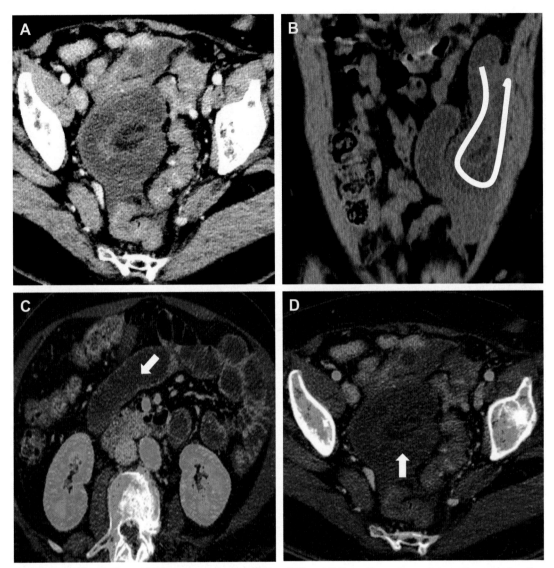

Fig. 8. Axial (*A*) and coronal (*B*) CT images demonstrating "C" and "U" configurations of closed-loop obstruction. Axial (*C, D*) IV contrast-enhanced CT images with iodine overlay demonstrates hypoenhancement of the obstructed bowel (*arrows*).

CAUSES OF SMALL BOWEL OBSTRUCTION

To determine the cause of the obstruction, the best place to look is at the transition point. The cause of the obstruction is almost always located at or around the transition point. The causes of bowel obstruction are categorized as extrinsic, intrinsic, and intraluminal. Extrinsic causes of SBO exert external pressure on the bowel causing the obstruction. If the underlying cause of obstruction is due to or arising from the bowel wall itself, it is categorized as an intrinsic cause. Intraluminal causes include blockages from gallstones, bezoars, and foreign bodies.[26,32] A summary of causes of bowel obstruction ids presented in **Table 4**. Once the cause of obstruction is limited to a category, the clinical history can be incorporated with additional diagnostic clues to further narrow down the possible causes of the obstruction.

Extrinsic Causes

By far the most common cause of bowel obstruction is adhesions, causing 60% to 85% of cases of SBO.[25,32,33] Although most adhesions form following prior abdominal surgery,

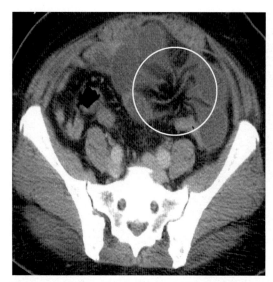

Fig. 9. Axial IV contrast-enhanced CT image demonstrating a spoke-wheel sign from volvulus with radial distribution of fluid-filled dilated loops of bowel around a single point.

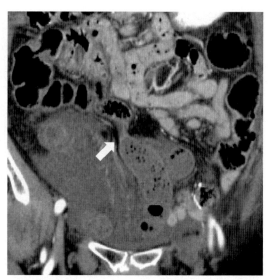

Fig. 10. Coronal IV contrast-enhanced CT image demonstrating adhesion as a cause of SBO, diagnosed by excluding other causes of obstruction (arrow).

approximately 10% to 15% of patients with adhesive SBO do not have a surgical history, so these adhesions are most likely due to prior episodes of peritonitis.[32] Since the adhesive bands are not directly visible on MDCT, the diagnosis is made by excluding other causes of obstruction (Fig. 10).

Hernias cause an estimated 10% to 20% of all cases of SBO.[32,33] External hernias can be easily identified by locating the transition point at the neck of the hernia with proximal bowel dilation. Fig. 11 demonstrates an example of a parastomal hernia. Internal hernias occur when small bowel protrudes through an opening in the mesentery or peritoneum into another cavity. Identifying internal hernias can be difficult on MDCT; however, the crowding of small bowel loops, swirling of mesenteric vessel or swirl sign, mushroom-shaped herniation of the mesenteric root and vessels or "mushroom sign", and the abnormal location of small bowel can indicate the presence of an internal hernia.[32,34,35]

Roux-en-Y gastric bypass

The increase in laparoscopic Roux-en-Y gastric bypass (LRYGB) surgery has resulted in an increased number of internal hernias causing SBO with an incidence rate of 1% to 4%.[34,36] Dilauro and colleagues[34] found that the swirl sign in LRYGB patients has a higher sensitivity for internal hernias than the typical criteria for SBO, 86% to 89% versus 22% to 25%. The presence of the swirl sign in LRYGB patients indicates an internal hernia even without the presence of dilated loops of small bowel. A proposed superior mesenteric vein (SMV) beaking sign, consisting of the tapering or beaking of the SMV, was also found to have high sensitivity of 80% to 88% for the presence of an internal hernia in LRYGB patients, as seen in Fig. 12.[34]

Intrinsic Causes

Crohn disease is a common cause of SBO with diagnostic characteristics of

Table 4 Causes of SBO	
Extrinsic	Adhesions
	Hernias (internal and external)
	Endometriosis
	Neoplasms (extraintestinal)
Intrinsic	Inflammatory/infectious diseases
	Neoplasms of the small bowel (primary and secondary)
	Vascular causes (mesenteric ischemia)
	Intramural hematoma
	Radiation enteritis
	Intussusception
Intraluminal	Gallstone ileus
	Bezoars
	Foreign bodies

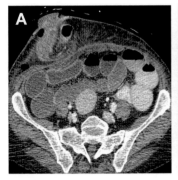

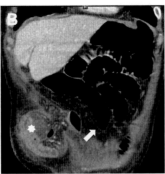

Fig. 11. Axial (*A*) and coronal (*B*) IV contrast-enhanced CT images demonstrating parastomal hernia (*asterisks*) as a cause of SBO (*arrows*).

narrowing of the bowel lumen, skip lesions, and transmural thickening.[25] Signs of active Crohn disease can mimic the target sign, a sign of bowel ischemia, with submucosal edema causing stratified mural enhancement.[25,37]

Mesenteric ischemia resulting from occlusion or a critical stenosis of the superior mesenteric artery (SMA) can cause SBO from ischemic changes including lack of peristalsis and wall thickening, as seen in **Fig. 13**. Diffuse decreased bowel wall enhancement of the small bowel should prompt an evaluation of the SMA for occlusion.

An estimated 80% to 92% of cases of intussusception in adults is secondary to an organic lesion, causing a lead point to initiate the invagination of a loop of bowel into another.[38] The presence of an intussusception in an adult should precipitate a search for a lesion. Benign and malignant lesions including adenomatous polyps, adenocarcinoma, lymphoma, metastases, and gastrointestinal stromal tumors can cause intussusception resulting in SBO or obstruction through the narrowing and occlusion of the bowel lumen.[38] An example of intrinsic small bowel lesion causing intussusception and obstruction is shown in **Fig. 14**.

Intramural hematoma is a rare cause of obstruction that is most often due to anticoagulant use. The typical presentation on MDCT is circumference thickening of the bowel wall with SBO on anticoagulation therapy.[39] A patient on warfarin with a supratherapeutic international normalized ratio should raise the suspicion of an intramural hematoma as a possible cause of obstruction.

Obstruction caused by radiation enteritis can present anywhere from 2 months to 30 years following radiation treatment.[40] Chronic radiation enteritis that causes SBO is really an occlusive vasculitis resulting in submucosal fibrosis with bowel wall thickening and luminal narrowing, as seen in **Fig. 15**.

Intraluminal Causes

Gallstone ileus is a rare cause of SBO whereby a passed gallstone becomes lodged in the small intestine, causing obstruction. Typical imaging features include Rigler's triad of pneumobilia, SBO, and a gallstone at the transition point, as seen in **Fig. 16**.[32]

Two additional rare intraluminal causes of SBO include foreign body ingestion and bezoars. Evaluating the transition point for the presence of an intraluminal mass is the key to identifying these causes.

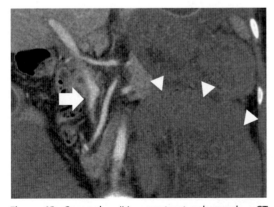

Fig. 12. Coronal IV contrast-enhanced CT image demonstrating a superior mesenteric vein beaking sign of a patient with a surgically confirmed internal hernia causing bowel obstruction after gastric bypass surgery (*arrow*). Also seen are ischemic loops of obstructed bowel with hypoenhancement of the bowel wall (*arrowheads*).

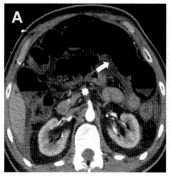

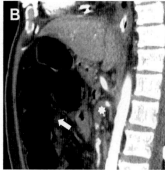

Fig. 13. Axial (*A*) and sagittal (*B*) IV contrast-enhanced CT images demonstrating mesenteric ischemia (*arrows*) as evidenced by lack of peristalsis and wall thickening caused by occlusion or critical stenosis of the SMA (*asterisks*).

SIGNS OF ISCHEMIA

Identifying the presence of ischemic or strangulated bowel is essential because its presence greatly increases the risk of mortality from 2% to 8% to up to 40% in cases of SBO.[9] MDCT has a sensitivity of 83% and specificity of 92% for the diagnosis of bowel ischemia.[25] Signs of ischemia as listed in **Table 5** include decreased bowel wall enhancement, mesenteric edema, bowel wall thickening greater than 3 mm that can present as a target sign, intraluminal hemorrhage, engorged mesenteric vessels, the whirl sign, pneumatosis, and mesenteric or portal venous gas.[9,11,25,26,37,41]

Decreased bowel wall enhancement is the most specific sign of bowel ischemia, with a specificity of 94% to 100%.[8,9,23–25] The presence of decreased bowel wall enhancement increases the likelihood of bowel ischemia by 11-fold.[9] **Fig. 17** shows an example of decreased bowel wall enhancement in a patient with ischemic bowel. The use of dual-energy CT has the potential to make identifying bowel ischemia easier. Iodine overlay maps make the difference in bowel wall enhancement more prominent and easier to detect.[42]

Mesenteric edema or fluid presents as haziness in the mesentery adjacent to a loop of obstructed bowel, as seen in **Fig. 18**; this has a sensitivity of 84% and specificity of 40% for ischemia.[23] Abundant ascites can confound or mimic mesenteric edema, which can be problematic in cirrhotic patients.

Less specific and sensitive signs of bowel ischemia including the target sign, pneumatosis, mesenteric and portal venous gas, engorged mesenteric vessels, and the whirl sign need to be viewed in conjunction with the patient's overall clinical picture and additional imaging findings on the MDCT. Numerous mimics of these signs decrease their value when they are seen in isolation.

Circumferential bowel wall thickening >3 mm, also known as the target sign, is a relatively nonspecific sign with numerous possible causes. Active inflammation in Crohn disease can cause submucosal edema, which can mimic ischemia. In addition, deposition of fat within the submucosa, which can be due to chronic Crohn disease or benign intramural fat deposition, can also cause bowel wall thickening with a stratification of enhancing layers mimicking ischemia, as seen in **Fig. 19**.[37]

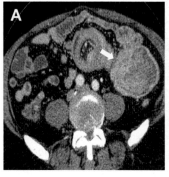

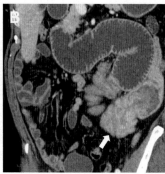

Fig. 14. Axial (*A*) and coronal (*B*) IV contrast-enhanced CT images demonstrating intrinsic small bowel lesion, a jejunal adenocarcinoma, causing intussusception and obstruction (*arrows*).

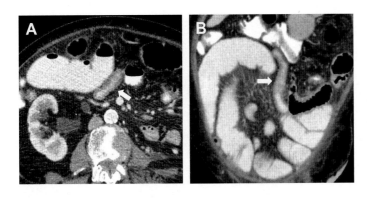

Fig. 15. Axial (*A*) and coronal (*B*) IV contrast-enhanced CT images demonstrating radiation enteritis causing occlusive vasculitis and submucosal fibrosis with small bowel wall thickening and luminal narrowing (*arrows*).

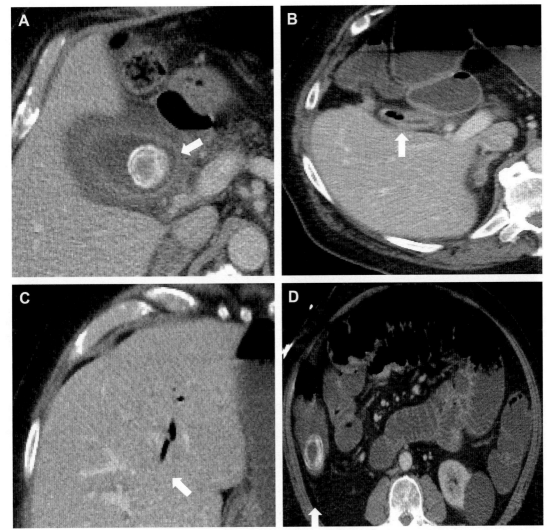

Fig. 16. Axial (*A*) IV contrast-enhanced CT image demonstrating acute gallstone cholecystitis. Axial (*B, C*) and coronal (*D*) IV contrast-enhanced CT images after a few months, demonstrating collapsed gallbladder with foci of air, pneumobilia, and gallstone ileus (*arrows*).

Table 5
Signs and mimics of bowel ischemia

Sign of Bowel Ischemia	Mimics of the Sign
Decreased bowel wall enhancement	None
Mesenteric edema	Ascites
Occlusion of a mesenteric vessel (typically the SMA)	None
Intraluminal hemorrhage	Retained fecal material or contrast
Target sign (bowel wall thickening)	Crohn disease Infectious enteritis Benign intramural fat deposition
Whirl sign	Internal hernia without ischemia Whirl sign without ischemia or an internal hernia
Engorged mesenteric vessels	Internal hernia without ischemia
Pneumatosis intestinalis	Pneumatosis cystoides intestinalis Pseudopneumatosis
Mesenteric or portal venous gas	Pneumobilia

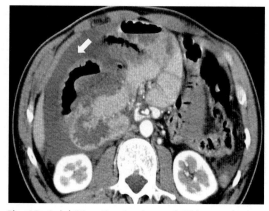

Fig. 18. Axial IV contrast-enhanced CT image demonstrating mesenteric fluid (*arrow*).

The whirl sign, which consists of swirling mesentery, and the engorgement of mesenteric vessels are important signs of volvulus and internal hernia, especially in LRYGB patients.[34,43] Visualization of either of these signs should prompt a careful search for additional signs of ischemia. When seen in isolation, they are highly suspicious for an internal hernia or volvulus and should be reported as such.

Pneumatosis and mesenteric and portal venous gas are important late-stage signs of bowel ischemia, indicating transmural bowel necrosis. As such, additional signs of ischemia should be present to make the diagnosis of strangulated bowel. Portal venous gas is seen as tubular air-filled structures within the liver. Portal venous gas can be distinguished from pneumobilia by the peripheral extent of gas within the liver, whereas pneumobilia typically remains centrally located within the large intrahepatic biliary ducts as seen in Fig. 20.[44]

Pneumatosis intestinalis caused by ischemia, which is characterized by air within the bowel wall, can be confused with pneumatosis cystoides intestinalis, a rare benign condition of air-filled cysts within the bowel wall.[45,46] Pneumatosis cystoides intestinalis is associated with chronic obstructive pulmonary disease, prior intestinal surgeries, and connective tissue disorders.[45] Furthermore, pneumatosis intestinalis is only associated with life-threatening

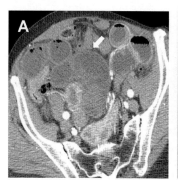
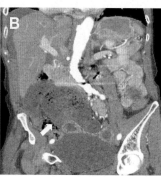

Fig. 17. Axial (*A*) and coronal (*B*) IV contrast-enhanced CT images demonstrating decreased bowel wall enhancement from bowel ischemia (*arrows*).

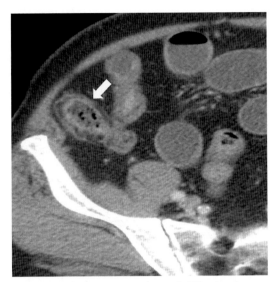

Fig. 19. Axial IV contrast-enhanced CT image demonstrating chronic terminal ileitis causing a bowel wall thickening with intramural fat deposition and a stratification of enhancing layers mimicking ischemia (*arrow*).

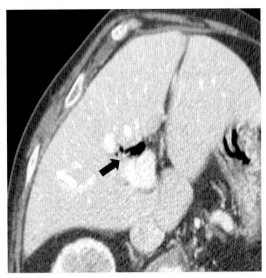

Fig. 20. Axial CT images demonstrating pneumobilia (*arrow*).

bowel ischemia 30% of the time, with the remaining causes representing benign processes.[47] Benign nonischemic pneumatosis is theorized to be caused by increased intraluminal pressure, gas diffusion, bacterial invasion of the bowel wall, mucosal injury, and a defective immune barrier.[47] Pseudopneumatosis is gas trapped with stool and fluid along the bowel wall that can mimic pneumatosis, but respects fluid levels and does not occur in air-filled areas. Fig. 21 shows examples of pneumatosis and its mimics.

WHAT THE REFERRING PHYSICIAN NEEDS TO KNOW

- CT of the abdomen and pelvis with IV contrast only is the best and most efficient method to evaluate suspected SBO.

- Including pertinent clinical history when ordering the examination, especially history of any prior abdominal surgery (particularly Roux-en-Y gastric bypass), is essential for raising the suspicion of an internal hernia causing obstruction.
- Most obstructions can be treated conservatively with nonoperative management. The role of MDCT is to diagnose, find the cause, and look for complications of SBO that can lead to the failure of nonoperative treatment.
- The presence of a closed-loop obstruction or signs of ischemia, particularly reduced bowel wall enhancement, are surgical emergencies that require immediate evaluation by the surgical team.

SUMMARY

SBO is a common condition that often results in ischemia, which carries a high risk of mortality if

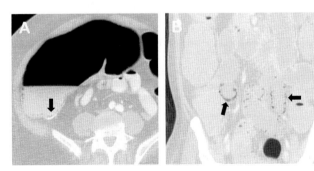

Fig. 21. Axial (*A*) and coronal (*B*) IV contrast-enhanced CT images in lung window demonstrate 2 examples of ischemic pneumatosis mimics, with (*A*) showing pseudopneumatosis (*arrow*) and (*B*) showing benign pneumatosis intestinalis (*arrows*) without bowel ischemia. Pseudopneumatosis is air that is trapped with stool and fluid along the bowel wall, whereas pneumatosis would be seen along the bowel wall that does not abut the intraluminal contents, including antidependent wall.

there is a delay in diagnosis. MDCT of the abdomen and pelvis with IV contrast only has become the standard in diagnosing and evaluating SBO. It is the radiologist's job to diagnosis SBO, find the transition point, determine the cause, and identify the presence of a closed-loop obstruction and any signs of ischemia. Answering these questions can help the clinical team determine which patient is likely to need surgical intervention.

REFERENCES

1. Millet I, Ruyer A, Alili C, et al. Adhesive small-bowel obstruction: value of ct in identifying findings associated with the effectiveness of nonsurgical treatment. Radiology 2014;273(2):425–32.
2. Frasure SE, Hildreth A, Takhar S, et al. Emergency department patients with small bowel obstruction: What is the anticipated clinical course? World J Emerg Med 2016;7(1):35–9.
3. Ten Broek RPG, Krielen P, Di Saverio S, et al. Bologna guidelines for diagnosis and management of adhesive small bowel obstruction (ASBO): 2017 update of the evidence-based guidelines from the world society of emergency surgery ASBO working group. World J Emerg Surg 2018;13:24.
4. Ellis H, Moran BJ, Thompson JN, et al. Adhesion-related hospital readmissions after abdominal and pelvic surgery: a retrospective cohort study. Lancet 1999;353(9163):1476–80.
5. ten Broek RP, Issa Y, van Santbrink EJ, et al. Burden of adhesions in abdominal and pelvic surgery: systematic review and met-analysis. BMJ 2013;347: f5588.
6. Berman DJ, Ijaz H, Alkhunaizi M, et al. Nasogastric decompression not associated with a reduction in surgery or bowel ischemia for acute small bowel obstruction. Am J Emerg Med 2017;35(12):1919–21.
7. Barkan H, Webster S, Ozeran S. Factors predicting the recurrence of adhesive small-bowel obstruction. Am J Surg 1995;170(4):361–5.
8. Burkill G, Bell J, Healy J. Small bowel obstruction: the role of computed tomography in its diagnosis and management with reference to other imaging modalities. Eur Radiol 2001;11(8):1405–22.
9. Millet I, Taourel P, Ruyer A, et al. Value of CT findings to predict surgical ischemia in small bowel obstruction: a systematic review and meta-analysis. Eur Radiol 2015;25(6):1823–35.
10. Jancelewicz T, Vu LT, Shawo AE, et al. Predicting strangulated small bowel obstruction: an old problem revisited. J Gastrointest Surg 2009;13(1):93–9.
11. Paulson EK, Thompson WM. Review of small-bowel obstruction: the diagnosis and when to worry. Radiology 2015;275(2):332–42.

12. Maglinte DDT, Kelvin FM, Rowe MG, et al. Small-bowel obstruction: optimizing radiologic investigation and nonsurgical management. Radiology 2001;218(1):39–46.
13. Foster NM, McGory ML, Zingmond DS, et al. Small bowel obstruction: a population-based appraisal. J Am Coll Surg 2006;203(2):170–6.
14. Thompson WM, Kilani RK, Smith BB, et al. Accuracy of abdominal radiography in acute small-bowel obstruction: does reviewer experience matter? AJR Am J Roentgenol 2007;188(3):W233–8.
15. Ros PR, Huprich JE. ACR appropriateness criteria on suspected small-bowel obstruction. J Am Coll Radiol 2006;3(11):838–41.
16. Thompson WM. Gasless abdomen in the adult: what does it mean? AJR Am J Roentgenol 2008;191(4): 1093–9.
17. Lappas JC, Reyes BL, Maglinte DDT. Abdominal radiography findings in small-bowel obstruction. AJR Am J Roentgenol 2001;176(1):167–74.
18. Boudiaf M, Soyer P, Terem C, et al. Ct evaluation of small bowel obstruction. Radiographics 2001; 21(3):613–24.
19. Anderson SW, Soto JA, Lucey BC, et al. Abdominal 64-MDCT for suspected appendicitis: the use of oral and IV Contrast material versus IV contrast material only. AJR Am J Roentgenol 2009;193(5):1282–8.
20. Uyeda JW, Yu H, Ramalingam V, et al. Evaluation of acute abdominal pain in the emergency setting using computed tomography without oral contrast in patients with body mass index greater than 25. J Comput Assist Tomogr 2015;39(5):681–6.
21. Wang ZJ, Chen KS, Gould R, et al. Positive enteric contrast material for abdominal and pelvic CT with automatic exposure control: what is the effect on patient radiation exposure? Eur J Radiol 2011;79(2): e58–62.
22. Chou CK, Wu RH, Mak C-W, et al. Clinical significance of poor CT enhancement of the thickened small-bowel wall in patients with acute abdominal pain. AJR Am J Roentgenol 2006;186(2):491–8.
23. Millet I, Boutot D, Faget C, et al. Assessment of strangulation in adhesive small bowel obstruction on the basis of combined ct findings: implications for clinical care. Radiology 2017;285(3):798–808.
24. Ha HK, Kim JS, Lee MS, et al. Differentiation of simple and strangulated small-bowel obstructions: usefulness of known CT criteria. Radiology 1997;204(2): 507–12.
25. O'Malley RG, Al-Hawary MM, Kaza RK, et al. MDCT findings in small bowel obstruction: implications of the cause and presence of complications on treatment decisions. Abdom Imaging 2015;40(7): 2248–62.
26. Silva AC, Pimenta M, Guimaraes LS. Small bowel obstruction: what to look for. Radiographics 2009; 29(2):423–39.

27. Gazelle GS, Goldberg MA, Wittenberg J, et al. Efficacy of CT in distinguishing small-bowel obstruction from other causes of small-bowel dilatation. AJR Am J Roentgenol 1994;162(1):43–7.

28. Khaled W, Millet I, Corno L, et al. Clinical relevance of the feces sign in small-bowel obstruction due to adhesions depends on its location. AJR Am J Roentgenol 2018;210(1):78–84.

29. Deshmukh SD, Shin DS, Willmann JK, et al. Nonemergency small bowel obstruction: assessment of CT findings that predict need for surgery. Eur Radiol 2011;21(5):982–6.

30. Rocha FG, Theman TA, Matros E, et al. Nonoperative management of patients with a diagnosis of high-grade small bowel obstruction by computed tomography. Arch Surg 2009;144(11):1000–4.

31. Rudloff U. The spoke wheel sign: bowel. Radiology 2005;237(3):1046–7.

32. Tirumani H, Vassa R, Fasih N, et al. Small bowel obstruction in the emergency department: MDCT features of common and uncommon causes. Clin Imaging 2014;38(5):580–8.

33. Szeliga J, Jackowski M. Laparoscopy in small bowel obstruction—current status—review. Wideochir Inne Tech Maloinwazyjne 2017;12(4):455–60.

34. Dilauro M, McInnes MDF, Schieda N, et al. Internal hernia after laparoscopic Roux-en-Y gastric bypass: optimal CT signs for diagnosis and clinical decision making. Radiology 2017;282(3):752–60.

35. Miller PA, Mezwa DG, Feczko PJ, et al. Imaging of abdominal hernias. Radiographics 1995;15(2):333–47.

36. Champion JK, Williams M. Small bowel obstruction and internal hernias after laparoscopic Roux-en-Y gastric bypass. Obes Surg 2003;13(4):596–600.

37. Ahualli J. The target sign: bowel wall. Radiology 2005;234(2):549–50.

38. Marinis A, Yiallourou A, Samanides L, et al. Intussusception of the bowel in adults: a review. World J Gastroenterol 2009;15(4):407–11.

39. Pimenta JM, Saramet R, Pimenta de Castro J, et al. Overlooked complication of anticoagulant therapy: the intramural small bowel hematoma-A case report. Int J Surg Case Rep 2017;39:305–8.

40. Harb AH, Abou Fadel C, Sharara AI. Radiation enteritis. Curr Gastroenterol Rep 2014;16(5):383.

41. Zielinski MD, Eiken PW, Bannon MP, et al. Small bowel obstruction—who needs an operation? A multivariate prediction model. World J Surg 2010;34(5):910–9.

42. Wortman JR, Uyeda JW, Fulwadhva UP, et al. Dual-energy CT for abdominal and pelvic trauma. Radiographics 2018;38(2):586–602.

43. Blachar A, Federle MP, Dodson SF. Internal hernia: clinical and imaging findings in 17 patients with emphasis on CT criteria. Radiology 2001;218(1):68–74.

44. Sebastià C, Quiroga S, Espin E, et al. Portomesenteric vein gas: pathologic mechanisms, CT findings, and prognosis. Radiographics 2000;20(5):1213–24.

45. Azzaroli F, Turco L, Ceroni L, et al. Pneumatosis cystoides intestinalis. World J Gastroenterol 2011;17(44):4932–6.

46. Wang YJ, Wang YM, Zheng YM, et al. Pneumatosis cystoides intestinalis: six case reports and a review of the literature. BMC Gastroenterol 2018;18(1):100.

47. Torres US, Fortes C, Salvadori PS, et al. Pneumatosis from esophagus to rectum: a comprehensive review focusing on clinico-radiological differentiation between benign and life-threatening causes. Semin Ultrasound CT MR 2018;39(2):167–82.

Utility of MR Imaging in Abdominopelvic Emergencies

Jennifer W. Uyeda, MD

KEYWORDS

- MR imaging • Acute abdominal pain • Acute abdomen • Acute pelvic pain • Appendicitis
- Pregnancy

KEY POINTS

- MR imaging may be performed in the emergency setting as an alternative to computed tomography, particularly in pediatric and pregnant populations.
- Use of magnetic resonance in the acute setting is performed for specific indications with the use of tailored protocols focused on rapid image acquisition.
- Lack of ionizing radiation, ability to provide excellent tissue contrast, and an established and proven track record make MR imaging an attractive imaging modality for evaluating acute abdominopelvic emergencies.

INTRODUCTION

Acute abdominal pain is one of the most common symptoms in patients who present to the emergency department (ED). Of all patients who present to the ED, approximately 8% have acute abdominal pain with an estimated seven million visits a year.[1,2] Acute abdominal pathologic conditions account for more than half of all nontrauma-related surgical interventions performed in the emergency setting.[3,4] Acute abdominopelvic pain can be a diagnostic challenge given the large differential diagnosis with a wide spectrum of pathologic conditions encompassing multiple organ systems. Moreover, there is a broad range of pathologic conditions that can produce acute abdominopelvic pain, ranging from benign self-limiting to life-threatening and emergent diseases. Of all patients presenting with acute abdominopelvic pain, one-third have acute appendicitis, one-third never have a diagnosis, and one-third will have pain secondary to a diagnosis in the category of so-called other. Within this other category, the most common diagnoses causing acute abdominopelvic pain include acute cholecystitis, small bowel obstruction, pancreatitis, renal colic, perforated peptic ulcer disease, and diverticulitis.[5]

Diagnostic imaging plays a critical role in the treatment of patients with acute abdominopelvic pain given the high diagnostic accuracy in making a confident and accurate diagnosis and in guiding management.[6,7] A recent study by Pandharipande and colleagues[8] found that the leading diagnosis changed in more than half of all patients undergoing computed tomography (CT) scan in the ED, and the decision to admit changed in 25% of patients who presented with abdominal pain after receiving a CT scan in the ED. About 16% of all patients who present to the ED receive a CT scan.[2] According to the American College of Radiology (ACR) appropriateness criteria, a contrast-enhanced CT scan is the preferred imaging given the widespread availability and speed of imaging acquisition.[9] MR imaging may be appropriate in evaluating acute abdominopelvic pain and is usually performed for specific indications with the use of tailored protocols.[9–11] Magnetic resonance (MR) has been shown to be accurate for

Disclosure Statement: The author has no relevant financial disclosures.
Department of Radiology, Brigham and Women's Hospital, 75 Francis Street, Boston, MA 02115, USA
E-mail address: JUyeda@bwh.harvard.edu

Radiol Clin N Am 57 (2019) 705–715
https://doi.org/10.1016/j.rcl.2019.02.010

diagnosing a range of pathologic conditions in the abdomen and pelvis, and may be used as an alternative to CT.[9,11] The major advantages of MR imaging are the lack of ionizing radiation and the high inherent tissue contrast resolution, which may obviate intravenous (IV) contrast administration. MR imaging is an attractive and commonly used imaging modality in evaluating acute abdominopelvic pain, particularly in the pediatric and pregnant populations, and offers several advantages. The purpose of this article is to provide an overview of the advantages and disadvantages of MR imaging in evaluating acute abdominopelvic pain in the emergency setting; to review MR imaging protocols, focusing on rapid image acquisition techniques; and to discuss the MR imaging appearances of the most common diagnoses encountered in acute abdominopelvic pain.

ADVANTAGES AND DISADVANTAGES OF MR IMAGING

Overall, MR imaging costs more than other cross-sectional imaging modalities, such as ultrasound (US) and CT.[12,13] Saini and colleagues[12] showed the technical cost per examination for a US, CT, and MR at a tertiary care academic center was $50.28, $112.32, and $266.96, respectively. However, the cost per technical relative value unit for US, CT, and MR imaging were $28.74, $20.95, and $17.69, respectively.

From a patient perspective, because MR is more susceptible to motion artifact, this requires patients to cooperate and lie still for the duration of the MR acquisition. Additionally, patients are confined to the MR bore, which may not be suitable for claustrophobic patients. Compatibility with the equipment used for patient monitoring can be an issue given the high magnetic field of MR in addition to other implants and devices, such as cardiac devices, cochlear implants, and contraceptive devices.

Consistent availability of MR and institutional expertise are potential drawbacks of MR imaging in the acute setting. Although many large academic institutions have MR readily available 24 hours, 7 days a week, this may not be feasible for all institutions. Furthermore, many radiologists and other physicians are familiar with various pathologic conditions on CT examinations and are less attune to the imaging appearances on MR.

The lack of ionizing radiation exposure gives MR a major advantage in imaging pediatric and pregnant patients in whom radiation is of particular concern. MR has superior contrast resolution and increased tissue characterization that aid in making an accurate diagnosis, especially in patients with allergy to iodinated contrast material or renal failure. The feasibility of using MR for acute abdominopelvic pain depends on institutional availability and expertise, as well as adoption of tailored MR imaging protocols.

MR IMAGING PROTOCOLS

Although traditional MR examinations can be time-consuming, imaging protocols in the emergency setting should be optimized and tailored to address specific indications and should be aimed at rapid acquisition and multiorgan assessment.[10,11,14] Oral contrast use is optional and dilute barium sulfate is most commonly used. Gadolinium-based contrast agents are routinely administered, except in pregnant patients and patients with severe renal failure, and there is a general trend in clinical practice to administer macrocyclic gadolinium contrast agents. Gadolinium-based contrast agents cross the placental barrier and are not routinely administered. Per the ACR, gadolinium-based contrast agents should "only be administered when there is a potential significant benefit to the patient or fetus that outweighs the possible but unknown risk of fetal exposure to free gadolinium ions.[15]

Image acquisition should be focused on minimizing image acquisition time and motion-related artifacts in the acute setting. Free-breathing or respiratory-triggering MR sequences are preferred to a breath-hold technique because patients may have difficulty with breath holding and image quality may be compromised by respiratory motion. The main sequences obtained include gradient-recalled echo (GRE) T1-weighted sequences and single-excitation half-Fourier T2-weighted single-shot turbo spin-echo (HASTE) sequences. Fluid-sensitive sequences are also helpful and include short inversion time inversion-recovery (STIR) and respiratory-triggered T2-weighted chemically fat-suppressed turbo spin-echo techniques. Coherently balanced steady-state sequences may also be used. These are sensitive to the T2 to T1 ratio, provide a clear delineation of the anatomy, and can serve as a white-blood imaging technique to evaluate major vessels without using IV contrast, as well as evaluate fluid-filled bowel.[14] Three-dimensional isotropic volumetric T1-weighted sequences allow coverage of a single organ with a 15-second to 20-second breath hold. Dynamic phase images after IV contrast injection of gadolinium-based contrast agents can be obtained.

A typical MR imaging protocol for evaluating acute abdominopelvic pain includes axial and coronal HASTE; axial STIR; axial GRE T1-weighted in-phase and out-of-phase; axial steady-state free precession; unenhanced and contrast-enhanced dynamic phase volumetric acquisitions; and, if needed, thick-slab MR cholangiopancreatographic respiratory-triggered T2-weighted images. The typical duration of the examination is 20 to 30 minutes. Byott and Harris[11] have shown that a rapid acquisition MR examination consisting of axial and coronal T2-HASTE sequences is effective in evaluating acute abdominal pain with an estimated acquisition time of less than 2 minutes.

CLINICAL APPLICATIONS
Acute Appendicitis

Acute appendicitis is the most common abdominal emergency and the most common nonobstetric surgical emergency in pregnant patients.[2,4,16] Diagnosing acute appendicitis during pregnancy can be challenging because the classic manifestations, including fever, leukocytosis, and right lower quadrant pain, are nonspecific and the appendix is typically displaced from the typical right lower quadrant location by the gravid uterus.

In nonpregnant adults, CT is the primary diagnostic imaging modality in evaluating patients with suspected acute appendicitis given the high sensitivity of 86% to 100% and specificity of 95% to 100%.[17,18] In a pregnant patient, a targeted right lower quadrant US and MR abdomen and pelvis without IV contrast are the most appropriate imaging modalities to evaluate for acute appendicitis; a CT abdomen and pelvis with IV contrast may be obtained if the appendix is not seen on US or MR.[15] Currently, there are no known short-term or long-term detrimental effects from fetal exposure to high magnetic fields, radiofrequency energy deposition, and rapid gradient shifts.[4,19,20] However, the benefits and potential risks are discussed with the patient and written consent is obtained.

At the author's institution, axial, coronal, and sagittal HASTE sequences without fat saturation are obtained of the abdomen and pelvis, as well as axial STIR, axial diffusion-weighted images, and axial T1-weighted in-phase and out-of-phase GRE images.

MR imaging has a sensitivity of 85% to 95%, a specificity of 93% to 99%, a positive predictive value of 94%, a negative predictive value of 100%, and an accuracy of 94% to 96%.[11,21–26] The imaging appearances of acute appendicitis are similar regarding of the imaging modality and include a blind-ending tubular structure with a diameter of 7 mm or larger and a wall thickness of more than 2 mm. HASTE sequences are

particularly helpful in identifying the appendix, and STIR sequences are useful in depicting edema and inflammation within the appendiceal wall and surrounding mesentery, which is seen as T2-hyperintense signal (Fig. 1). Diffusion-weighted imaging has been a valuable technique by increasing the conspicuity and sensitivity of an inflamed appendix. The appendix is usually in the right lower quadrant, caudal to the iliac crests during the first trimester; however, during the third trimester, the appendix is displaced out of the pelvis and often is located cranial to the iliac crests.[27] MR can also detect periappendiceal T2-hyperintense fluid collections in cases of perforated appendicitis (Fig. 2).

Acute Cholecystitis, Choledocholithiasis, and Acute Pancreatitis

Right upper quadrant pain is commonly seen in the emergency setting and acute cholecystitis is one of the most frequent causes for hospital admission.[28] US is the imaging modality of choice for diagnosing acute cholecystitis; however, MR can confirm or exclude acute cholecystitis and is a reliable alternative diagnostic imaging modality, particularly in patients with a difficult or indeterminate US.[29–32] MR and MR cholangiopancreatography (MRCP) are the preferred imaging tests for pregnant patients with right upper quadrant pain and an inconclusive US.[33] Complications, including gangrenous cholecystitis, gallbladder perforation, hemorrhagic cholecystitis, obstructive jaundice, and cholangitis, can be assessed on MR, which aids in determining the treatment, including endoscopic biliary drain, percutaneous drainage, or surgical management.[14,32,34] Stones impacted in the cystic duct resulting in Mirizzi syndrome or choledocholithiasis can be readily detected on MRCP[30,35] (Fig. 3).

The MR findings of acute cholecystitis mirror those on US and include gallbladder distension greater than 4 mm and a thickened wall greater than 3 mm. The low T2-signal intensity of the gallbladder wall increases and may appear stratified on T2-weighted imaging. Pericholecystic fluid is also seen as a T2-hyperintense signal around the gallbladder and stones are a low T2-signal. After the administration of IV gadolinium, transient hepatic enhancement can be seen adjacent to the gallbladder on the arterial-dominant phase, which becomes isointense to hepatic parenchyma in the portal and interstitial phases[30] (Fig. 4). Gallbladder necrosis is seen as asymmetric foci of intramural T2-hyperintensity due to ulceration and microabscess formation in the wall, whereas gangrenous cholecystitis will show little to no enhancement after IV contrast administration.[14,32] MR findings of

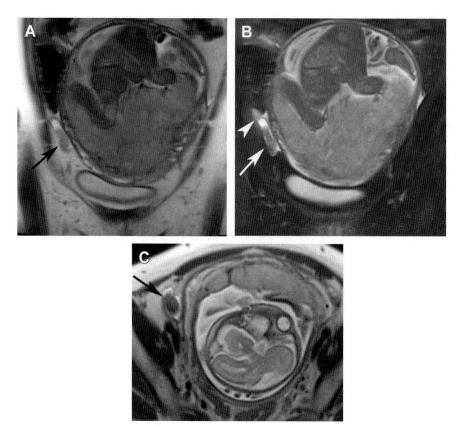

Fig. 1. A 30-year-old woman with a 32-week pregnancy presents with right lower quadrant pain with acute appendicitis. Coronal T2-HASTE without (A) and with (B) fat saturation shows a dilated appendix measuring 12 mm with intraluminal T2-hypointense appendicoliths (arrows) with surrounding T2-hyperintense fluid (arrowhead). Axial HASTE (C) shows an appendicolith at the tip of the appendix (arrow).

gallbladder perforation are disruption of the gallbladder wall, which are best delineated on postcontrast images, as well as irregular or asymmetric wall thickening with heterogeneous T2-signal.[14,34]

Choledocholithiasis is seen in 10% to 15% of acute cholecystitis cases and are usually depicted on MRCP as a round signal defect. Artifacts on HASTE sequences can be seen in the common bile duct and careful interpretation of single-section MRCP, axial fat-suppressed T2-weighted images is important.

Acute pancreatitis is caused by gallstones in 50% of patients and occurs when gallstones

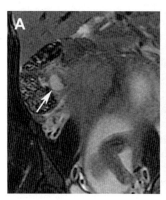
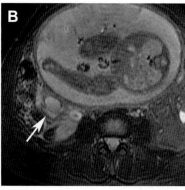

Fig. 2. A 38-year-old woman with a 30-week pregnancy presents with right lower quadrant pain. She is found to have perforated appendicitis with periappendiceal abscess. Coronal (A) and axial (B) T2-weighted IMAGES with fat saturation show a 2.7 cm fluid collection in the right lower quadrant adjacent to the base of the cecum (arrows) in the expected location of the appendix. The patient was initially treated conservatively but failed and was taken for a laparoscopic appendectomy, which was subsequently complicated by a postoperative collection at the appendectomy site.

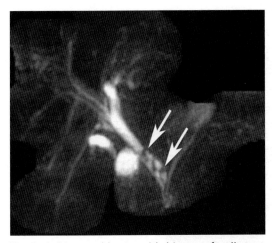

Fig. 3. A 51-year-old man with history of gallstones who presents with nausea, vomiting, and elevated liver function tests with choledocholithiasis. Maximum intensity projection MRCP image shows multiple stones in the distal common bile duct (*arrows*).

migrate into the common bile duct and obstruct the ampulla of Vater.[36] Gallstone-induced pancreatitis necessitates endoscopic sphincterotomy and retrieval of impacted stones. Although endoscopic retrograde cholangiopancreatography (ERCP) is highly successful, complications can occur and accurate detection of gallstones causing pancreatitis is imperative. Acute pancreatitis on MR is depicted as glandular enlargement, periglandular inflammation, and peripancreatic and intrapancreatic fluid collections, all of which can be seen on hyperintense on T2-weighted images. The inherent high T1-signal intensity of normal pancreatic parenchyma decreases with acute pancreatitis and, in cases of hemorrhagic pancreatitis, high T1-signal intensity is seen within and around the pancreas. Additionally, MR-MRCP is useful in acute pancreatitis for monitoring and following the disease and its complications.

Adnexal Torsion

Adnexal torsion frequently involves the ovary and adjacent fallopian tubes. This leads to vascular compromise, initially venous, followed by arterial compromise, and (potentially) gangrene and hemorrhagic necrosis if untreated. Early and accurate diagnosis is crucial to conserve normal ovarian tissue and function. US is the imaging modality of choice in evaluating patients with acute pelvic pain but sonographic findings are nonspecific.[37,38] MR is helpful in cases in which the US is indeterminate, when the presence of acute torsion with a suspected pelvis mass is suspected, or to detect the twisted pedicle or thickened fallopian tube in subacute or chronic cases.[3,38]

Imaging findings of adnexal torsion on MR include fallopian tube thickening, wall thickening of a twisted cystic ovarian mass, ascites, and ipsilateral deviation of the uterus. T2-weighted imaging best delineates the imaging findings with enlargement of the ovary and increased T2-signal with peripherally oriented follicles (**Fig. 5**). Ischemia may progress to hemorrhagic infarct of the ovary and this can be seen as a progression from normal low T1-signal to increasing T1-signal intensity. As torsion progresses, there will be decreased to absence of enhancement of ovarian parenchyma, indicating interruption of blood flow to the ovary, leading to the diagnosis of torsion (see **Fig. 5**).

Crohn Disease

Crohn disease (CD) is a chronic inflammatory disease involving the gastrointestinal tract with involvement of any portion of the bowel from the mouth to the anus; the small bowel is involved in 80% of cases, mostly involving the terminal ileum, and the colon is involved in up to 50% of cases.[39] This disease is characterized by episodic flares with intermittent times of remission. Histologically, CD is characterized by transmural inflammation of bowel wall, ulceration, strictures, and

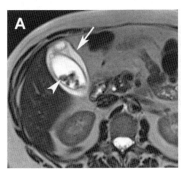
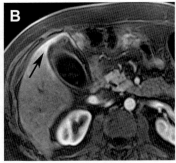

Fig. 4. A 58-year-old woman with epigastric pain and acute cholecystitis. Axial T2-weighted image (*A*) shows gallbladder wall thickening (*arrow*) and multiple T2-hypointense gallstones in the gallbladder (*arrowhead*). Axial T1 postgadolinium (*B*) demonstrates transient pericholecystic enhancement in the hepatic parenchyma on the early arterial phase (*arrow*) in this case of surgically confirmed acute cholecystitis.

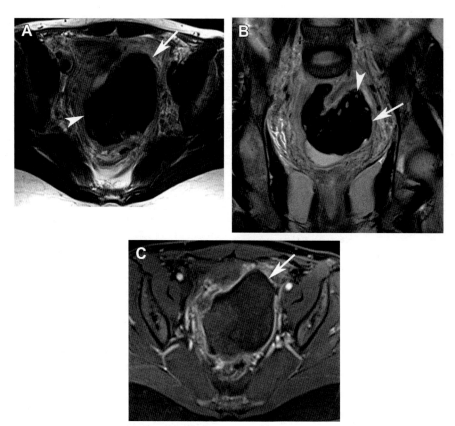

Fig. 5. A 38-year-old woman presented with pelvic pain and vomiting. She was found to have a torsed ovary with infarction. Axial (*A*) and coronal (*B*) T2-weighted images show an enlarged left ovary with T2-hypointense parenchyma (*arrows*) and peripherally oriented follicles (*arrowhead*). The ovary shows no enhancement (*arrow*) on the postgadolinium T1-weighted image with fat saturation (*C*). The patient was taken to the operating room where a necrotic ovary and fallopian tube were found.

discontinuous involvement with skip areas of normal bowel adjacent to diseased bowel.[40]

CT and MR enterography (MRE) are used to diagnose CD, determine the distribution of disease involvement, detect complications of the disease, assess response to treatment, and monitor disease progression.[41–44] The lack of ionizing radiation with MR is advantageous in this patient population because CD is episodic and recurrent with a need for multiple subsequent studies. The diagnostic performance for MRE is high, with sensitivities and specificities of 77% to 82% and 80% to 100%, respectively.[45,46] Detection of active inflammation and complications such as obstruction, abscess, or fistula is comparable to CT.[47–49] It is recommended that the initial evaluation of patients with suspected CD undergo CT due to potential respiratory and bowel motion artifact on MR.[50]

Accurate detection and evaluation of imaging findings of CD are crucial in determining management options by gastroenterologists and intestinal surgeons.[43] Imaging findings suggestive of CD include segmental mural hyperenhancement, bowel wall thickening, mural stratification, and intramural edema,[43] and asymmetric involvement of bowel (hyperenhancement, wall thickening, or stratification) is a specific feature of this disease.[43,51] On MR, mural enhancement is seen as increased intensity after the administration of gadolinium and the degree of enhancement correlates with the severity of inflammatory lesion activity.[52] Bowel wall thickening is best detected in a distended loop of bowel at the site of most severe inflammation on T2-weighted images[43] (**Fig. 6**). The normal small and large bowel wall thickness is 1 to 2 mm and 3 mm, respectively; bowel wall greater than 4 to 5 mm in thickness is abnormal.[39,53] Mural stratification (double-halo or target appearance) is seen as alternating areas of high and low signal intensity with inner-wall hyperenhancement, and may be due to submucosal edema, intramural fat deposition, or inflammatory infiltration.[43] Intramural edema manifests as T2-

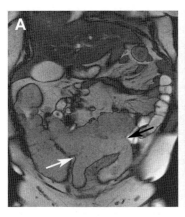

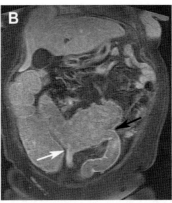

Fig. 6. A 74-year-old woman with CD complicated by enterocolonic fistulae. Coronal steady-state free precession (A) and T1 postgadolinium (B) images demonstrate an enterocolonic fistula between the transverse colon and distal ileum in the mid-abdomen (white arrow), and an additional fistula between the transverse colon and mid to distal ileum in the left hemiabdomen (black arrow).

hyperintense signal in the bowel wall and is associated with more severe inflammation.[43,54] Most strictures associated with CD have both inflammation and fibrosis, and can be reliably detected by the presence of both luminal narrowing and upstream dilation of small bowel greater than 3 cm.[55] Strictures may also be diagnosed without upstream dilation when fixed luminal narrowing is seen on multiple pulse sequences or on serial imaging examinations.[43] Identifying inflammation within a stricture is critical for management because medical treatment can alleviate inflammation and delay surgery, whereas fibrotic strictures require surgical excision or endoscopic dilatation.[43]

Imaging findings of penetrating CD can be seen on MR, including fistula, inflammatory mass, perianal fistula, sinus tract, and abscess. Sinus tracts are blind-ending tracts arising from bowel that can extend to the mesentery or fascial planes, and are seen as high T2-signal tracts.[43,56] Fistulae are described by the epithelial structures they connect (eg, enteroenteric, enterocolic, enterovesical, enterocutaneous, or rectovaginal) and can be simple or complex, whereas complex fistulae tether loops of small and/or large bowel[43,56] are typically

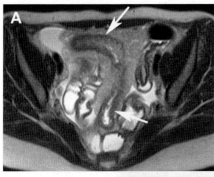

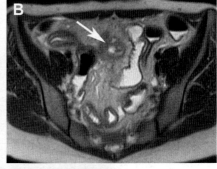

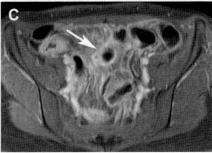

Fig. 7. A 22-year-old man with diffuse abdominal pain with CD. Axial T2-weighted image (A) shows a long 20 to 30 cm segment of terminal ileum in the right lower quadrant and central pelvis with wall thickening (arrows). Axial T2-weighted image (B) shows a fluid collection (arrow) adjacent to the thickened loop of terminal ileum, which shows rim enhancement (arrow) on the axial T1 postgadolinium image (C).

seen as T2-hyperintense tracts, which avidly enhance after gadolinium administration[43,56] (see **Fig. 6**). Approximately 25% of patients with CD present with an anorectal fistula; adequate imaging and close scrutiny of the perineum and anal sphincters are recommended.[43] Dedicated MR planes and sequences are often required to fully characterize perianal fistulae and abscesses, which are not typically included in MRE examinations. In clinical care, evaluating the presence of absence of perianal disease is sufficient.[43] On MR, the sphincter anatomy is best delineated on T2-weighted imaging and fistulae are hyperintense tracts that avidly enhance after gadolinium administration.[57] An abscess is a peripherally enhancing fluid collection seen as a T2-hyperintense

collection with surrounding enhancement (**Fig. 7**). The 4 fistula classifications based on the Parks classification are intersphincteric, transsphincteric, extrasphincteric, and suprasphincteric.[58] The St. James University Hospital classification system is another classification of perianal fistulas that is based on pelvic MR imaging radiologic anatomy, correlates with long-term outcome, and uses reproducible anatomic landmarks.[59,60] There are 5 grades, which describe the primary fistulous tract and secondary extensions, along with associated abscesses.[59,60]

Nephroureterolithiasis

Approximately 1.2 million Americans are affected with urinary stones with up to 14% of men and

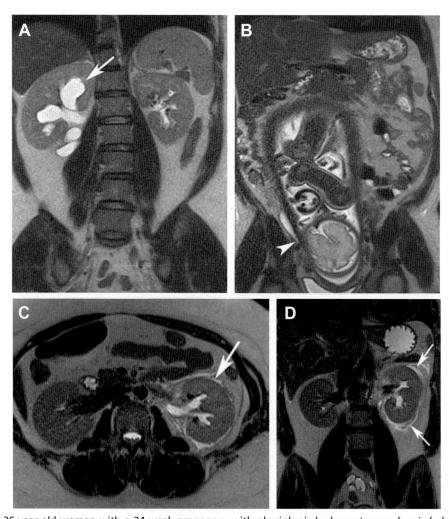

Fig. 8. A 26-year-old woman with a 34-week pregnancy with physiologic hydroureteronephrosis (*white arrow*) related to pregnancy seen on coronal T2-HASTE (*A, B*) with a change in caliber in the distal ureter (*arrowhead*) due to compression by the gravid uterus. A 35-year-old woman with an early pregnancy (pregnancy is not shown) with MR findings concerning for obstructing hydronephrosis on axial (*C*) and coronal (*D*) T2-HASTE with perinephric inflammation and mild perinephric enlargement (*arrows*).

6% of women developing stones in their lifetime.[61] Urolithiasis is the most common nonobstetric reason for hospitalization of pregnant patients.[59,62] Evaluating pregnant patients with suspected urolithiasis can be diagnostically challenging because conventional CT is avoided due to radiation exposure to the fetus. Renal US is the initial imaging modality of choice in evaluating for stones in pregnant patients; however, US offers indirect clues to urinary tract obstruction and lacks sensitivity and specificity to reliably direct therapeutic decision-making.[62,63] Physiologic hydronephrosis and/or ureteral dilatation occur during pregnancy and can limit accurate detection of hydronephrosis.[62,63] Prior studies report a negative ureteroscopy rate of 50% in pregnant patients when solely evaluated with renal US.[64] Thus many pregnant patients undergo stent or nephrostomy tube placement unnecessarily.

MR urography (MRU) should be considered when US does not provide a diagnosis in the symptomatic pregnant patient. MRU offers highly accurate anatomic detail of the urinary tract without exposing the patient to ionizing radiation, and the diagnostic accuracy has been shown to be comparable to CT.[65,66] MRU sequences should include T2-weighted images with multiple acquisitions (cine MRU) to visualize the entire ureters and to assess for fixed ureteral narrowing or filling defects.[67] On MR, stones are seen as filling defects on T2-weighted images and renal enlargement and perirenal fluid are suggestive of obstruction rather than physiologic dilatation (**Fig. 8**). Additionally, physiologic dilatation is due to extrinsic compression by the gravid uterus at the middle third of the ureter, whereas obstruction can occur at any level[62] (see **Fig. 8**). Physiologic renal and/or ureteral dilatation more frequently occurs on the right.[62] MRU has limited evaluation of small stones and institutional availability.

SUMMARY

Use of MR in the emergency setting is useful in specific clinical settings and in patient populations, including pregnant patients in whom exposure to ionizing radiation is concerning. MR has been shown to be accurate for diagnosing a range of pathologic conditions in the abdomen and pelvis, and may be used as an alternative to CT. MR limitations, such as availability; patient cooperation; including respiratory motion and claustrophobia; and acquisition times, may limit use of MR in the emergency setting; however, MR examinations should be tailored to evaluate specific indications with the use of tailored MR protocols. This article has provided an overview of the advantages and disadvantages of MR imaging

in evaluating acute abdominopelvic pain in the emergency setting; reviewed MR imaging protocols, focusing on rapid image acquisition techniques; and discussed the MR imaging appearances of the most common diagnoses encountered in acute abdominopelvic pain.

REFERENCES

1. Ditkofsky NG, Singh A, Avery L, et al. The role of emergency MRI in the setting of acute abdominal pain. Emerg Radiol 2014;21:615–24.
2. National Hospital Ambulatory Medical Care Survey: 2010 Emergency department summary tables. Available at: http://www.cdc.gov/nchs/data/ahcd/nhamcs_emergency/2010_ed_web_tables.pdf. Accessed January 1, 2019.
3. Singh A, Danrad R, Hahn PF, et al. MR imaging of the acute abdomen and pelvis: acute appendicitis and beyond. Radiographics 2007;27:1419–31.
4. Ciesla DJ, Moore EE, Moore JB, et al. The academic trauma center is a model for the future trauma and acute care surgeon. J Trauma 2005;58(4):657–62.
5. Mindelzun RE, Jeffrey RB. Unenhanced helical CT for evaluating acute abdominal pain: a little more cost, a lot more information. Radiology 1997;205:43–5.
6. Stoker J, Van Randen A, Lameris W, et al. Imaging patients with acute abdominal pain. Radiology 2009;254:31–46.
7. Otoni JC, Noschang J, Okamoto TY, et al. Role of computed tomography at a cancer center emergency department. Emerg Radiol 2017;24:113–7.
8. Pandharipande PV, Reisner AT, Binder WD, et al. CT in the emergency department: a real-time study of changes in physician decision making. Radiology 2016;278:812–21.
9. ACR appropriateness criteria, 2018. American College of Radiology Web site. Acute nonlocalized abdominal pain. Available at: https://acsearch.acr.org/docs/69467/Narrative/. Accessed January 1, 2019.
10. Siddiki H, Fidler J. MR imaging of the small bowel in Crohn's disease. Eur J Radiol 2009;69:409–17.
11. Byott S, Harris I. Rapid acquisition axial and coronal T2 HASTE MR in the evaluation of acute abdominal pain. Eur J Radiol 2016;85:286–90.
12. Saini S, Seltzer SE, Bramson RT, et al. Technical cost of radiologic examinations: analysis across imaging modalities. Radiology 2000;216(1):269–72.
13. Sistrom CL, McKay NL. Costs, charges, and revenues for hospital diagnostic imaging procedures: differences by modality and hospital characteristics. J Am Coll Radiol 2005;2:511–9.
14. Tkacz JN, Anderson SA, Soto JA. MR Imaging in gastrointestinal emergencies. Radiographics 2009;29:1767–80.

15. American CollegBe of Radiology. Manual on contrast media. Available at: https://www.acr.org/Clinical-Resources/Contrast-Manual. Accessed October 1, 2018.

16. Buckius MT, McGrath B, Monk J, et al. Changing epidemiology of acute appendicitis in the United States: study period 1993-2008. J Surg Res 2012; 175:185–90.

17. Chiu YH, Chen JD, Wang SH, et al. Whether intravenous contrast is necessary for CT diagnosis of acute appendicitis in adult ED patients? Acad Radiol 2013;20:73–8.

18. Drake FT, Alfonso R, Bhargava P, et al. Enteral contrast in the computed tomography diagnosis of appendicitis: comparative effectiveness in a prospective surgical cohort. Ann Surg 2014;260: 311–6.

19. Hand JW, Li Y, Thomas EL, et al. Prediction of specific absorption rate in mother and fetus associated with MRI examinations during pregnancy. Magn Reson Med 2006;55:883–93.

20. Kanal E, Barkovich AJ, Bell C, et al. ACR guidance document for safe MR practices: 2007. AJR Am J Roentgenol 2007;188:1447–74.

21. Avcu S, Cetin FA, Arslan H, et al. The value of diffusion-weighted imaging and apparent diffusion coefficient quantification in the diagnosis of perforated and nonperforated appendicitis. Diagn Interv Radiol 2013;19:106–10.

22. Petkovska I, Martin DR, Covington MF, et al. Accuracy of unenhanced MR imaging in the detection of acute appendicitis: single-institution clinical performance review. Radiology 2016;270:451–60.

23. Heverhagen JT, Pfestroff K, Heverhagen AE. Diagnostic accuracy of magnetic resonance imaging: a prospective evaluation of patients with suspected appendicitis. J Magn Reson Imaging 2012;35: 617–23.

24. Leeuwenburgh MM, Wiarda BM, Jensch S, et al. Accuracy and interobserver agreement between MR-non-expert radiologists and MR-experts in reading MRI for suspected appendicitis. Eur J Radiol 2014; 83:103–10.

25. Leeuwenburgh MM, Wiarda BM, Wiezer MJ, et al. Comparison of imaging strategies with conditional contrast-enhanced CT and unenhanced MR imaging in patients suspected of having appendicitis; a multicenter diagnostic performance study. Radiology 2013;268:135–43.

26. Pedrosa I, Levine D, Eyvazzadeh AD, et al. MR imaging evaluation of acute appendicitis in pregnancy. Radiology 2006;238:891–9.

27. Oto A, Srinivasan PN, Ernest RD, et al. Revisiting MRI for appendix location during pregnancy. AJR Am J Roentgenol 2006;186:883–7.

28. O'Connor OJ, Maher MM. Imaging of cholecystitis. AJR Am J Roentgenol 2011;196:W367–74.

29. Akpinar E, Turkbey B, Karcaaltincaba M, et al. Initial experience on utility of gadobenate dimeglumine (Gd-BOPTA) enhanced T1-weighted MR cholangiography in diagnosis of acute cholecystitis. J Magn Reson Imaging 2009;30:578–85.

30. Altun E, Semelka RC, Elias J Jr, et al. Acute cholecystitis: MR findings and differentiation from chronic cholecystitis. Radiology 2007;244:174–83.

31. Oh KY, Gilfeather M, Kennedy A, et al. Limited abdominal MRI in the evaluation of acute right upper quadrant pain. Abdom Imaging 2003;28:643–51.

32. Watanabe Y, Nagayama M, Okumura A, et al. MR imaging of acute biliary disorders. Radiographics 2007;27:477–95.

33. ACR appropriateness criteria, 2018. American College of Radiology Web site. Acute right upper quadrant pain. Available at: https://acsearch.acr.org/docs/69467/Narrative/. Accessed January 1, 2019.

34. Adusumilli S, Siegelman ES. MR imaging of the gallbladder. Magn Reson Imaging Clin N Am 2002;10: 165–84.

35. Park MS, Yu JS, Kim YH, et al. Acute cholecystitis: comparison of MR cholangiography and US. Radiology 1998;209:781–5.

36. Stimac D, Miletic D, Radic M, et al. The role of non-enhanced magnetic resonance imaging in the early assessment of acute pancreatitis. Am J Gastroenterol 2007;102:997–1004.

37. Rosado WM Jr, Trambert MA, Gosink BB, et al. Adnexal torsion: diagnosis by using Doppler sonography. AJR Am J Roentgenol 1992;159:1251–3.

38. Rha SE, Byun JY, Jun SE, et al. CT and MR imaging features of adnexal torsion. Radiographics 2002;22: 283–94.

39. Furukawa A, Saotome T, Yamasaki M, et al. Cross-sectional imaging on Crohn Disease. Radiograhics 2004;24:689–702.

40. Baugmgart DC, Sandborn WJ. Crohn's disease. Lancet 2012;9853:1590–605.

41. Fletcher JG, Fidler JL, Bruining DH, et al. New concepts in intestinal imaging for inflammatory bowel diseases. Gastroenterology 2011;140:1795–806.

42. Panes J, Bouhnik Y, Reinisch W, et al. Imaging techniques for assessment of inflammatory bowel disease: joint ECCO and ESGAR evidence-based consensus guidelines. J Crohns Colitis 2013;7: 556–85.

43. Bruining DH, Zimmermann EM, Loftus EV, et al. Consensus recommendations for evaluation, interpretation, and utilization of computed tomography and magnetic resonance enterography in patients with small bowel Crohn's disease. Radiology 2018; 286:776–99.

44. Deepak P, Fletcher JG, Fidler JL, et al. Radiological response is associated with better long-term outcomes and is a potential treatment target in patients

with small bowel Crohn's disease. Am J Gastroenterol 2016;111:997–1006.

45. Pilleul F, Godefroy C, Yzebe-Beziat D, et al. Magnetic resonance imaging in Crohn's disease. Gastroenterol Clin Biol 2005;29:803–8.

46. Borthen AS, Abdelnoor M, Rugtveit J, et al. Bowel magnetic resonance imaging of pediatric patients with oral mannitol MRI compared to endoscopy and intestinal ultrasound. Eur Radiol 2006;16: 207–14.

47. Lee SS, Kim AY, Yang SK, et al. Crohn disease of the small bowel: comparison of CT enterography, MR enterography, and small-bowel follow-through as diagnostic techniques. Radiology 2009;251(3): 751–61.

48. Schmidt S, Guibal A, Meuwly JY, et al. Acute complications of Crohn's disease: comparison of multidetector-row computed tomographic enterography with magnetic resonance enterography. Digestion 2010;82(4):229–38.

49. Fiorino G, Bonifacio C, Peyrin-Biroulet L, et al. Prospective comparison of computed tomography enterography and magnetic resonance enterography for assessment of disease activity and complications in ileocolonic Crohn's disease. Inflamm Bowel Dis 2011;17(5):1073–80.

50. Kim DH, Carucci LR, Baker ME, et al. ACR appropriateness criteria, 2018. American College of Radiology Web site. Crohn disease.

51. Meyers MA, McGuire PV. Spiral CT demonstration of hypervascularity in Crohn disease: "vascular jejunization of the ileum" or the "comb sign". Abdom Imaging 1995;20:327–32.

52. Gore RM, Balthazar EJ, Ghahremani GG, et al. CT features of ulcerative colitis and Crohn's disease. AJR Am J Roentgenol 1996;167:3–15.

53. Low RN, Sebrechts CP, Politoske DA, et al. Crohn disease with endoscopic correlation: single-shot fast spin-echo and gadolinium-enhanced fat-suppressed spoiled gradient-echo MR imaging. Radiology 2002;222:652–60.

54. Levine A, Griffiths A, Markowitz J, et al. Pediatric modification of the Montreal classification for inflammatory bowel disease: the Paris classification. Inflamm Bowel Dis 2011;17:1314–21.

55. Barkmeier DT, Dillman JR, Al-Hawary M, et al. MR enterography-histology comparison in resected pediatric small bowel Crohn disease strictures: can imaging predict fibrosis? Pediatr Radiol 2016;46: 498–507.

56. Tolan DJM, Greenhalgh R, Zealley IA, et al. MR enterographic manifestations of small bowel Crohn disease. Radiographics 2010;30:367–84.

57. Sheedy SP, Bruining DH, Dozois EJ, et al. MR imaging of perianal Crohn disease. Radiology 2017;282: 628–45.

58. Parks AG, Gordon PH, Hardcastle JD. A classification of fistula-in-ano. Br J Surg 1976; 63(1):1–12.

59. McAleer SJ, Loughlin KR. Nephrolithiasis and pregnancy. Curr Opin Urol 2004;14:123–7.

60. Morris J, Spencer JA, Ambrose NS. MR imaging classification of perianal fistulas and its implications for patient management. Radiographics 2000;20(3): 623–35 [discussion: 635–37].

61. Kambadakone AR, Eisner BH, Catalano OA, et al. New and evolving concepts in the imaging and management of urolithiasis: urologists' perspective. Radiographics 2010;30:603–23.

62. Patel SJ, Reede DL, Katz DS, et al. Imaging the pregnant patient for nonobstetric conditions: algorithms and radiation dose considerations. Radiographics 2007;27:1705–22.

63. White WM, Johnson EB, Zite NB, et al. Predictive value of current imaging modalities for the detection of urolithiasis during pregnancy: a multicenter, longitudinal study. J Urol 2013;189:931–4.

64. Srirangam SJ, Hickerton B, Van Cleynenbreugel B. Management of urinary calculi in pregnancy: a review. J Endourol 2008;22:867.

65. Regan F, Bohlman ME, Khazan R, et al. MR urography using HASTE imaging in the assessment of ureteric obstruction. AJR Am J Roentgenol 1996; 167:1115–20.

66. Grenier N, Pariente JL, Trillaud H, et al. Dilatation of the collecting system during pregnancy: physiologic vs obstructive dilatation. Eur Radiol 2000;10:271–9.

67. Leyendecker JR, Barnes CE, Zagoria RJ. MR urography: techniques and clinical applications. Radiographics 2008;28:23–46.

Stroke Imaging

Shahmir Kamalian, MD*, Michael H. Lev, MD

KEYWORDS

- Stroke • CT • CT angiography • MR imaging • MR angiography • Intravenous thrombolysis
- Intra-arterial thrombectomy • Endovascular thrombectomy

KEY POINTS

- Abrupt onset of a focal neurologic deficit typically defines the clinical syndrome of stroke.
- Neuroimaging has an essential role in differentiating ischemic from hemorrhagic stroke and guiding patient selection for intravenous thrombolysis (IVT) and intra-arterial thrombectomy (IAT).
- Obtaining advanced imaging (CTA, DWI) for patient selection for IAT should never delay the administration of IVT when the patient is otherwise eligible, up to 4.5 hours post ictus.
- The recent DAWN and DEFUSE 3 trial results showed a strong benefit of IAT when performed within 24 hours post ictus, in appropriately selected patients using advanced imaging.

INTRODUCTION

It is estimated that 795,000 persons have a stroke each year in the United States, causing 140,000 deaths.[1,2] That said, stroke has moved from the third leading cause of death in 2007 to the fifth in 2017.[1–3] Although major recent advances in neuroimaging and stroke treatment have contributed to a decrease in mortality, stroke remains the leading cause of serious long-term disability in the United States and costs the health care system an estimated $34 billion each year.[1]

Abrupt onset of a focal neurologic deficit typically defines the clinical syndrome of stroke, although stroke mimics—which include but are not limited to seizure (20%), syncope (10%–20%), sepsis or hypo-/hyperglycemia (14%), subdural hematoma or tumor (10%–12%), somatization/anxiety and hyperventilation (5%–10%), transient global amnesia, and complex migraine (30%–35%)—have been estimated to occur as often as 10-fold more frequently as ischemic or hemorrhagic stroke.[4]

Most "true" stroke syndromes are ischemic, with a majority caused by an intracranial, circle of Willis large vessel occlusion (LVO) from an embolus (approximately 85%) and with only a small percentage attributable to global cerebral hypoperfusion (so-called low-flow or border-zone strokes); global anoxic injury from near-drowning, carbon monoxide poisoning, or other causes of suffocation are also less common. Approximately 10% of strokes are hemorrhagic resulting from intracerebral hemorrhage, with 3% being due to subarachnoid hemorrhage.[1,2]

Neuroimaging has a central role in the differential diagnosis of patients with suspected stroke, by differentiating ischemic from hemorrhagic stroke, identifying other causes of acute neurologic deficit (ie, stroke mimics), and helping in patient selection for intra-arterial thrombectomy (IAT). An estimated 9% to 30% of patients with suspected stroke—and 3% to 17% of patients treated with intravenous tissue plasminogen activator (IV-tPA)—have stroke mimics.[5–14] Current treatment options for acute embolic stroke include IV-tPA, IAT, or a combination of both. Therapeutic options for intracerebral hemorrhage, subarachnoid hemorrhage, and stroke mimics vary according to the etiology.

Ischemic stroke reflects neuronal dysfunction secondary to hypo-oxygenation and can be

Conflicts of Interest: S. Kamalian: None. M.H. Lev: Consultant for Takeda Pharm, GE Healthcare; institutional support for Siemens postprocessing software license.
Department of Radiology, Division of Emergency Radiology, Massachusetts General Hospital, Harvard Medical School, 55 Fruit Street, Blake SB Room 29A, Boston, MA 02114, USA
* Corresponding author.
E-mail address: skamalian@mgh.harvard.edu

Radiol Clin N Am 57 (2019) 717–732
https://doi.org/10.1016/j.rcl.2019.02.001

radiologic.theclinics.com

associated with temporary (transient ischemic attack) or permanent (infarction) neuronal injury. Because only a small number (<5%) of patients with signs and symptoms of acute stroke present to an emergency department within the 3- to 4.5-hour time window for treatment by "clot-busting" IV-rPA, timely advanced imaging with computed tomography (CT), CT angiography (CTA), and, whenever possible, diffusion-weighted MR imaging (DWI) remains essential to patient assessment, even in patients with transient ischemic attack or rapid clinical improvement (ie, "too good to treat"), to identify treatable causes of ischemia and prevent a stroke (eg, severe internal carotid artery stenosis or dissection).

Unenhanced CT (noncontrast CT) is required for all stroke patients to exclude hemorrhage. Advanced imaging requires, at minimum, CT angiography (CTA), to both identify a proximal LVO and access collaterals. To the greatest extent possible, DWI should be performed as the most accurate modality for determining irreversibly infarcted tissue "core"; additional CT or MR perfusion imaging (MRP) is increasingly obtained at many centers for determining potentially salvageable ischemic "penumbra." "Core" is brain tissue that has been irreversibly infarcted at presentation; "penumbra" is markedly hypoperfused "at-risk" tissue that has a high probability of infarction in the absence of timely reperfusion.

Recent prospective clinical trials published in The New England Journal of Medicine (NEJM) and other high-impact journals[15–20] have not only helped define the central role of advanced neuroimaging modalities—CTA, CTA collaterals, CT perfusion (CTP), MR imaging-DWI, MR imaging-fluid-attenuated inversion recovery (FLAIR), and magnetic resonance angiography (MRA)—in patient selection for IAT treatment but have also helped make possible extending the time window for this treatment up to 24 hours post ictus, as recently demonstrated in the DAWN and DEFUSE 3 trials.[21,22]

ETIOLOGY AND TIMELINE OF ISCHEMIC STROKE

Ischemic strokes are divided into 5 subtypes based on etiology: large-artery atherosclerosis (most commonly from the cervical carotid arteries), cardioembolism (secondary to clot formation in the heart), small-vessel occlusion (lacunar infarct, which is <20 mm diameter), stroke of other determined cause (such as dissection, nonatherosclerotic vasculopathies, or global hypoperfusion), and stroke of undetermined etiology.[23]

The most common causes of stroke vary in different age groups. Carotid disease (large artery) and atrial fibrillation (cardioembolism) are the most common causes of acute ischemic stroke in patients older than 40 years. Hypertensive and coronary heart diseases are the most common underlying disorders in patients with atrial fibrillation. Atrial fibrillation is highly associated with left atrium enlargement with 39% increase in risk per 5-mm increment.[24] Therefore, in an older patient with an enlarged left atrium, the stroke may be due to atrial fibrillation. The most common causes of ischemic stroke in patients younger than 40 years include dissection, nonatherosclerotic vasculopathies, and paradoxic stroke in conditions, such as a patent foramen ovale and arteriovenous shunts in the lungs.

Clinical history can provide important clues in determining the cause of stroke. For example, dissection should be considered in young patients (typically age <40) after yoga, weightlifting, or chiropractic manipulation, whereas paradoxic embolus from deep vein thrombosis through a patent foramen ovale is at the top of the differential diagnosis list as the cause of acute ischemic stroke in a pilot or a long-distance traveler presenting with abrupt onset of new neurologic deficit.[25,26]

Ischemic stroke is loosely classified as hyperacute, acute, subacute, and chronic, based on the time of symptom onset. Typically the hyperacute phase is within 6 to 8 hours of stroke onset, when patients are potentially eligible for various well-established reperfusion treatments (ie, IV-tPA and/or IAT). Acute stroke is considered stroke of less than 24 hours' duration, with the subacute and chronic stages ranging from 1 day to 1 month and greater than 1 month, respectively. Part of the problem with these loose definitions, however, is that stroke progression and infarct growth vary widely from patient to patient, largely attributable to the quality of the intracranial collateral blood flow around a site of proximal LVO. One of the overarching goals of patient selection using advanced imaging is to replace the concept of making treatment decisions based on an arbitrary "clock time" with the concept of making treatment decisions based on stroke physiology, as determined by the concurrent neuroimaging findings at the time of triage.

ROLE OF NEUROIMAGING IN DIAGNOSIS AND MANAGEMENT OF PATIENTS WITH ACUTE ISCHEMIC STROKE

Neuroimaging has 4 critical roles in the assessment of patients with an acute ischemic stroke: (1)

exclusion of an acute intracranial hemorrhage, (2) identification of a proximal LVO as a target for IAT, (3) determining the volume of already irreversibly dead brain at presentation (infarction core), and (4) estimating the volume of potentially salvageable ischemic tissue that is a target for treatment, which is likely to undergo irreversible injury in the absence of timely reperfusion (ischemic penumbra).

Presence of an acute intracranial hemorrhage is an absolute contraindication to IV-tPA therapy. Large-artery proximal occlusions of the middle cerebral artery (MCA) or other proximal circle of Willis vessels typically account for most of the morbidity and mortality of stroke; clot dissolution or retrieval to restore normal brain perfusion is therefore the goal of IV and/or intra-arterial thrombolysis. Determining the infarct core volume is important because patients with large cores—many studies have established 70 mL as a threshold beyond which a good clinical outcome is unlikely—are at higher risk for intraparenchymal hemorrhage after successful reperfusion.[27,28] Finally, in the absence

of a substantial volume of potentially salvageable ischemic target tissue (ie, penumbra), the risks of attempting reperfusion therapies may outweigh the benefits.

Imaging Findings in Acute Ischemic Stroke

Noncontrast computed tomography

Noncontrast CT is a specific but relatively insensitive modality for the detection of early ischemic changes. It has a pivotal role, however, in addressing the first critical question in treating acute stroke: is there an acute intracranial hemorrhage that is an absolute contraindication for IV-tPA or IAT therapy? Signs of early infarct on noncontrast head CT include loss of the gray matter-white matter differentiation along the cortical ribbon (especially in the insula) or lentiform nucleus, hyperdense vessel sign (which indicates an embolus in the vessel), and sulcal effacement from edema (**Fig. 1**A, B).[29] Presence of an obvious, well-established large hypodense infarct (more than one-third of MCA territory or 100 mL) is also

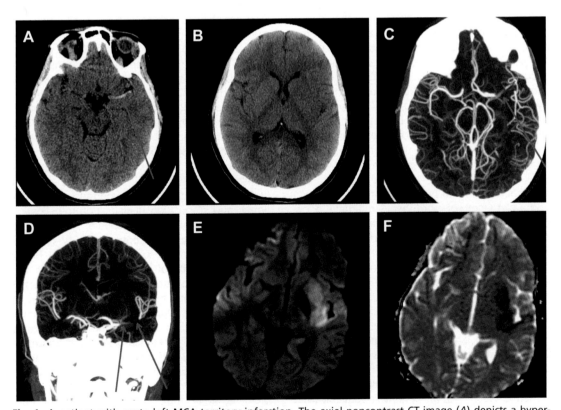

Fig. 1. A patient with acute left MCA territory infarction. The axial noncontrast CT image (A) depicts a hyperdense vessel sign (arrow). At the level of insula, CT (B) shows loss of gray matter-white matter differentiation in the posterior insula and lentiform nucleus and mild edema, which is evident by asymmetric effacement of the left sylvian fissure compared with the right side. The axial (C) and coronal (D) MIP CTA images depict an occlusive thrombus in the M1 segment of the left MCA (arrows). The MR images (DWI [E] and ADC [F]) show the posterior insula and lentiform nucleus, with restricted diffusion, consistent with acute infarct.

typically considered a contraindication to IV-tPA therapy. Noncontrast CT can also help identify a proximal thrombus and assess clot burden, by detection of a hyperdense vessel sign, a specific but insensitive marker for intravascular clot in the clinical setting of an abrupt-onset new neurologic deficit.

Computed tomography angiography

CTA is a quick and accurate method for addressing the second critical question in the imaging assessment of patients with acute ischemic stroke: is there a proximal circle of Willis LVO, which might be a target for IAT treatment? Maximum-intensity projection (MIP) images are helpful for rapid identification of more distal vascular stenosis or occlusions (eg, at the secondary [M2] or tertiary [M3] branch vessels) as well as for assessment of clot burden (ie, clot length) and leptomeningeal collateral status (Fig. 1C, D)[30,31] For optimal MIP image review and interpretation, the reformatting—which can be rapidly performed, typically in less than a minute, by the CT technologists at the scanner console—should be obtained as thick slab/thin overlapping intervals (3-cm thick at 5-mm overlapping intervals at the authors' institution). Moreover, to be certain that the observed collateral pattern reflects the true collateral status and is not an artifact of a delayed circulation time of contrast taking longer to reach the pial collateral circulation through a more circuitous pathway bypassing a proximal LVO, it is essential that delayed-phase CTA images be obtained routinely in acute stroke patients who are potential IAT candidates; some institutions use a multiphase CTA protocol for collateral assessment.[18]

Clot burden is an important marker that predicts response to IV-tPA.[30] Patients with LVO and a clot length of more than 8 mm have a low likelihood of successful recanalization by IV-tPA alone and hence may be good candidates for IAT treatment.[30,32]

The quality of the leptomeningeal collateral vasculature on CTA can also help distinguish patients most likely to benefit from IAT from those least likely to benefit.[33] Poor leptomeningeal collateralization has been associated with higher incidence and larger size of hemorrhage.[31,34,35] Patients with a proximal occlusion and good collateral vasculature usually have a small infarction core and a large potentially salvageable ischemic tissue (Fig. 2).[31] Likewise, patients with a proximal occlusion and poor collateral vasculature usually have a large infarction core and a small potentially salvageable ischemic penumbra (Fig. 3).[31] Hence, when DWI is unavailable or contraindicated as the modality to most accurately determine infarct core volume, the stratification of leptomeningeal CTA collaterals into robust (ie, symmetric), poor (absent in >30%–50% of the territory at risk), or intermediate categories can help in estimating the potential benefits versus risks of attempting IAT in any given individual patient (Fig. 4). Although patients with robust collaterals have higher odds of good clinical outcome after reperfusion than patients with poor collaterals, in the absence of robust complete or near-complete recanalization, the outcome of patients is similar, regardless of collateral status.[36]

Moreover, the preliminary results of one of our studies presented at the 56th Annual Meeting of the American Society of Neuroradiology in June 2008 showed that a simplified scoring approach combining the size of CTA source image hypodensity and leptomeningeal status may provide a more accurate method for estimation of the DWI lesion volume than CTP. This method is especially useful at primary stroke centers for making the decision to transfer the patient to comprehensive stroke centers.[37]

Computed tomography perfusion

CTP can visually depict and potentially measure several perfusion parameters at the microvascular level, such as cerebral blood flow (CBF), cerebral blood volume (CBV), and mean transit time (MTT). CTP has been the focus of many imaging research studies for identification of infarct core and ischemic penumbra. CBF and CBV maps can be used for infarct core measurement and CBF and MTT maps for ischemic penumbra measurement (see Fig. 4C).[38–41]

Although CTP findings may be useful for differential diagnosis of stroke, clinical management (notably for titration of antihypertensive medications), and disposition decisions/prognostication in acute ischemic stroke patients,[42] its specific role in the selection of patients for IV or intra-arterial reperfusion therapies remains highly controversial and hotly debated. Compared with a DWI reference standard, CTP may be insufficiently accurate for assessing core infarct volume in any given individual patient who is a potential IAT candidate; this is largely due to both image noise and lack of standardization, leading not only to potential inaccuracy but also to marked interscan variability in the quantification of perfusion parameter values as well as large measurement error in the estimation of infarct core volumes.[38,39,43–45] Moreover, using CTP to estimate penumbral volume may be unnecessary, in that patients who present within the time window for reperfusion therapy with a proximal LVO and a small infarct core almost always have a

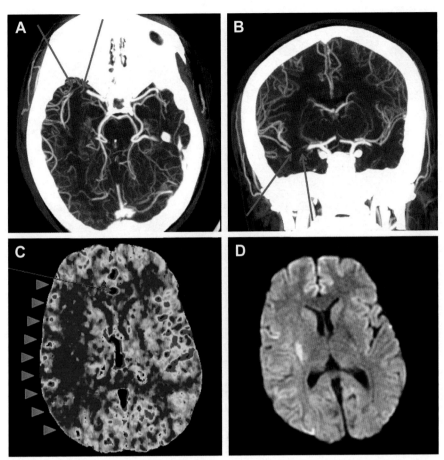

Fig. 2. A patient with CT/CTA acquired 1.5 hours after stroke onset: axial (*A*) and coronal (*B*) MIP CTA images depict a thrombus in the M1 segment of the right MCA (*arrows*), with good (symmetric) pial collateral vessels (*arrowheads*). Although the CBF map from the CTP data set (*C*) demonstrated a large area perfusion defect (*arrowheads*), DWI (*D*) showed a small infarct core, with an associated large area of at-risk tissue (penumbra). This combination of proximal LVO, small core, and large penumbra defines a cohort of patients most likely to benefit from IAT.

sufficiently large ischemic penumbra to warrant IAT if otherwise eligible.[46] Thus, using CTP might not only be unnecessary for triage of patients to appropriate IV or intra-arterial reperfusion therapies but may also inappropriately exclude patients who might otherwise benefit from such therapies by overestimating the infarct core or, at the other extreme, put patients at increased risk of hemorrhagic complications by underestimating the infarct core size. Hence, at several institutions CTP is not considered essential for the selection of patients for available revascularization therapies when MR imaging is contraindicated or unavailable; rather, both the presence of a proximal LVO and the quality of the pial CTA-collateral flow (robust, intermediate, or poor) are considered when making IAT decisions.

It should again be underscored, however, that perfusion imaging has other important potential applications in acute stroke management when MR imaging is unavailable or contraindicated, including (but not limited to) differential diagnosis (especially identifying distal branch occlusions that may not be evident on CTA thick-slab MIPs), hypertensive management, and disposition/prognosis.[47]

MR imaging

As with unenhanced CT, standard MR imaging sequences (T1-weighted, T2-weighted, and FLAIR) can be relatively insensitive for the detection of ischemia/infarction in the first few hours post ictus[29]; rather, the greatest value of MR imaging lies in the early detection and delineation of infarct core using DWI (**Fig.** 1E, F). DWI is highly sensitive (88%–100%), specific (95%–100%), and accurate (95%) for detecting and delineating ischemic brain tissue likely to be irreversibly infarcted despite

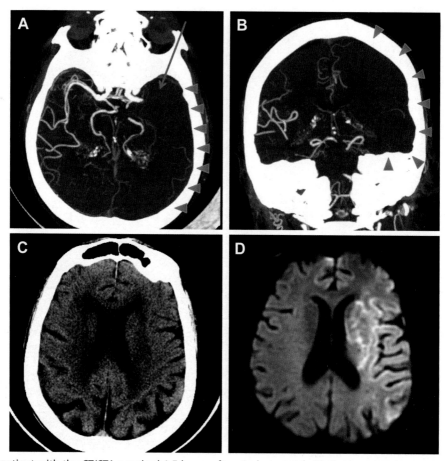

Fig. 3. A patient with the CT/CTA acquired 1.5 hours after stroke onset (with the same stroke onset to imaging time interval as the patient shown in **Fig. 2**). Axial (*A*) and coronal (*B*) MIP CTA images depict a thrombus in the M1 segment of the left MCA (*arrow*), with almost complete absence of collateral flow (*arrowheads*); a poor (or in this case, malignant collateral pattern). Although the noncontrast CT examination (*C*) shows no obvious hypodensity to suggest acute infarction, the DWI (*D*) depicts a large infarct core, involving almost the entire left MCA territory.

early, robust reperfusion. DWI can often detect ischemia even within minutes of onset; ischemia causes restricted free water diffusion in brain tissue, which results in a marked hyperintense (bright) signal on DWI sequences.

The DWI signal intensity is an exponential function of the random Brownian motion of water molecules within a voxel of tissue, with a linear component based on T2-weighted signal intensity, and with brighter signal reflecting lesser (ie, more restricted) diffusibility. The gray scale on the apparent diffusion coefficient (ADC) maps reflects a linear function of diffusibility, without the T2 component, and with brighter signal reflecting greater diffusibility (eg, CSF appears bright because the hydrogen atoms in water are more freely mobile). The ADC maps can, therefore, help distinguish a DWI-bright lesion as true restricted diffusion (ie, DWI bright, T2 bright, and

ADC dark) from T2 shine-through (DWI bright, T2 bright, and ADC bright).[29]

Infarct core size is a well-established and important marker for the likelihood of good outcome in MCA occlusive stroke. Infarct core volume on MR-DWI can be estimated with an acceptable level of accuracy by multiplying the largest cross-sectional dimensions on axial, sagittal, and coronal reconstructed images and dividing the product by 2 (length × width × height/2). Patients with small infarct core volumes (<70 mL) at presentation, in the setting of acute MCA occlusion, have the potential to derive the greatest benefit after successful reperfusion; conversely, those with initial large infarct core volumes (>100 mL) are at increased risk of hemorrhage after reperfusion and are unlikely to benefit from IAT.[48,49] Infarcts between 70 mL and 100 mL at presentation are uncertain to benefit from IAT.

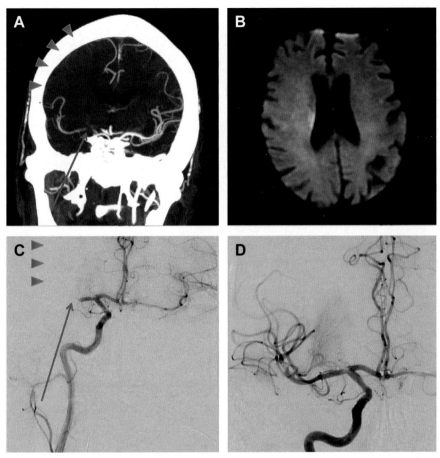

Fig. 4. A 75-year-old man with a medical history of atrial fibrillation who was off warfarin for thoracentesis. The patient presented 25 minutes after stroke onset. Despite an occlusive M1 thrombus in the right MCA (*arrow*) and poor collateral pattern (*arrowheads*), as depicted by coronal MIP CTA (*A*), the patient had a small infarct core (DWI [*B*]) in the right posterior caudate body. The patient underwent immediate IAT. The catheter angiogram (*C*) confirms the presence of a complete right M1-MCA occlusion (*arrow*) with poor collaterals (*arrowheads*). After a single pass of a "Penumbra" suction device, the patient had successful complete recanalization (*D*). The follow-up noncontrast CTP 24 hours later (not shown) was without significant abnormality in the right MCA territory.

In the posterior circulation, the correlation between initial infarct size and clinical outcome is poor, because even a tiny ischemic focus in a critical location in the brainstem can result in a devastating neurologic deficit.

MR angiography

Although CTA is considered the first-line imaging modality to rule in an LVO in setting of acute stroke, MRA provides a useful screening test to detect proximal LVO in patients who cannot receive iodinated CT IV contrast material because of allergy or acute renal failure.[50] The main limitations of MRA are overestimating the degree of stenosis and inaccuracy in detection of distal occlusions, given that MRA images are flow dependent rather than reflecting true intraluminal anatomy, as does CTA.[29]

MR perfusion

MRP can produce perfusion maps, including CBF, CBV, MTT, and time to peak/time to maximum. The role of MRP in the selection of patients for IV thrombolytic or IAT therapies is controversial and debated, as is the role of CTP. Arterial spin-labeled MRP is a method of estimating tissue-level perfusion in the brain without the need for IV gadolinium contrast; however, it too has several limitations; MRP methods are also notable for not requiring ionizing radiation.[29]

The Massachusetts General Hospital Stroke-Imaging Algorithm

The Massachusetts General Hospital stroke-imaging algorithm is an evidence-based tool to identify patients with severe ischemic strokes caused by anterior circulation occlusions who are candidates for IAT stroke therapy (**Fig. 5**). First, noncontrast CT is performed—with an expected door-to-CT time of less than 25 minutes per national "Get-With-The-Guidelines" criteria—to evaluate for hemorrhage (an absolute contraindication to IV-tPA or IAT) or a large well-established hypodensity (more than one-third MCA territory; a relative contraindication to IV thrombolysis or IAT). If neither is present and the patient is IV-tPA eligible, CTA is next performed and postprocessed during the 5 to 10 minutes it takes to prepare the tPA for IV administration; obtaining advanced imaging, however, should never slow the administration of definitive thrombolytic treatment in patients who are otherwise eligible. Next, in the setting of a proximal LVO (intracranial internal cerebral artery or MCA) and if there are no contraindications to MR imaging, a DW image is acquired. If DWI depicts a small (<70 mL) infarct, the patient is considered "likely to benefit" from IAT (assuming other criteria have been met) and immediately triaged to the interventional suite. If MR imaging is unavailable *and* the patient is not a candidate for IAT, CTP can be considered to help exclude stroke mimics or to help guide management decisions, such as the need for hypertensive therapy.[51]

In addition to detection of LVO, CTA is also useful for assessment of pial collateral flow. In the setting of a proximal LVO, a "malignant" collateral flow pattern (no contrast filling in >50% of the territory at risk on delayed CTA images) strongly correlates with DWI infarct volume greater than 70 to 100 mL.[52] Conversely, robust (ie, symmetric)

collaterals—although they do not necessarily guarantee a DWI infarct volume less than 70 mL—mean that a final infarct volume less than 70 mL is more likely in the setting of early, complete recanalization. Hence, patients with a poor collateral pattern are likely to have a poor

Table 1 Causes of restricted diffusion	
Na^+/K^+-ATPase Pump failure (ischemic and/ or excitotoxic injury)	Seizures, hypoglycemia, hyperglycemia, ketosis, transient global amnesia, drug-induced (eg, metronidazole or methotrexate) encephalopathies, necrotizing infections (eg, HSV), Wernicke encephalopathy
Tissue vacuolization or spongiform changes	Creutzfeldt-Jakob disease, heroin leukoencephalopathy, demyelination, diffuse axonal injury
High protein concentration or increased viscosity	Pyogenic infection, hemorrhage
Dense cell packing	High-grade glioma, lymphoma, small-blue-round-cell metastases such as small cell lung cancer

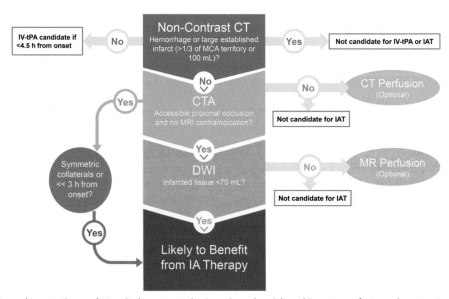

Fig. 5. Massachusetts General Hospital acute stroke-imaging algorithm. (*Courtesy of* Massachusetts General Hospital, Boston, MA; with permission.)

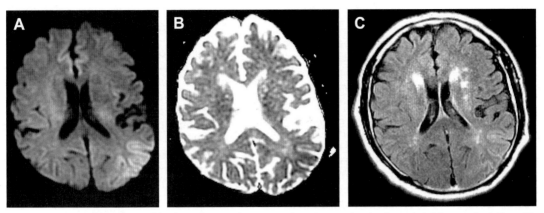

Fig. 6. A 66-year-old patient with altered mental status and acute-onset aphasia and right gaze deviation. The patient received IV-tPA for presumed stroke but was later found to have had a seizure. Admission MR imaging showed gyriform restricted diffusion (DWI [*A*], ADC map [*B*]) in the left parieto-occipital cortex, with cortical and subcortical white matter swelling (FLAIR [*C*]). The imaging findings completely resolved by the time of discharge (not shown).

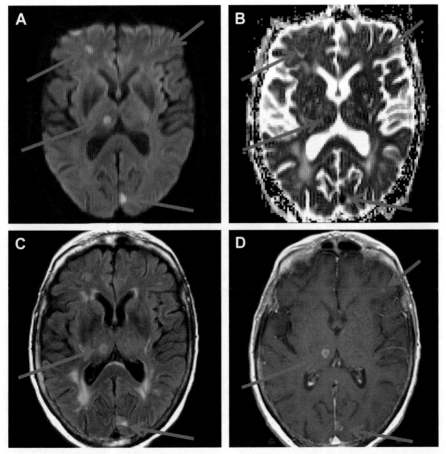

Fig. 7. A 69-year-old with small cell lung carcinoma presented with sudden onset of visual changes and gait imbalance. MR imaging depicted multiple foci of restricted diffusion (*arrows*) in the left occipital lobe, right thalamus, and bilateral frontal lobes (DWI [*A*] and ADC map [*B*]). All the lesions (*arrows*) demonstrate associated T2/FLAIR hyperintensity (*C*) and contrast enhancement on the postcontrast T1-weighted images (*D*). The lesion in the right frontal lobe is not included on the representative axial postcontrast T1-weighted image because of patient movement between the sequences.

clinical outcome, despite successful recanalization, whereas patients with robust (ie, symmetric) collaterals have the potential to benefit from IAT.[36,53] In the absence of recanalization, the outcome of patients with good versus poor collateral vasculature does not differ significantly.[36]

Acute Ischemic Stroke Differential Diagnosis ("Stroke Mimics")

It is estimated that 9% to 30% of patients suspected for stroke and 2.8% to 17% of patients treated with IV-tPA have stroke mimics.[5–14] Although several diverse entities can mimic stroke, most mimics are due to seizures, migraines, tumors, or toxic-metabolic disturbances. Imaging usually facilitates diagnosis, because "true" ischemic stroke typically has the imaging features previously described, although some of these features—even restricted diffusion (**Table 1**)—are not unique to stroke and can be associated with other entitities.[54] The topographic pattern of the DWI lesion, in combination with vascular imaging and CT or MRP findings, often helps diagnose these other entities (**Figs. 6–8**).

TREATMENT OF PATIENTS WITH ACUTE ISCHEMIC STROKE

The management of acute ischemic stroke (within the first few hours) differs from long-term management. The immediate goal of treatment is minimizing brain injury and preventing complications. In addition to IV-tPA and intra-arterial therapy, treatment of stroke requires stabilization of airway, breathing, and circulation; control of blood pressure; fluid management; treatment of hypoglycemia or hyperglycemia; and swallowing assessment.[55,56] The IV and intra-arterial treatment is discussed here.

Intravenous Thrombolysis

The goal of IV-tPA thrombolysis is timely restoration of blood flow and salvaging the ischemic brain tissue not already infarcted. In 1995, the National Institute of Neurologic Disorders and Stroke trial showed the benefit of IV thrombolytic therapy given during the first 3 hours after stroke onset.[57] Later in 2008, the European Cooperative Acute Stroke Study III—a double-blinded, parallel-group, randomized trial—showed that the benefit of

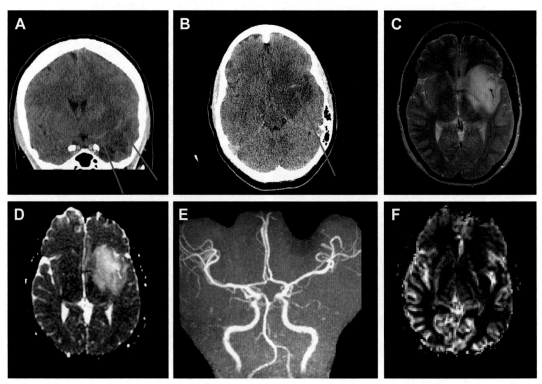

Fig. 8. A 49-year-old with sudden-onset aphasia. The initial noncontrast CT (*A*, *B*) was interpreted as a left MCA infarction with a hyperdense left MCA sign (*arrows*). MR imaging showed a T2 hyperintense expansile lesion (T2-weighted imaging [*C*]) with elevated diffusion (ADC map [*D*]). MRA showed patency of the left MCA (*E*), and MRP (CBF [*F*]) showed no areas of decreased CBF. The patient underwent biopsy, which subsequently showed an anaplastic oligoastrocytoma.

IV-tPA thrombolysis extends up to 4.5 hours after stroke onset.[58]

All data suggest that the sooner IV-tPA therapy is initiated, the more likely it is to be beneficial and that this benefit extends up to 4.5 hours after stroke onset. Therefore, all eligible patients (Table 2) should be treated with IV-tPA as soon as possible, even if IAT is considered.

As discussed previously, if hyperdense vessel clot length is greater than 8 mm, the likelihood that IV-tPA alone will result in complete recanalization approaches zero, and these patients should be considered for IAT if possible.[30,59]

Intra-Arterial Thrombolysis

In 2015, 5 multicenter randomized clinical trials (MR CLEAN, ESCAPE, REVASCAT, EXTEND-IA, and SWIFT PRIME) were published in NEJM, all of which showed the benefit of IAT treatment after IV-tPA compared with IV-tPA alone, in patients with acute ischemic stroke (Table 3).[15,17–20]

Despite the success of these recent IAT trials, several prior studies from 2013 failed to show a benefit of IAT. The success of these more recent studies can be attributed both to the availability of more effective "current-generation" clot retriever

---

Table 2
Eligibility criteria for intravenous tissue plasminogen activator administration

Inclusion Criteria
- Clinical diagnosis of ischemic stroke
- Symptom onset <4.5 h before start of treatment
- Age ≥18 y

Absolute Exclusion Criteria

Historical	• Stroke or head trauma in the last 3 months • Previous intracranial hemorrhage • Intracranial neoplasm, arteriovenous malformation, or aneurysm • Recent intracranial or intraspinal surgery • Arterial puncture at a noncompressible site in the previous 7 d
Clinical	• Symptoms suggestive of subarachnoid hemorrhage • Persistent hypertension (systolic ≥185 or diastolic ≥110 mm Hg) • Serum glucose <50 mg/dL (<2.8 mmol/L) • Active internal bleeding • Acute bleeding diathesis, including but not limited to conditions defined in "Hematologic"
Hematologic	• Platelet count <100,000/mm^{3a} • Current anticoagulant use with an INR >1.7 or PT >15 s[a] • Heparin use within 48 h and an abnormally elevated aPTT[a] • Current use of a direct thrombin inhibitor or direct factor Xa inhibitor with evidence of anticoagulant effect by laboratory tests
Head CT	• Evidence of hemorrhage • Extensive well-established hypodensity (>1/3 of MCA territory)

Relative Exclusion Criteria
- Minor and isolated neurologic signs or rapidly improving stroke symptoms
- Seizure at the onset of stroke with postictal neurologic impairments
- Major surgery or serious trauma in the previous 14 d
- Gastrointestinal or urinary tract bleeding in the previous 21 d
- Myocardial infarction in the previous 3 mo
- Pregnancy

Additional, Relative Exclusion Criteria for Treatment 3–4.5 h Post Ictus
- Age >80 y
- Severe stroke (NIHSS score >25)
- Combination of both previous ischemic stroke and diabetes mellitus

Abbreviations: aPTT, activated partial thromboplastin time; INR, international normalized ratio; NIHSS, National Institutes of Health Stroke Scale; PT, prothrombin time.

[a] It is desirable to have the results of these tests, but thrombolytic therapy should not be delayed for the test results unless (1) there is clinical suspicion of a bleeding abnormality or thrombocytopenia, or (2) the patient is currently on or has recently received anticoagulants.

Table 3
Summary of 5 *The New England Journal of Medicine* 2015 randomized clinical trials showing efficacy of intra-arterial thrombectomy plus intravenous thrombolysis over that of intravenous thrombolysis alone in patients with acute ischemic stroke secondary to proximal large vessel occlusion

	MR CLEAN	ESCAPE	REVASCAT	SWIFT PRIME	EXTEND-IA
Subjects	PIACO	PIACO	PIACO	PIACO	PIACO + salvageable tissue on CTP
No. of patients	500	315	206	196	70
Imaging	CT, CTA	CT, CTA	CT, CTA/MRA	CT, CTA, CTP/MRP	CT, CTA, CTP
Intervention group	Any IA method	Any IA method	IA treatment with a stent retriever device	IA treatment with a stent retriever device	IA treatment with a stent retriever device
Control group	Medical treatment (± IV-tPA)	Medical treatment (± IV-tPA)	Medical treatment (± IV-tPA)	IV-tPA	IV-tPA
Time to intervention	<6 h	<12 h	<8 h	<6 h	<4.5 h
Median time to groin puncture	260 min	241 min	269 min	224 min	210 min
90-d mRS improvement	I: 32.6%[a] C: 22.1%	I:53%[a] C: 29.3%	I: 43.7%[a] C: 28.2%	I: 60.2%[a] C: 35.5%	I: 71.4%[a] C: 40%
90-d mortality reduction	I: 21% C: 22.1%	I: 10.4%[a] C: 19%	I: 21% C: 22.1%	I: 9.2% C: 12.4%	I: 18.4% C: 15.5%
Conclusion	IA therapy within 6 h of stroke onset is effective and safe	Rapid IA therapy in patients with small infarct and moderate-to-good collaterals improves functional outcome and mortality	IA therapy with a stent retriever improves functional outcome	IA therapy with a stent retriever within 6 h improves functional outcomes	Early IA therapy with a stent retriever, compared with IV-tPA alone, improves reperfusion, early neurologic recovery, and functional outcome

Abbreviations: C, control group; I, intervention group; IA, intra-arterial; PIACO, proximal intracranial anterior circulation occlusion.
[a] Statistically significant.
Data from Refs.[15,17–20]

devices (stent retriever and penumbra devices versus older-generation concentric MERCI retriever device) and to the use of advanced imaging (CTA plus some measure of "infarct core") for patient selection.[60,61]

In patients with anterior circulation occlusion stroke and contraindications to IV-tPA, endovascular therapy with stent retriever devices within 6 hours of stroke onset is a reasonable option.[56] Most recently, the DAWN and DEFUSE 3 trials, published in NEJM in November 2017 and February 2018, respectively, have shown that, with advanced imaging selection, patients can be safely treated with IAT up to 24 hours post ictus.[21,22] DAWN patients achieved 49% functional independence at 90 days versus 13% in controls; for every 2.8 treated patients, 1 additional patient was functionally independent at 90 days. Inclusion criteria used in the DAWN trial were complex and required a mismatch between the infarction core volume and clinical deficit in addition to LVO (**Table 4**). In the DEFUSE 3 trial, the treated patients achieved 47% functional independence at 90 days versus 17% in the control group; for every 3.3 treated patients, 1 additional patient was functionally independent at 90 days. Clinical deficit was not used as an inclusion criterion in DEFUSE 3, and patients were enrolled up to 16 hours post ictus if the infarct core volume was less than 70 mL and the ratio of the ischemic tissue volume on perfusion imaging to infarct volume was $\geq$1.8. The DAWN and DEFUSE 3 trials raise doubt against use of a rigid time window for IAT. In addition, a few nonrandomized and retrospective studies and case reports have suggested that IAT appears to be safe and feasible beyond 24 hours post ictus and, in the presence of potentially salvageable brain tissue, patients may benefit from thrombectomy even up to 6 days after stroke onset.[62–65] Therefore, it is expected that future trials will potentially simplify the inclusion criteria and decision making for "late window" IAT and extend the time window for treatment even beyond 24 hours.

SUMMARY

Abrupt onset of a focal neurologic deficit typically defines the clinical syndrome of stroke. Neuroimaging has an essential role in the assessment of patients with suspected stroke, by differentiating ischemic from hemorrhagic stroke, identifying stroke mimics, and guiding patient selection for available therapies. Improved awareness of the neuroimaging findings highlighted in recent stroke clinical trials as well as their role in patient selection for novel treatment options, including "late window" (8–24 hours post ictus) IAT, has become increasingly important as advanced neuroimaging methods (ie, head and neck CTA, MRA, and perfusion and diffusion techniques) are gaining widespread acceptance for evaluation of acute stroke.

REFERENCES

1. Benjamin EJ, Blaha MJ, Chiuve SE, et al. Heart disease and stroke statistics—2017 update: a report from the American heart association. Circulation 2017;135:e146–603.
2. Xu J, Murphy SL, Kochanek KD, et al. Mortality in the United States, 2015. NCHS Data Brief 2016;1–8.
3. Xu J, Kochanek KD, Murphy SL, et al. Deaths: final data for 2007. Natl Vital Stat Rep 2010;58:1–19.
4. Kidwell CS, Saver JL, Schubert GB, et al. Design and retrospective analysis of the los angeles prehospital stroke screen (LAPSS). Prehosp Emerg Care 1998;2:267–73.
5. Hand PJ, Kwan J, Lindley RI, et al. Distinguishing between stroke and mimic at the bedside: the brain attack study. Stroke 2006;37:769–75.
6. Hemmen TM, Meyer BC, McClean TL, et al. Identification of nonischemic stroke mimics among 411 code strokes at the University of California, San Diego, Stroke center. J Stroke Cerebrovasc Dis 2008;17:23–5.
7. Allder SJ, Moody AR, Martel AL, et al. Limitations of clinical diagnosis in acute stroke. Lancet 1999;354: 1523.
8. Moritani T, Smoker WR, Sato Y, et al. Diffusion-weighted imaging of acute excitotoxic brain injury. AJNR Am J Neuroradiol 2005;26:216–28.
9. Libman RB, Wirkowski E, Alvir J, et al. Conditions that mimic stroke in the emergency department. Implications for acute stroke trials. Arch Neurol 1995; 52:1119–22.
10. Merino JG, Luby M, Benson RT, et al. Predictors of acute stroke mimics in 8187 patients referred to a stroke service. J Stroke Cerebrovasc Dis 2013;22: e397–403.
11. Chernyshev OY, Martin-Schild S, Albright KC, et al. Safety of TPA in stroke mimics and

Table 4 DAWN trial criteria used for thrombectomy decisions	
Group A	Age $\geq$80 y, NIHSS $\geq$10, and DWI infarct volume <21 mL
Group B	Age <80 y, NIHSS $\geq$10, and DWI infarct volume <31 mL
Group C	Age <80 y, NIHSS $\geq$20, and DWI infarct volume <51 mL

neuroimaging-negative cerebral ischemia. Neurology 2010;74:1340–5.

12. Multicenter Acute Stroke Trial–Europe Study Group, Hommel M, Cornu C, Boutitie F, et al. Thrombolytic therapy with streptokinase in acute ischemic stroke. N Engl J Med 1996;335:145–50.

13. Winkler DT, Fluri F, Fuhr P, et al. Thrombolysis in stroke mimics: Frequency, clinical characteristics, and outcome. Stroke 2009;40:1522–5.

14. Guillan M, Alonso-Canovas A, Gonzalez-Valcarcel J, et al. Stroke mimics treated with thrombolysis: further evidence on safety and distinctive clinical features. Cerebrovasc Dis 2012;34:115–20.

15. Berkhemer OA, Fransen PS, Beumer D, et al. A randomized trial of intraarterial treatment for acute ischemic stroke. N Engl J Med 2015;372:11–20.

16. Bracard S, Ducrocq X, Mas JL, et al. Mechanical thrombectomy after intravenous alteplase versus alteplase alone after stroke (THRACE): a randomised controlled trial. Lancet Neurol 2016;15:1138–47.

17. Campbell BC, Mitchell PJ, Kleinig TJ, et al. Endovascular therapy for ischemic stroke with perfusion-imaging selection. N Engl J Med 2015;372:1009–18.

18. Goyal M, Demchuk AM, Menon BK, et al. Randomized assessment of rapid endovascular treatment of ischemic stroke. N Engl J Med 2015;372:1019–30.

19. Jovin TG, Chamorro A, Cobo E, et al. Thrombectomy within 8 hours after symptom onset in ischemic stroke. N Engl J Med 2015;372:2296–306.

20. Saver JL, Goyal M, Bonafe A, et al. Stent-retriever thrombectomy after intravenous t-PA vs. t-PA alone in stroke. N Engl J Med 2015;372:2285–95.

21. Jovin TG, Saver JL, Ribo M, et al. Diffusion-weighted imaging or computerized tomography perfusion assessment with clinical mismatch in the triage of wake up and late presenting strokes undergoing neurointervention with trevo (DAWN) trial methods. Int J Stroke 2017;12:641–52.

22. Albers GW, Marks MP, Kemp S, et al. Thrombectomy for stroke at 6 to 16 hours with selection by perfusion imaging. N Engl J Med 2018;378:708–18.

23. Adams HP Jr, Bendixen BH, Kappelle LJ, et al. Classification of subtype of acute ischemic stroke. Definitions for use in a multicenter clinical trial. TOAST. Trial of org 10172 in acute stroke treatment. Stroke 1993;24:35–41.

24. Kannel WB, Wolf PA, Benjamin EJ, et al. Prevalence, incidence, prognosis, and predisposing conditions for atrial fibrillation: population-based estimates. Am J Cardiol 1998;82:2N–9N.

25. Miley ML, Wellik KE, Wingerchuk DM, et al. Does cervical manipulative therapy cause vertebral artery dissection and stroke? Neurologist 2008;14:66–73.

26. Biller J, Sacco RL, Albuquerque FC, et al. Cervical arterial dissections and association with cervical manipulative therapy: a statement for healthcare professionals from the american heart association/

american stroke association. Stroke 2014;45:3155–74.

27. Sanak D, Nosal V, Horak D, et al. Impact of diffusion-weighted MRI-measured initial cerebral infarction volume on clinical outcome in acute stroke patients with middle cerebral artery occlusion treated by thrombolysis. Neuroradiology 2006;48:632–9.

28. Yoo AJ, Verduzco LA, Schaefer PW, et al. MRI-based selection for intra-arterial stroke therapy: value of pretreatment diffusion-weighted imaging lesion volume in selecting patients with acute stroke who will benefit from early recanalization. Stroke 2009;40:2046–54.

29. Kidwell CS, Hsia AW. Imaging of the brain and cerebral vasculature in patients with suspected stroke: advantages and disadvantages of CT and MRI. Curr Neurol Neurosci Rep 2006;6:9–16.

30. Kamalian S, Morais LT, Pomerantz SR, et al. Clot length distribution and predictors in anterior circulation stroke: implications for intra-arterial therapy. Stroke 2013;44:3553–6.

31. Berkhemer OA, Jansen IG, Beumer D, et al. Collateral status on baseline computed tomographic angiography and intra-arterial treatment effect in patients with proximal anterior circulation stroke. Stroke 2016;47:768–76.

32. Meyne JK, Zimmermann PR, Rohr A, et al. Thrombectomy vs. systemic thrombolysis in acute embolic stroke with high clot burden: a retrospective analysis. Rofo 2015;187:555–60.

33. Tan IY, Demchuk AM, Hopyan J, et al. CT angiography clot burden score and collateral score: correlation with clinical and radiologic outcomes in acute middle cerebral artery infarct. AJNR Am J Neuroradiol 2009;30:525–31.

34. Puetz V, Dzialowski I, Hill MD, et al. Intracranial thrombus extent predicts clinical outcome, final infarct size and hemorrhagic transformation in ischemic stroke: the clot burden score. Int J Stroke 2008;3:230–6.

35. Puetz V, Dzialowski I, Hill MD, et al. Malignant profile detected by CT angiographic information predicts poor prognosis despite thrombolysis within three hours from symptom onset. Cerebrovasc Dis 2010;29:584–91.

36. Tong E, Patrie J, Tong S, et al. Time-resolved CT assessment of collaterals as imaging biomarkers to predict clinical outcomes in acute ischemic stroke. Neuroradiology 2017;59(11):1101–9.

37. McWilliams SR, Kamalian S, Raymond SB, et al. CTA collaterals versus CT perfusion CBF maps for core infarct volume assessment in patient selection for intra-arterial thrombectomy. Presented in annual meeting of American Society of Neuroradiology 2018.

38. Kamalian S, Kamalian S, Konstas AA, et al. CT perfusion mean transit time maps optimally

distinguish benign oligemia from true "at-risk" ischemic penumbra, but thresholds vary by postprocessing technique. AJNR Am J Neuroradiol 2012; 33:545–9.

39. Kamalian S, Kamalian S, Maas MB, et al. CT cerebral blood flow maps optimally correlate with admission diffusion-weighted imaging in acute stroke but thresholds vary by postprocessing platform. Stroke 2011;42:1923–8.

40. Campbell BC, Christensen S, Levi CR, et al. Cerebral blood flow is the optimal CT perfusion parameter for assessing infarct core. Stroke 2011;42:3435–40.

41. Bivard A, McElduff P, Spratt N, et al. Defining the extent of irreversible brain ischemia using perfusion computed tomography. Cerebrovasc Dis 2011;31:238–45.

42. Lev MH. CT perfusion. AJNR News Digest 2016.

43. Copen WA, Morais LT, Wu O, et al. In acute stroke, can ct perfusion-derived cerebral blood volume maps substitute for diffusion-weighted imaging in identifying the ischemic core? PLoS One 2015;10:e0133566.

44. Schaefer PW, Souza L, Kamalian S, et al. Limited reliability of computed tomographic perfusion acute infarct volume measurements compared with diffusion-weighted imaging in anterior circulation stroke. Stroke 2015;46:419–24.

45. Copen WA, Deipolyi AR, Schaefer PW, et al. Exposing hidden truncation-related errors in acute stroke perfusion imaging. AJNR Am J Neuroradiol 2015;36:638–45.

46. Copen WA, Rezai Gharai L, Barak ER, et al. Existence of the diffusion-perfusion mismatch within 24 hours after onset of acute stroke: dependence on proximal arterial occlusion. Radiology 2009;250:878–86.

47. Wintermark M, Sanelli PC, Albers GW, et al. Imaging recommendations for acute stroke and transient ischemic attack patients: a joint statement by the American Society of Neuroradiology, the American College of Radiology, and the Society of Neurointerventional Surgery. AJNR Am J Neuroradiol 2013;34:E117–27.

48. Lev MH, Segal AZ, Farkas J, et al. Utility of perfusion-weighted CT imaging in acute middle cerebral artery stroke treated with intra-arterial thrombolysis: prediction of final infarct volume and clinical outcome. Stroke 2001;32:2021–8.

49. Leslie-Mazwi TM, Hirsch JA, Falcone GJ, et al. Endovascular stroke treatment outcomes after patient selection based on magnetic resonance imaging and clinical criteria. JAMA Neurol 2016;73:43–9.

50. Nederkoorn PJ, van der Graaf Y, Hunink MG. Duplex ultrasound and magnetic resonance angiography compared with digital subtraction angiography in carotid artery stenosis: a systematic review. Stroke 2003;34:1324–32.

51. Gonzalez RG, Copen WA, Schaefer PW, et al. The Massachusetts General Hospital acute stroke imaging algorithm: an experience and evidence based approach. J Neurointerv Surg 2013;5(Suppl 1):i7–12.

52. Souza LC, Yoo AJ, Chaudhry ZA, et al. Malignant CTA collateral profile is highly specific for large admission DWI infarct core and poor outcome in acute stroke. AJNR Am J Neuroradiol 2012;33:1331–6.

53. Bouslama M, Bowen MT, Haussen DC, et al. Selection paradigms for large vessel occlusion acute ischemic stroke endovascular therapy. Cerebrovasc Dis 2017;44:277–84.

54. Kamalian S, Boulter DJ, Lev MH, et al. Stroke differential diagnosis and mimics: part 1. Appl Radiol 2015;44:26–39.

55. Jauch EC, Saver JL, Adams HP Jr, et al. Guidelines for the early management of patients with acute ischemic stroke: a guideline for healthcare professionals from the American Heart Association/American Stroke Association. Stroke 2013;44:870–947.

56. Powers WJ, Derdeyn CP, Biller J, et al. 2015 American Heart Association/American Stroke Association focused update of the 2013 guidelines for the early management of patients with acute ischemic stroke regarding endovascular treatment: a guideline for healthcare professionals from the American Heart Association/American Stroke Association. Stroke 2015;46:3020–35.

57. National Institute of Neurological Disorders and Stroke rt-PA Stroke Study Group. Tissue plasminogen activator for acute ischemic stroke. N Engl J Med 1995;333:1581–7.

58. Hacke W, Kaste M, Bluhmki E, et al. Thrombolysis with alteplase 3 to 4.5 hours after acute ischemic stroke. N Engl J Med 2008;359:1317–29.

59. Riedel CH, Zimmermann P, Jensen-Kondering U, et al. The importance of size: successful recanalization by intravenous thrombolysis in acute anterior stroke depends on thrombus length. Stroke 2011;42:1775–7.

60. Broderick JP, Palesch YY, Demchuk AM, et al. Endovascular therapy after intravenous t-PA versus t-PA alone for stroke. N Engl J Med 2013;368:893–903.

61. Ciccone A, Valvassori L, Nichelatti M, et al. Endovascular treatment for acute ischemic stroke. N Engl J Med 2013;368:904–13.

62. Jovin TG, Liebeskind DS, Gupta R, et al. Imaging-based endovascular therapy for acute ischemic stroke due to proximal intracranial anterior circulation occlusion treated beyond 8 hours from time last seen well: retrospective multicenter analysis of 237 consecutive patients. Stroke 2011;42:2206–11.

63. Aguilar-Salinas P, Santos R, Granja MF, et al. Revisiting the therapeutic time window dogma: successful thrombectomy 6 days after stroke onset. BMJ Case Rep 2018;2018 [pii:bcr-2018-014039].

64. Lansberg MG, Cereda CW, Mlynash M, et al. Response to endovascular reperfusion is not time-dependent in patients with salvageable tissue. Neurology 2015;85:708–14.

65. Desai SM, Haussen DC, Aghaebrahim A, et al. Thrombectomy 24 hours after stroke: beyond DAWN. J Neurointerv Surg 2018;10: 1039–42.

Imaging of Brain Trauma

Mariza O. Clement, MD, MSE

Mariza O. Clement, MD, MSE

KEYWORDS

- Traumatic brain injury • Neurovascular injury • Dissection • Radiology • Brain hemorrhage
- Diffuse axonal injury

KEY POINTS

- Brain Trauma is an epidemic affecting up to 2.8 million Americans a year and mortality rates of moderate to severe brain trauma are 21% to 46%.
- Rapid recognition of epidural hematoma "swirl sign," subdural hematoma, subarachnoid hemorrhage, cortical contusions, intraparenchymal hemorrhage "spot sign," intraventricular hemorrhage, vascular injuries, and herniation is imperative.
- MR imaging is most sensitive for detection and grading of diffuse axonal injury, where CT may even be negative.
- Secondary injuries result from complications developing typically within the first 24 hours of the primary injury and include ischemic injury, herniation, and edema.

An estimated 69 million people worldwide experience brain trauma.[1] In the United States, a reported 2.8 million Americans were seen in the emergency room in 2013 for brain trauma; most injuries were related to falls, particularly in the elderly and children, followed by motor vehicle accidents and violence.[2,3] The incidence of traumatic brain injury is likely underreported because of potential impact on professional careers where injuries are prevalent, such as the military and athletes. Increasingly, evidence is emerging of long-term functional decline and staggering suicide rates of 1.5 to 1.9 times the general population in patients who have experienced traumatic brain injury.[4,5]

In the initial clinical setting, the Glasgow Coma Scale (GCS) is typically used to grade the severity of traumatic injury. The scale grades injury based on level of consciousness. In severe brain injury (score of 3–8), the patient is essentially comatose and at risk for immediate secondary complications of brain injury including cerebral edema, hypoxic injury, hypotension.[6] In moderate injury (GCS of 9–13), the patient is essentially lethargic. In mild injury (GCS of 13–15), there is immediate

neurologic recovery. Most injuries are classified as mild.[6] Mortality rates with moderate or severe brain injury demonstrated 6-month mortality rates of 21% and 46%, respectively.[7,8]

Imaging plays numerous roles in the management of patients with traumatic brain injury: from the immediate triage, serial imaging for neurologic deterioration, to prognostication. Noncontrast head computed tomography (CT), supported by class I evidence, is the most appropriate initial imaging test and subsequent follow-up on patients with neurologic deterioration. Class I evidence is defined by at least one large random controlled trial with proper randomization and clear results.[9] Imaging findings are dependent on the mechanism of injury, which includes blunt trauma, penetrating trauma, acceleration/deceleration, and blast injuries. Primary injuries are the direct manifestation of the initial trauma, such as intra-axial and extra-axial hemorrhages, skull fractures, and vascular injury. Secondary injuries result from complications developing typically within the first 24 hours of the primary injury and include ischemic injury, herniation, and edema.[10]

No disclosures.
Department of Radiology, Boston Medical Center of Boston University, 820 Harrison Avenue FGH3, Boston, MA 02118, USA
E-mail address: Mariza.Clement@bmc.org

Radiol Clin N Am 57 (2019) 733–744
https://doi.org/10.1016/j.rcl.2019.02.008

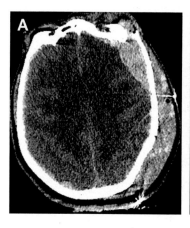

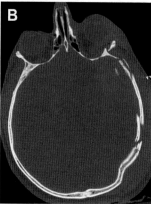

Fig. 1. Epidural hematoma. Noncontrast CT demonstrates (A) hyperdense lenticular extraxial collection with the "swirl sign" along the left frontotemporal convexity and associated (B) calvarial fracture.

PRIMARY INJURIES
Epidural Hematoma

Epidural hematoma is a collection of hemorrhage contained between the dura and inner table of the skull, which typically does not cross suture lines forming a lenticular biconvex shape. In children, epidural hematomas have been found to cross suture lines because they are associated with sutural diastases and fractures involving the sutures.[11] Epidural hematoma may be arterial or venous in origin. Most often epidural hematomas result from injury of a branch of the middle meningeal artery; however, approximately 10% are a result of injury to a dural venous sinus.[12,13] The "swirl sign" (Fig. 1) is a salient prognostic sign indicative of active bleeding and retrospectively found to be independently associated with 1-month mortality rates of up to 61%.[14] On CT, a hypoattenuating lucent ovoid or irregular foci appear within a heterogeneously hyperdense crescent. Rapid expansion of an epidural hematoma can lead to secondary complications of herniation and ischemia.[14]

Subdural Hematoma

Subdural hematomas are formed from injury of bridging veins and result in the accumulation of blood between the dura and arachnoid membrane, and are bound by the falx. Morphologically subdural hematomas appear crescentic and do not cross midline but may cross suture lines (Fig. 2). Although subdural hematomas may be seen in a wide variety of mechanism of trauma, they are frequently encountered in the elderly and pediatric populations. Even mild injury in the elderly, such as fall from standing height, is associated with a subdural hematoma. As the brain ages, there is volume loss and increased fragility and stretching of the bridging veins leading to increased susceptibility to injury.[15] Moreover, in

children subdural hematomas are most often caused by injury of bridging veins during rapid acceleration and deceleration injuries, such as shaken baby syndrome. In a prospective study of nonaccidental trauma in the pediatric population, subdural hemorrhage was found in 90% of patients with shaken baby syndrome.[16]

Elderly patients are also vulnerable to solitary interhemispheric subdural hematomas,[15] which result from tearing of bridging veins draining into the superior sagittal sinus or straight sinus (Fig. 3). Large interhemispheric subdural hematomas may result in monoparesis of a lower extremity, known

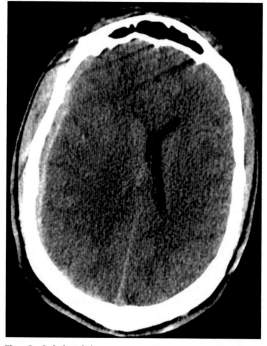

Fig. 2. Subdural hematoma. Noncontrast CT shows hyperdense crescentic collection along right frontoparietal convexity crossing suture lines.

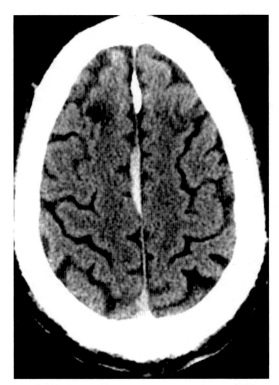

Fig. 3. Interhemispheric hematoma. Noncontrast CT shows hyperdense hemorrhage layering along the falx.

as "falx syndrome."[15] Furthermore, subdural hematomas are associated with vasogenic edema, which can cause shift of the midline structures. The degree of midline shift in conjunction with hematoma thickness is being investigated to optimize neurosurgical management. Some studies have shown that a midline shift of greater than 1 cm or greater than 3 mm than the maximum thickness of the subdural hematoma may warrant immediate intervention.[17,18]

Subarachnoid Hemorrhage

Subarachnoid hemorrhage results from stretching and tearing of veins within the subarachnoid space, redistribution of intraventricular hemorrhage, or perforation of the subarachnoid space by adjacent intraparenchymal hemorrhage/cortical contusions. On CT, subarachnoid hemorrhage appears as hyperdense hemorrhage conforming to the sulci, fissures, and cisterns as the cerebrospinal fluid communicates these regions of the brain (Fig. 4).[19]

The role of CT angiography (CTA) in the setting of traumatic subarachnoid hemorrhage is controversial and potentially overused.[20] A pattern approach to subarachnoid hemorrhage may help reduce overuse of CTA, where central subarachnoid hemorrhage (Fig. 5) within the cisterns and sylvian fissures are more typically associated with an

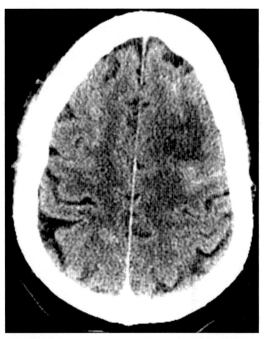

Fig. 4. Traumatic subarachnoid hemorrhage. Noncontrast CT shows hyperdense hemorrhage conforming to the sulci of the bifrontal cerebrum in a typical peripheral pattern.

underlying aneurysm compared with peripheral hemorrhages. In a multivariate study of 617 patients with post-traumatic subarachnoid hemorrhage, 186

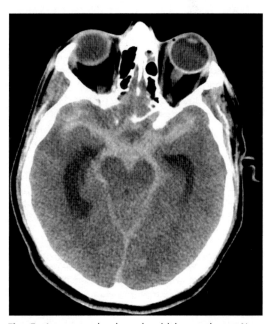

Fig. 5. Aneurysmal subarachnoid hemorrhage. Noncontrast CT shows subarachnoid hemorrhage in a central pattern within the cisterns and sylvian fissures often associated with an underlying aneurysm.

underwent CTA, and only patients with subarachnoid hemorrhage localized centrally had an underlying aneurysm (eight patients).[20]

Isolated subarachnoid hemorrhage in the setting of mild injury (GCS >13), despite a high rate of intensive care unit admissions, is associated with a low level of neurosurgical intervention or neurologic deterioration, with adult reported rates of 0.0017% to 0.24%.[21,22] A retrospective study was conducted in the pediatric population, where 317 children with isolated subarachnoid hemorrhage, no midline shift, and a GCS greater than 13 were admitted to intensive care units but had no neurologic deterioration.[23]

Intraventricular Hemorrhage

Intraventricular hemorrhage is a rare finding in brain injury (reported prevalence of approximately 3%–4%), but associated with a high mortality rate (22%–62%). Hemorrhage results from injury to local vascularity, the subependymal/corpus colossal vessels, injury to the paraventricular structures (septum pellucidum, fornix, corpus collosum), and redistribution of hemorrhage from the subarachnoid space or direct penetration of intraparenchymal hematomas.[24] Intraventricular hemorrhage can in turn lead to acute obstructive hydrocephalus and increased intracranial pressure. In a large prospective observational cohort, 63% of patients with intraventricular hemorrhage were associated with moderate disability to brain death. Children had worse outcomes, with approximately 50% resulted in severe disability or death.[25]

Cortical Contusions

Hemorrhagic contusions are petechial hemorrhages originating in the vascular gray matter that may extend into the white matter. Morphologically they can appear as wedge-shaped hyperdensities on CT conforming to the gyral crests. They frequently occur at the site of injury (coup) and opposed within the cerebrum (contre coup). Head motion against the inner surfaces of skull, such as the anterior cranial fossa, sphenoid wings, and petrous, creates a propensity for contusions to form along the inferior, anterior, and lateral frontal temporal lobes (**Fig. 6**).[19]

Intraparenchymal Hematoma and "Spot Sign"

Injury to the intraparenchymal vessels results in an intraparenchymal hematoma that in turn leads to dysregulation of the local microvasculature.[26] A cascade can cause ischemia, edema, vasoconstriction/vasospasm, and increased hemorrhage within the primary lesion. Microvascular dysregulation is also thought to lead to new intraparenchymal

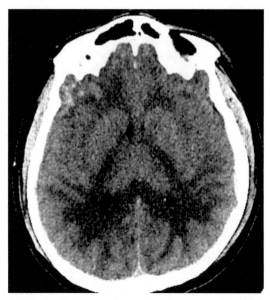

Fig. 6. Cortical contusions. Noncontrast CT shows hyperdense hemorrhage conforming to the gyral crests along the anterior temporal lobes and inferior frontal lobes.

hemorrhage in separate site. Retrospective studies have found that approximately 51% of contusions expand within the first 24 hours, most commonly in the first few hours, but may show delayed progression 3 to 4 days after the initial injury.[26]

Furthermore, increased edema can compound ischemia leading to rapid increases in intracranial pressure that can result in herniation.[24] Pediatric patients are particularly susceptible to secondary complications of increased intracranial pressure caused by limited confined space in comparison with adults.

On CTA, a "spot sign" describes active extravasation and is used to predict hematoma expansion. The "spot sign" within the hematoma appears as a hyperdense spot or serpiginous foci (**Fig. 7**) with a few caveats: no connection to a vessel, less than 1.5 mm, and at least double the Hounsfield units (>120 HU) of adjacent hematoma. Swirl and spot signs are indicative of active bleeding on noncontrast CT and CTA, respectively.[27] Hematoma expansion is theoretically the result of secondary hemorrhage from shearing of vessels by mass effect, inflammation, and local injury from the primary hemorrhage.

Furthermore, CTA techniques in the setting of trauma are implemented to accentuate detection of extravasated contrast by using 90-second delayed CT or dual-energy early arterial CTA.[28] In a recent study, conspicuity of contrast enhancement or leakage of contrast was superior in dual-energy CTA compared with delayed CT imaging.[29]

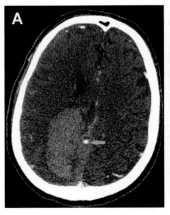 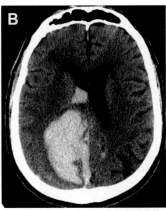

Fig. 7. Intraparenchymal hematoma. (A) CTA demonstrates the "spot sign" (arrow) indicative of active extravasation in a large right parietal hematoma. (B) Follow-up shows hematoma expansion and penetration into the adjacent ventricle.

Also, detection of iodine leakage on dual-energy CT is more detectable than the traditional spot sign on CTA.[30] Spot sign on CTA has a reported sensitivity of 53% and reported specificities of 88% to 96%; with mimickers leading to false positives including microaneurysms, partially thrombosed aneurysms, moyamoya disease, and calcifications.[28] Ninety-second delayed CTA increased sensitivity from 53% to 64%.[28] By comparison, in a recent study dual-energy CTA has a reported sensitivity of 94% for detection of extravasation.[29]

MR imaging not only has better sensitivity than CT in detecting intraparenchymal hemorrhage and ischemia, but also may play a valuable role in the initial evaluation of pediatric patients with mild brain injury while minimizing exposure to ionizing radiation.[31] In a retrospective cohort of 109 pediatric patients with head trauma, MR imaging was able detect three times as many lesions (hemorrhage, ischemia, diffuse axonal injury [DAI]) compared with CT.[31] Six out of eight patients with a negative head CT were found to have post-traumatic lesions conspicuous only on MR imaging.[31] There is class I evidence to support the use of MR imaging in acute/subacute traumatic brain injury in the setting of a negative head CT with unexplained neurologic findings.[9]

There is conflicting data regarding follow-up of anticoagulated patients with mild trauma and an initial negative head CT. In a meta-analysis of seven studies of 1594 patients anticoagulated with vitamin K antagonist, the incidence of delayed intracranial hemorrhage on 24 hour follow up CT was minimal at 0.6%.[32] Similar studies of patients chronically medicated with warfarin, clopidogrel, or aspirin showed up to 2.5% of patients had delayed hemorrhage on 24- to 48-hour follow-up.[33,34] Elderly patients on anticoagulation or antiplatelet medicines with an initial negative head CT are also not found to have delayed hemorrhage on 24-hour follow-up head CT.[35]

Diffuse Axonal Injury

DAI is a stress injury resulting from the rotational acceleration/deceleration movement of the head, shearing the axons and adjacent capillaries.[19] Regions of the brain that receive the maximum shear strain in descending order include: gray/white matter junctions, corpus callosum (splenium), brainstem, superior cerebellar peduncles, and internal capsule.[19] Concurrent shear-strain may also produce cortical contusions and hemorrhage in the deep gray matter.[19] Three grades have been pathologically correlated with degree of neurologic impairment (Table 1) based on anatomic location of sheer injury[36]; MR imaging can detect the presence of microhemorrhages, edema, or restricted diffusion in these regions (Figs. 8 and 9).

Microhemorrhages in DAI are used as a biomarker for neurologic prognosis. Microbleeds are paramagnetic and detected by T2*-weighted sequences in a linear fashion related to field strength, where 3-T magnets are twice as sensitive to 1.5-T magnets.[37] Furthermore, the location of lesions within the brainstem has been found to be an independent prognosticator, where posterior lateral lesions have a worse outcome and are more highly correlated with the persistent vegetative state.[38] More recently in the acute stage,

Table 1
Adams Classification of diffuse axonal injury grading based on location of lesions

Grade	Location
I	White matter
II	Corpus collosum
III	Brainstem (dorsolateral, worse prognosis)

From Adams JH, Doyle D, Ford I, et al. Diffuse axonal injury in head injury: definition, diagnosis and grading. Histopathology 1989;15(1):49–59; with permission.

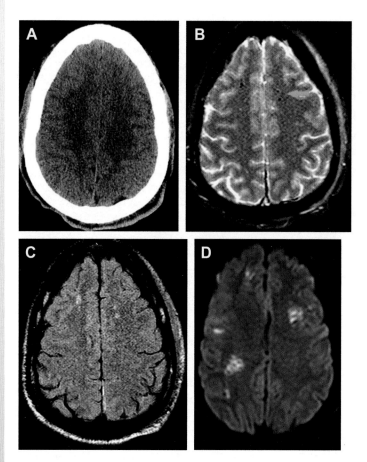

Fig. 8. Grade I diffuse axonal injury. (*A*) Noncontrast CT appears normal. MR imaging T2*-weighted sequence (*B*) demonstrates punctate blooming foci (*arrow*) in the bilateral subcortical white matter with FLAIR signal abnormality (*C*) and restricted diffusion (*D*).

lesions on MR imaging in the thalami, basal ganglia, and brainstem have been proposed as biomarkers of worse grades of DAI and have been associated with low levels of consciousness without mass lesions.[39]

Vascular Injury

Class IIb evidence supports the use of CTA if there is suspected vascular injury.[9] Direct intracranial vascular injury is rare, occurring in approximately 1% of blunt cerebral trauma and is most often associated with fractures of the skull base and craniofacial structures.[40] These injuries have a high mortality rate secondary to hemorrhagic shock.[40] Since 1999, the Denver group developed the Biffl scale, which is widely used to systemically grade vascular injury on digital subtraction angiography and been modified to apply to CTA and magnetic resonance angiography (MRA) (**Table 2**).[41] Application of this scale has been associated with high interreader reliability.[42] CTA compared with digital subtraction angiography has reported sensitivities of 74% to 97%, specificities of 86% to 100%, positive predictive value of 65% to 99.3%, and negative predictive value of 90% to 90.3%.[42–44]

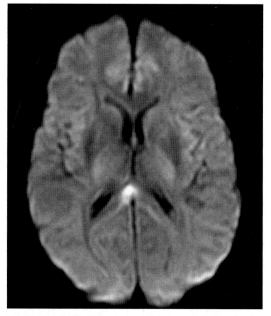

Fig. 9. Grade II diffuse axonal injury. A lesion in the splenium of the corpus collosum is restricting diffusion (ADC map not shown).

Table 2
Modified Biffl scale

Grade	Degree of Occlusion
I	Luminal irregularity, dissection flap, or intramural hematoma Vessel lumen stenosis <25%
II	Dissection flap or intramural hematoma Vessel lumen stenosis 25%–50%
III	Vessel lumen stenosis >50% or pseudoaneurysm
IV	Occlusion
V	Complete transection

From Biffl WL, Moore EE, Offner PJ, et al. Blunt carotid arterial injuries: implications of a new grading scale. J Trauma 1999;47:845–53; with permission.

A dissection flap may not always be visualized by CTA technique and differentiating a dissection from atherosclerotic disease or vasculitis can sometimes be challenging. Vessel wall MR imaging techniques may be helpful to detect intracranial dissection.[40,45] Increased signal to noise ratio of 3-T scanners in conjunction with fat, blood flow, and cerebrospinal fluid suppression techniques are used to image the intracranial vessel walls, which are only 0.2 to 0.3 mm in thickness. The intimal flap, separating the true and false lumen, appears as curvilinear T2. T1 fat suppressed black blood imaging can detect the presence of an intramural hematoma and wall morphology. Eccentric arterial wall thickening may demonstrate enhancement along the luminal and peripheral margins of the artery.[45]

An intramural hematoma appears as T1 hyperintensity eccentrically layering within the vessel wall (**Fig. 10**). In a study of 107 patients with suspected intracranial arterial dissection, the intimal flap was detected in more than twice the patients compared with CTA.[46] There is variability in the presence of intramural hematoma (evident on 59%–83%) and wall enhancement (evident in 51% of patients). Intramural hematomas are an evolving process where T1 shortening depends on the presence of methemoglobin in early and late subacute blood products (3–14 days). Studies have confirmed presence of an intramural hematoma on repeat imaging approximately 1 week after the initial insult up to 2 months on T1 black blood fat-saturated MR imaging.[40,46] Furthermore, the dissection itself is an evolving process and may be progressing or resolving.[46]

In intracranial cerebral artery dissection, the vertebral and basilar artery were the most common vessels affected with the posterior circulation affected more commonly than the anterior circulation.[46] Findings of acute dissection on CTA, MRA, and digital subtraction angiography include double lumen (**Fig. 11**), intramural hematoma, pearl and string sign, aneurysmal dilatation (**Fig. 12**), occlusion, stenosis, and saccular aneurysm. Of note, the double lumen sign was more often identified on MRA than CTA in cerebral artery dissection.[46]

Other less common vascular injuries include dural arterial venous fistula and carotid cavernous fistula.[47,48] A dural arteriovenous fistula is an abnormal communication between a meningeal artery and dural sinus or cortical vein.[47] Dural arterial venous fistulas are located in the dura or arachnoid membrane, not intraparenchymal, such as an

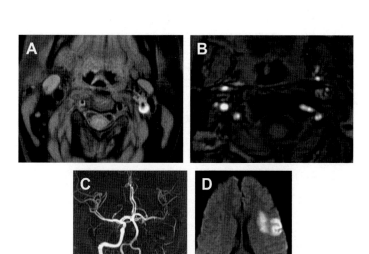

Fig. 10. Left internal carotid artery (ICA) dissection. MRA black blood fat-suppressed imaging (*A*) demonstrates T1 hyperintense intramural hematoma layering posteriorly within the left ICA wall. Time of flight (*B*) shows occlusion of the left ICA at the level of the dissection and distally on maximum intensity projection reformats (*C*). Diffusion imaging with restricted diffusion displaying infarcted left middle cerebral artery (*D*).

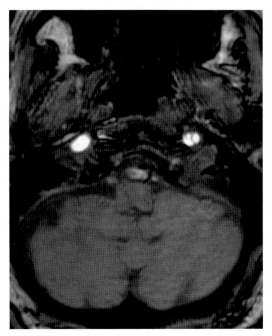

Fig. 11. Time-of-flight MRA demonstrates double lumen sign of dissection in left ICA in another patient.

arteriovenous malformation. The Borden classification entails three types of connections: type I, the most common, is a direct communication between a meningeal artery and a vein or dural venous sinus with antegrade flow; type II is communication between a meningeal artery and dural sinus with retrograde flow into the subarachnoid veins; and type III, the most rare, is venous drainage into the subarachnoid veins.[47] The high-pressure arterial system connecting to the low pressure subarachnoid veins may cause venous hypertension and/or hemorrhage. The radiographic appearance demonstrates prominent cluster of vessels near a dural sinus (Fig. 13). On CTA, this appears as hyperintensity from associated hemorrhage.[47]

Proptosis may be a secondary sign of venous congestion, with a dilated ophthalmic vein and cavernous sinus, which is seen in dural arteriovenous fistula and carotid cavernous fisutula.[47,48] Trauma is the most common cause of a carotid cavernous fistula.[48] Carotid cavernous fistulas occur in approximately 0.2% of brain trauma injuries and in 4% of patients with basilar skull fracture and should be suspected in trauma patients with abnormal enhancement of small tortuous vessels on CTA/MRA near the cavernous sinus.[48] If a dural venous arterial fistula or carotid cavernous fistula is suspected, then the patient should be referred to conventional diagnostic angiogram for confirmation and endovascular embolization.[47,48]

SECONDARY INJURIES AND COMPLICATIONS

Secondary injuries in the setting of brain trauma include territorial infarctions, local ischemia, diffuse hypoxic injury, diffuse cerebral edema, and herniation.[49] The Traumatic Brain Injury Model Systems National Database is funded by the National Institute of Disability and Rehabilitation research, which has currently enrolled more than 15,000 participants in a multicenter longitudinal study of outcome in traumatic brain injury, following participants for up to 25 years after injury.[50] From 2007 to 2015, at total of 6488 patients with traumatic brain injury were recorded in the Traumatic Brain Injury Model Systems National Database; 2.5% of patients were found to have an ischemic stroke, most often from cervical carotid of vertebral dissection caused by high velocity motor vehicle accidents.[51] Currently stroke guidelines issued by the American Heart Association and American Stroke Association contraindicate the use of tissue plasminogen activator after major head trauma because of the theoretic increased risk of hemorrhage; with a caveat that there is little evidence to support the current guidelines.[51]

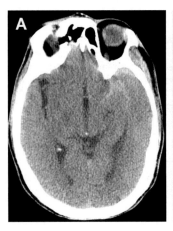
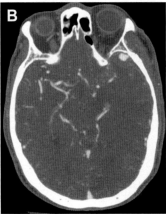

Fig. 12. Post-traumatic pseudoaneurysm. Noncontrast CT (A) demonstrates a left temporal epidural hematoma and subarachnoid hemorrhage in the left sylvian fissure. CTA (B) shows a pseudoaneurysm arising from a branch of the left meningeal artery.

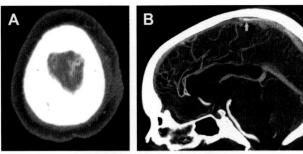

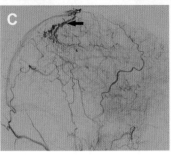

Fig. 13. Dural arteriovenous fistula. Axial CTA (A) shows serpiginous vessels near the vertex. Sagittal reformats demonstrates dense arterial-like enhancement (arrow) in this region (B). Anomalous connection between a branch of the left meningeal artery and the superior sagittal sinus (arrow) was confirmed on diagnostic angiogram (C).

Endovascular thrombectomy in the treatment of post-traumatic ischemic infarctions may be a useful alternative that needs to be explored.

Severe diffuse hypoxic injury can present as the ominous "reversal sign" on noncontrast CT, characterized by diffusely decreased density; loss of gray/white matter differentiation; and hyperdense thalami, brainstem, and cerebellum (Fig. 14).[52] The pathophysiology is not well understood but autopsies have correlated diffuse acute neuronal necrosis and edema. Prognosis is poor and correlated with the persistent vegetative state. Most severely, the entire supratentorial hemisphere infarcts leaving only the hyperdense cerebellum ("white cerebellum sign").[52]

Effacement of the cisterns is often associated with failure of nonoperative management in the presence of intra-axial and/or extra-axial hemorrhages and DAI.[53] The ambient, quadrigeminal plate, interpeduncular, and cerebellar medullary cistern should be carefully evaluated for impending herniation (Fig. 15).

Duret hemorrhages, are delayed secondary hemorrhages thought to be caused by evolving descending transtentorial herniation and are consequently associated with a mortality rate. These hemorrhages occur in the ventral and central areas of the upper brainstem (mesencephalon and pons) and appear as small linear hyperdense foci on CT (Fig. 16). The origin is unclear and may be related to injury of basilar artery pontine perforators, venous thrombosis, intractable hypertension, or even contusions related to cervical spine injury.[54]

At the other end of the spectrum, mild injury, such as concussions, may not have any apparent imaging findings during the acute phase.[55,56]

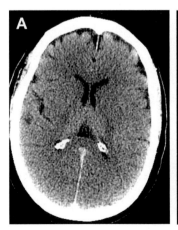

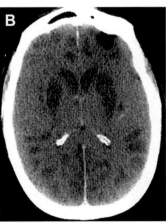

Fig. 14. Hypoxic injury "reversal sign." Noncontrast axial CT (A) diffuse loss of gray white matter differentiation with preservation of dense thalami. Follow-up imaging 24 hours later (B) shows progression and "reversal sign" where the white matter appears hypodense and cortical gray matter is dense, the basal ganglia are infarcted.

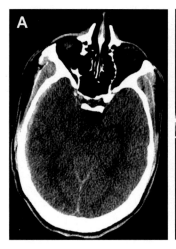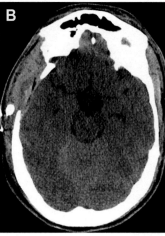

Fig. 15. Bilateral uncal herniation. Noncontrast CT shows effacement of the basilar cisterns (A). Follow-up imaging after immediate decompressive craniectomy for evacuation of a right subdural hematoma in a young patient shows patent cisternal spaces (B).

However, imaging findings in the chronic phase are becoming apparent with advanced MR imaging techniques. susceptibility weighted imaging is the most sensitive imaging sequence for detecting hemosiderin deposition from microhemorrhages, which may have occurred in areas vulnerable to shear stress, the corpus collosum, basal ganglia and deep white matter, up to two times more sensitive that T2*-weighted imaging.[55] In addition,

cerebral atrophy manifests in many patients with mild to severe injury. Atrophy may be diffuse or focal localizing to anatomic regions of high shear stress: corpus collosum, fornix, and brainstem. Degree of atrophy has been correlated with degree of injury.[56]

Overall, the prompt recognition of primary injuries related to brain trauma and their secondary complications can substantially guide clinical

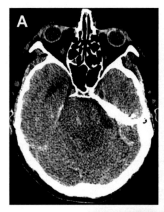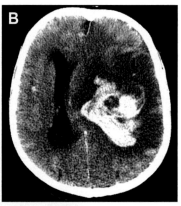

Fig. 16. Duret hemorrhages and developing transtentorial herniation. Noncontrast axial CT (A) shows linear hyperdense hemorrhage in the pons in this patient with subfalcine (B) and uncal herniation (C).

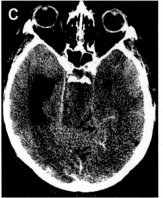

management. Noncontrast CT is the workhorse of emergent brain imaging. CTA/MRA should be used when vascular injury is suspected. MR imaging has increased sensitivity for detecting traumatic brain injury and should be used for prognostication and to explain deterioration of neurologic symptoms unexplained by CT.

REFERENCES

1. Dewan MC, Rattani A, Gupta S, et al. Estimating the global incidence of traumatic brain injury. J Neurosurg 2018. [Epub ahead of print].
2. Center for Disease Control. Traumatic brain injury and concussion get the facts website. Available at: https://www.cdc.gov/traumaticbraininjury/get_the_facts.html. Accessed September 15, 2018.
3. Peeters W, van den Brande R, Polinder S, et al. Epidemiology of traumatic brain injury in Europe. Acta Neurochir (Wien) 2015;157(10):1683–96.
4. Brenner LA, Ignacio RV, Blow FC. Suicide and traumatic brain injury among individuals seeking Veterans Health Administration services. J Head Trauma Rehabil 2011;26(4):257–64.
5. Madsen T, Erlangsen A, Orlovska S, et al. Association between traumatic brain injury and risk of suicide. JAMA 2018;320(6):580–8.
6. Mckee AC, Daneshvar DH. The neuropathology of traumatic brain injury. Handb Clin Neurol 2015;127:45–66.
7. Andriessen TM, Horn J, Franschman G, et al. Epidemiology, severity classification, and outcome of moderate and severe traumatic brain injury: a prospective multicenter study. J Neurotrauma 2011; 28(10):2019–31.
8. Raj R, Skrifvars MB, Bendel S, et al. Predicting six-month mortality of patients with traumatic brain injury: usefulness of common intensive care severity scores. Crit Care 2014;18(2):R60.
9. Wintermark M, Sanelli PC, Anzai Y, et al, ACR Head Injury Institute, ACR Head Injury Institute. Imaging evidence and recommendations for traumatic brain injury: conventional neuroimaging techniques. J Am Coll Radiol 2015;12(2):e1–14.
10. Lolli V, Pezzullo M, Delpierre I, et al. MDCT imaging of traumatic brain injury. Br J Radiol 2016;89(1061): 20150849.
11. Huisman TA, Tschirch FT. Epidural hematoma in children: do cranial sutures act as a barrier? J Neuroradiol 2009;36(2):93–7.
12. Heit JJ, Iv M, Wintermark M. Imaging of intracranial hemorrhage. J Stroke 2017;19(1):11–27.
13. Zimmerman RA, Bilaniuk LT. Computed tomographic staging of traumatic epidural bleeding. Radiology 1982;144(4):809–12.
14. Selariu E, Zia E, Brizzi M, et al. Swirl sign in intracerebral haemorrhage: definition, prevalence, reliability and prognostic value. BMC Neurol 2012;12:109.
15. Karibe H, Hayashi T, Narisawa A, et al. Clinical characteristics and outcome in elderly patients with traumatic brain injury: for establishment of management strategy. Neurol Med Chir (Tokyo) 2017;57(8):418–25.
16. Fanconi M, Lips U. Shaken baby syndrome in Switzerland: results of a prospective follow-up study, 2002-2007. Eur J Pediatr 2010;169(8):1023–8.
17. D'Amato L, Piazza O, Alliata L, et al. Prognosis of isolated acute post-traumatic subdural haematoma. J Neurosurg Sci 2007;51(3):107–11.
18. Bartels RH, Meijer FJ, van der Hoeven H, et al. Midline shift in relation to thickness of traumatic acute subdural hematoma predicts mortality. BMC Neurol 2015;15:220.
19. Grossman RI, Yousem DM. Neuroradiology: the requisites. 2nd edition. Philadelphia: Elsevier Inc; 2003. p. 243–70.
20. Balinger KJ, Elmously A, Hoey BA, et al. Selective computed tomographic angiography in traumatic subarachnoid hemorrhage: a pilot study. J Surg Res 2015;199(1):183–9.
21. Nassiri F, Badhiwala JH, Witiw CD, et al. The clinical significance of isolated traumatic subarachnoid hemorrhage in mild traumatic brain injury: a meta-analysis. J Trauma Acute Care Surg 2017;83(4):725–31.
22. Witiw CD, Byrne JP, Nassiri F, et al. Isolated traumatic subarachnoid hemorrhage: an evaluation of critical care unit admission practices and outcomes from a North American perspective. Crit Care Med 2018;46(3):430–6.
23. Dalle Ore CL, Rennert RC, Schupper AJ, et al. The identification of a subgroup of children with traumatic subarachnoid hemorrhage at low risk of neuroworsening. J Neurosurg Pediatr 2018;22(5):559–66.
24. Araki T, Yokota H, Morita A. Pediatric traumatic brain injury: characteristic features, diagnosis, and management. Neurol Med Chir (Tokyo) 2017;57(2): 82–93.
25. Lichenstein R, Glass TF, Quayle KS, et al, Traumatic Brain Injury Study Group of the Pediatric Emergency Care Applied Research Network (PECARN). Presentations and outcomes of children with intraventricular hemorrhages after blunt head trauma. Arch Pediatr Adolesc Med 2012;166(8):725–31.
26. Kurland D, Hong C, Aarabi B, et al. Hemorrhagic progression of a contusion after traumatic brain injury: a review. J Neurotrauma 2012;29(1):19–31.
27. Wada R, Aviv RI, Fox AJ, et al. CT angiography "spot sign" predicts hematoma expansion in acute intracerebral hemorrhage. Stroke 2007;38(4):1257–62.
28. Peng WJ, Reis C, Reis H, et al. Predictive value of CTA spot sign on hematoma expansion in intracerebral hemorrhage patients. Biomed Res Int 2017; 2017:4137210.
29. Watanabe Y, Tsukabe A, Kunitomi Y, et al. Dual-energy CT for detection of contrast enhancement or leakage within high-density haematomas in

patients with intracranial haemorrhage. Neuroradiology 2014;56(4):291–5.

30. Orito K, Hirohata M, Nakamura Y, et al. Leakage sign for primary intracerebral hemorrhage: a novel predictor of hematoma growth. Stroke 2016;47(4):958–63.

31. Buttram SD, Garcia-Filion P, Miller J, et al. Computed tomography vs magnetic resonance imaging for identifying acute lesions in pediatric traumatic brain injury. Hosp Pediatr 2015;5(2):79–84.

32. Chauny JM, Marquis M, Bernard F, et al. Risk of delayed intracranial hemorrhage in anticoagulated patients with mild traumatic brain injury: systematic review and meta-analysis. J Emerg Med 2016;51(5):519–28.

33. Swap C, Sidell M, Ogaz R, et al. Risk of delayed intracerebral hemorrhage in anticoagulated patients after minor head trauma: the role of repeat cranial computed tomography. Perm J 2016;20(2):14–6.

34. Hill JH, Bonner P, O'Mara MS, et al. Delayed intracranial hemorrhage in the patient with blunt trauma on anticoagulant or antiplatelet agents: routine repeat head computed tomography is unnecessary. Brain Inj 2018;32(6):735–8.

35. Mann N, Welch K, Martin A, et al. Delayed intracranial hemorrhage in elderly anticoagulated patients sustaining a minor fall. BMC Emerg Med 2018;18(1):27.

36. Adams JH, Doyle D, Ford I, et al. Diffuse axonal injury in head injury: definition, diagnosis and grading. Histopathology 1989;15(1):49–59.

37. Scheid R, Ott DV, Roth H, et al. Comparative magnetic resonance imaging at 1.5 and 3 Tesla for the evaluation of traumatic microbleeds. J Neurotrauma 2007;24(12):1811–6.

38. Hilario A, Ramos A, Millan JM, et al. Severe traumatic head injury: prognostic value of brain stem injuries detected at MRI. AJNR Am J Neuroradiol 2012;33:1925–31.

39. Moe HK, Moen KG, Skandsen T, et al. The influence of traumatic axonal injury in thalamus and brainstem on level of consciousness at scene or admission: a clinical magnetic resonance imaging study. J Neurotrauma 2018;35(7):975–84.

40. Kobata H. Diagnosis and treatment of traumatic cerebrovascular injury: pitfalls in the management of neurotrauma. Neurol Med Chir (Tokyo) 2017;57(8):410–7.

41. Biffl WL, Moore EE, Offner PJ, et al. Blunt carotid arterial injuries: implications of a new grading scale. J Trauma 1999;47:845–53.

42. Foreman PM, Griessenauer CJ, Kicielinski KP, et al. Reliability assessment of the Biffl scale for blunt traumatic cerebrovascular injury as detected on computer tomography angiography. J Neurosurg 2017;127(1):32–5.

43. Malhotra AK, Camacho M, Ivatury RR, et al. Computed tomographic angiography for the diagnosis of blunt carotid/vertebral artery injury: a note of caution. Ann Surg 2007;246:632–42 [discussion: 642–3].

44. Eastman AL, Chason DP, Perez CL, et al. Computed tomographic angiography for the diagnosis of blunt cervical vascular injury: is it ready for primetime? J Trauma 2006;60:925–9 [discussion: 929].

45. Mandell DM, Mossa-Basha M, Qiao Y, et al, Vessel Wall Imaging Study Group of the American Society of Neuroradiology. Intracranial vessel wall MRI: principles and expert consensus recommendations of the American Society of Neuroradiology. AJNR Am J Neuroradiol 2017;38(2):218–29.

46. Kanoto M, Hosoya T. Diagnosis of intracranial artery dissection. Neurol Med Chir (Tokyo) 2016;56(9):524–33.

47. Sun L, Tang W, Liu L, et al. Dural arteriovenous fistula disguised as cerebral venous sinus thrombosis. J Zhejiang Univ Sci B 2017;18(8):733–6.

48. Ellis JA, Goldstein H, Connolly ES Jr, et al. Carotid-cavernous fistulas. Neurosurg Focus 2012;32(5):E9.

49. Gentry LR, Godersky JC, Thompson B. MR imaging of head trauma: review of the distribution and radiopathologic features of traumatic lesions. AJR Am J Roentgenol 1988;150(3):663–72.

50. Mayo Clinic. Clinical trials website. Available at: https://www.mayo.edu/research/clinical-trials/cls-20312410. Accessed September 28, 2018.

51. Kowalski RG, Haarbauer-Krupa JK, Bell JM, et al. Acute ischemic stroke after moderate to severe traumatic brain injury: incidence and impact on outcome. Stroke 2017;48(7):1802–9.

52. Han BK, Towbin RB, De Courten-Myers G, et al. Reversal sign on CT: effect of anoxic/ischemic cerebral injury in children. AJNR Am J Neuroradiol 1989;10(6):1191–8.

53. Chang EF, Meeker M, Holland MC. Acute traumatic intraparenchymal hemorrhage: risk factors for progression in the early post-injury period. Neurosurgery 2007;61(1 Suppl):222–30 [discussion: 230–1].

54. Nguyen HS, Doan NB, Gelsomino MJ, et al. Good outcomes in a patient with a Duret hemorrhage from an acute subdural hematoma. Int Med Case Rep J 2016;9:15–8.

55. Wintermark M, Sanelli PC, Anzai Y, et al, American College of Radiology Head Injury Institute. Imaging evidence and recommendations for traumatic brain injury: advanced neuro- and neurovascular imaging techniques. AJNR Am J Neuroradiol 2015;36(2):E1–11.

56. Shinoday J, Asano Y. Disorder of executive function of the brain after head injury and mild traumatic brain injury – neuroimaging and diagnostic criteria for implementation of administrative support in Japan. Neurol Med Chir (Tokyo) 2017;57(5):199–209.

Imaging of Neck Visceral Trauma

Clint W. Sliker, MD

KEYWORDS

- Trauma • Neck • Larynx • Trachea • Pharynx • Esophagus • Thyroid

KEY POINTS

- Injuries to neck visceral organs are uncommon but clinically important.
- Aerodigestive injuries are associated with significant mortality and morbidity. Although generally less severe, thyroid gland injuries may also lead to poor patient outcomes.
- Computed tomography and endoscopy are complementary, rather than exclusive, diagnostic tools and are the most important diagnostic modalities used to evaluate patients with potential neck visceral injury caused by either blunt or penetrating trauma.
- Soft tissue gas is a sensitive but nonspecific sign of penetrating aerodigestive injuries. However, although gas absent from deep neck soft tissue spaces virtually excludes penetrating aerodigestive injury, its absence does not exclude a blunt injury.
- In addition to recognizing the various imaging manifestations of injuries, radiologists must also recognize the clinical scenarios and ancillary imaging findings that should prompt a high index of suspicion for neck visceral injury, promoting prompt diagnosis, thereby facilitating early treatment, which improves clinical outcomes.

INTRODUCTION

The neck is a complex region that houses many important structures from many different organ systems, including the vascular, respiratory, digestive, neurologic, musculoskeletal, and endocrine systems.[1] Although significant traumatic injury to the neck is uncommon, both blunt and penetrating neck injuries may have devastating consequences to the patient.

Described generally, the neck is the region between the skull base and the chest (Fig. 1).[2] The superior boundary can be better localized to the inferior/mandibular margin and superior nuchal line,[2–4] whereas the inferior boundary is demarcated by the suprasternal notch, superior clavicular borders, and T1 vertebral body.[3,4] Based on the complexity of the anatomy, many organs and structures of the neck may either overlap or extend into the chest or face.[2,5] There are multiple ways the neck may be anatomically compartmentalized, but, when considering related groups of injury, it is useful to divide the neck into 4 gross anatomic compartments: midline visceral, posterior musculoskeletal, and 2 bilateral neurovascular compartments (Table 1).

Given their frequency and their potentially devastating neurologic consequences, trauma to the musculoskeletal compartment injuries, in particular cervical spine injuries, have historically drawn much of the attention of radiologists in both the medical literature and clinical practice. For similar reasons, injuries to the neurovascular compartments and vertebral arteries (posterior compartment) also engender academic and clinical interest.

Despite the understandable attention given to the cervical musculoskeletal and neurovascular compartments, trauma to the neck visceral

Disclosures: None.
Department of Diagnostic Radiology and Nuclear Medicine, Division of Emergency and Trauma Imaging, University of Maryland Medical Center, 22 South Greene Street, Baltimore, MD 21201, USA
E-mail address: csliker@umm.edu

radiologic.theclinics.com

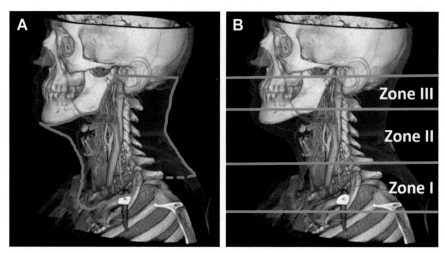

Fig. 1. (*A*, *B*) Neck anatomy. (*A*) Gross anatomic boundaries of the neck (*blue lines*). (*B*) Zonal anatomy of the neck.

compartment may also have potentially devastating consequences. Visceral compartment injuries, especially aerodigestive, may lead to death or long-term morbidity if not rapidly diagnosed and treated accordingly. However, they may be easily overlooked by both radiologists and clinicians.[6,7]

Aerodigestive Injuries

Both blunt and penetrating aerodigestive injuries, those involving the larynx, pharynx, cervical

trachea, or cervical esophagus, are rare. Although more frequently resulting from penetrating trauma than blunt trauma,[8] the incidence of penetrating aerodigestive injury is only 5% to 7% of penetrating neck injuries,[1,5,9] whereas penetrating neck trauma, in general, is very uncommon, accounting for 1% of all patients with trauma in the United States.[1] Regardless of injury mechanism, laryngotracheal injuries are more common than pharyngoesophageal injuries.[10]

Despite being more common than blunt injuries, penetrating laryngotracheal injuries, like all aerodigestive injuries, are rare and encountered in only 1% to 7% of all patients with penetrating neck injuries.[5] Although more common than cervical tracheal injuries, blunt laryngeal injuries are rare, diagnosed in 0.06% of all patients with trauma in one series.[11] Supported by reports indicating that blunt laryngeal injuries are frequently missed during both the initial clinical[7] and imaging[6] evaluations, Becker and colleagues[12] suggested the true incidence may be closer to 1% of all patients with blunt trauma.

Pharyngoesophageal injuries are rare. More commonly resulting from penetrating neck trauma than blunt trauma,[8] they are still seen in only 0.9% to 6.6% of patients with penetrating neck injuries.[5] Blunt esophageal injuries have a reported incidence of 0.001% to 0.08% of all patients with blunt trauma,[8,13] whereas there are only scattered case reports and series of blunt pharyngeal injuries in the medical literature.[14–18]

Both laryngotracheal and pharyngoesophageal injuries may result in either short-term death or

Table 1		
Gross anatomic compartments of the neck		
Compartment	**Location**	**Contents**
Visceral	Midline	Pharynx Esophagus Larynx Trachea Thyroid gland Parathyroid glands
Musculoskeletal	Posterior	Spine and spinal cord Prevertebral and paravertebral muscles Vertebral arteries
Neurovascular (bilateral)	Lateral	Common and internal carotid arteries Internal jugular vein Vagus nerve

Data from Berkovitz B, Neck. In: Stranding S, editor. Gray's anatomy: the anatomical basis of clinical practice, 39th edition. Philadelphia: Elsevier Churchill Livingstone; 2005. p. 531, 560–1.

long-term morbidity. Death caused by laryngotracheal injuries is virtually always related to loss of the airway.[12] However, although up to 80% of patients with laryngotracheal injuries may die before establishment of a secure airway, either prehospital or at the trauma bay, mortality is only 5% after a secure airway is established.[12] With regard to blunt pharyngoesophageal injuries, there is a paucity of data regarding outcomes in the medical literature, although pharyngeal injuries typically do well with prompt treatment. In contrast, penetrating esophageal injuries have significant mortalities, even when treated, ranging from 12.5% to 50%.[5,19] Patients who survive aerodigestive trauma risk recurrent aspiration, vocal cord paralysis, and hypoglossal nerve (cranial nerve [CN] XII) paralysis.[20] For both laryngotracheal[12] and pharyngoesophageal injuries,[15,19] early diagnosis and treatment (<24 hours), but not necessarily definitive repair, decrease mortality and improve long-term outcomes.

Several clinical signs and symptoms are associated with acute aerodigestive injuries (**Table 2**). Although aerodigestive injuries may have a wide range of clinical manifestations, it is important to note that, with the probable exception of signs of impending airway collapse,[23] the number and severity of clinical signs and symptoms shown do not directly correlate with the severity of the underlying injury.[7,23] In addition, clinical manifestations of injury, which may be difficult or impossible to identify in unconscious or intubated patients,[12] may not develop until hours after the initial trauma.[23] Consequently, aerodigestive injuries may initially be missed by clinicians, and radiologists may be the first to suspect, if not definitively make, the diagnosis.

Endocrine Glands

Thyroid gland injuries are uncommon. Blunt thyroid injury is particularly rare[24] and most commonly affects abnormal glands (ie, goiter, adenoma, cyst) than normal glands.[25] Thyroid gland injuries are potentially lethal because of airway compromise caused by either compression by hematoma or vocal cord paralysis related to recurrent laryngeal nerve injury.[26]

Clinically, thyroid gland injuries may manifest similar to aerodigestive injuries (see **Table 2**).[25,26] In addition, rupture of a thyroid lobe may result in a hematoma that causes noticeable neck swelling and/or tracheal deviation.[25] It is notable that significant signs and symptoms may either progress or occur 24 hours or more after the initial injury.[26] Therefore, it has been recommended that patients with thyroid injuries should be carefully monitored for at least 24 hours.[26]

There is virtually nothing in the medical literature regarding acute parathyroid gland traumatic injury. A single case report discusses blunt trauma–induced hematoma caused by a ruptured adenoma.[27] To the author's knowledge, there are no reports of acute trauma to the normal parathyroid glands. Possibly, the small size of parathyroid glands, averaging 5 mm × 3 mm × 1 mm, which are rarely depicted by routine diagnostic imaging,[28] either protects them from injury or results in them being obscured by hemorrhage from adjacent structures (eg, thyroid gland).

DIAGNOSTIC WORK-UP
General Considerations

Although knowing whether a patient has relevant clinical signs and symptoms may alert both radiologists and clinicians to underlying aerodigestive injury, improving the odds of correct diagnosis,[6] there are other factors that may facilitate prompt, accurate diagnosis.

First, blunt aerodigestive injuries tend to occur as the result of one of several mechanisms of injury, all of which involve either a blow to the anterior neck or crushing injury:

- Usually, a blow to the anterior neck during hyperextension (eg, sports injury, assault, handlebar injury) either causes direct injury or pins the pharynx against the spine, leading to barotrauma caused by forced exhalation against the closed airway.[15,17,18,20]
- Pinning of the larynx against the spine (eg, clothesline injury) may lead to shearing injury.[20]
- The pharynx may be directly punctured by the intact hyoid bone,[17,18] a fracture fragment,[20] or cervical spine osteophyte.[29]

Consequently, the possibility of an aerodigestive injury should be expected in patients with a history of anterior neck blunt trauma.

Table 2 Clinical signs and symptoms of aerodigestive injuries	
Hoarseness	Aphonia
Soft tissue emphysema and crepitance	Dyspnea
Pain	Stridor
Dysphagia	Hemoptysis
Odynophagia	Glomus sensation

Data from Refs.[7,20–22]

When evaluating patients with penetrating neck trauma, knowing the anatomic zone of the entry/exit wounds can be helpful. In penetrating trauma, traumatologists localize the entry wound to 1 of 3 anatomic zones[5] (see **Fig. 1**):

- Zone I: sternal notch to cricoid cartilage
- Zone II: cricoid cartilage to mandibular angle
- Zone III: mandibular angle to skull base

Zonal anatomy was once used to guide management decisions, but its role has been superseded by the widespread adoption of computed tomography (CT) angiography.[5,30] However, the terminology remains in use, and understanding zonal anatomy facilitates communication with traumatologists. Although knowing the zone of the entry/exit wounds may guide radiologists to an area of suspicion, it must be stressed that areas of clinically significant injury may be remote from the entry wound[5,30] (**Fig. 2**). Usually done with CT, identifying the trajectory of the wound tracts may allow a significant injury to be excluded[5,9] if the tract clearly extends away from a vital structure. In contrast, identification of the tract allows radiologists to determine what structures may be injured, as well as which diagnostic tool should be used for further evaluation.

Patient age should also influence the degree of suspicion for an aerodigestive injury and the type of injury. Aerodigestive injuries are more common with advancing age. Because the mandible and chest provide greater protection to the neck in children than in adults, aerodigestive injuries are less common in children.[11,31] In addition, with increasing age, typically beginning in the second decade of life[12,32] (**Fig. 3**), progressive mineralization and ossification of the larynx decrease its pliability, making it more prone to fracture with increasing age.[11] Therefore, diagnostic imaging of older patients with neck trauma should be closely scrutinized for aerodigestive injuries, especially those involving the larynx.

In addition, 50% of patients with aerodigestive injuries have other severe injuries.[32] Laryngotracheal injuries are frequently associated with a craniofacial, cervical spine, and cervical vascular injuries:

- Mandible and/or midface fractures (37%)[6] (**Fig. 4**)
- Traumatic brain injury (13%–15%)[12]
- Cervical spine injuries (8%–13%)[6,12]
- Internal or common carotid injuries (7%)[6]

Similarly, 37% and 16% of hypopharyngeal injuries are associated with mandible fractures and laryngeal injuries, respectively.[17] Ironically, although these coexisting (ie, distracting) injuries are one potential reason for delayed diagnosis of aerodigestive injuries,[6,7] they should heighten suspicion for aerodigestive injury, which should decrease possibility of a missed injury.

Aerodigestive Injuries

In some instances, especially in patients with penetrating neck trauma and airway compromise, emergent neck exploration is diagnostic as well as therapeutic. However, in most instances, diagnostic imaging and/or endoscopy are needed to diagnose and fully characterize acute aerodigestive injuries.

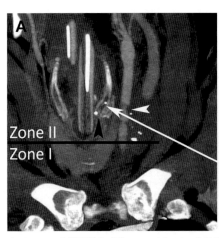
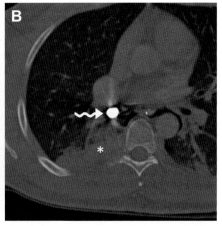

Fig. 2. Gunshot wound (GSW) in 36-year-old man. (*A*) CT slab maximum intensity projection (MIP). Wound tract (*white arrow*) extends from supraclavicular entry (not shown) through zone I into zone II, where there are left common carotid (*white arrowhead*) and laryngeal injuries, with the latter isolated to the left thyroid lamina (*black arrowhead*) injuries. (*B*) Chest CT. Aspirated bullet (*wavy arrow*) in right lower lobe bronchus causes obstructive atelectasis.

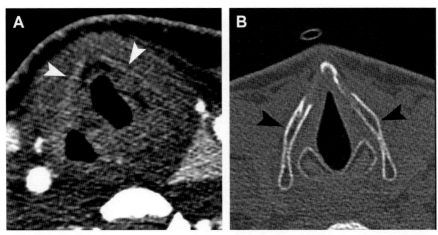

Fig. 3. CT images of normal unossified thyroid laminae (*white arrowheads*) of a 16-year-old boy (*A*) and partially ossified thyroid laminae (*black arrowheads*) of a 42-year-old man (*B*).

Computed tomography

Computed tomography imaging protocol: general considerations In contemporary practice, CT is the mainstay diagnostic tool for evaluating patients with either blunt or penetrating neck injuries. It is the current diagnostic standard in the initial evaluation of patients with suspected acute injury to the cervical spine and neck arteries. In addition, it can be used to evaluate for aerodigestive injuries. Regardless of the specific protocol and scanner used for image acquisition, several factors related to image reconstruction and interpretation are vital for maximizing the accuracy of CT for identifying aerodigestive injuries:

- Cross-sectional images should be reconstructed with thickness of, at most, 1 mm with an overlap of at least 50%.[12,22]
- Axial, sagittal, and coronal cross-sectional multiplanar reformation (MPR) images should all be routinely reconstructed.[12,22]
- Off-axis MPR images should be reconstructed in relation to the long axis of the neck to best show normal anatomic relationships. When necessary, additional MPRs reconstructed relative to the long axis of the larynx should also be reconstructed.[12,22,33]
- Three-dimensional (3D) reconstructions (eg, volume rendered, virtual endoscopic) images should be used liberally, because some laryngeal injuries are only identified with 3D reconstructions.[33]

Although not used at the author's institution, Conradie and Gebremariam[34] reported that CT esophagography, performed 5 minutes after the patient ingests 50 mL of oral contrast (50% solution of iohexol 300 mg I/mL and water) can be used to accurately diagnose injuries. However, as with fluoroscopic esophagography,[5] a controlled swallow may be difficult or impossible in some acutely injured, uncooperative, or unconscious patients.

Although some investigators state that intravenous (IV) contrast is necessary only if a CT angiogram is being performed to assess for coexisting vascular injury,[22] there is no consensus in the medical literature about the use of IV contrast for detecting aerodigestive injuries.[12] However, the author finds IV contrast useful to assess active mucosal bleeding, a sign of aerodigestive injury,[9] and to differentiate normal soft tissue from hemorrhage and devascularized tissue.

Computed tomography image interpretation: general considerations Window and level settings used to evaluate CT scans for potential aerodigestive injuries are important, particularly when evaluating the larynx. It is vital to review images with both bone and soft tissue settings,[12,22,32] because bone settings may better depict fractures of mineralized cartilage (**Fig. 5**), whereas soft tissue settings are necessary to assess the unossified laryngeal cartilage (**Fig. 6**).

Direct CT signs of injury include regions of cartilage discontinuity, representing laryngeal fractures[12,32] (see **Figs. 5** and **6**) and full-thickness mucosal or transmural defects[9,12,15,35] (**Fig. 7**). Indirect signs of injury include deep compartment soft tissue emphysema,[9,13,14,18,32,34,35] intralaryngeal soft tissue emphysema caused by mucosal disruption,[12] and intralaryngeal or paralaryngeal hemorrhage[12] (see **Fig. 6**).

Soft tissue gas as an indirect CT sign of an aerodigestive injury must be used with caution.

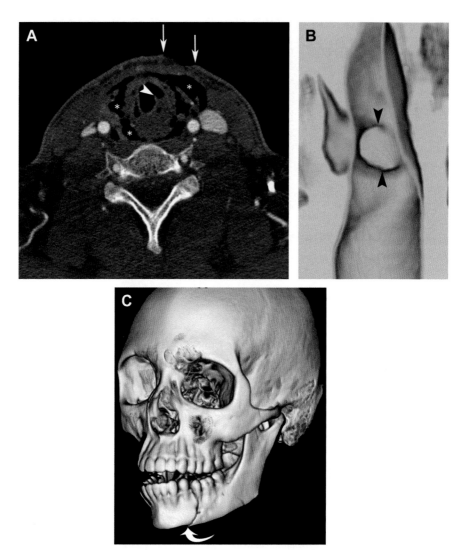

Fig. 4. Partial tracheal disruption in 16-year-old girl struck in neck with wooden post in motor vehicle collision (MVC). (*A*) Axial CT angiogram (CTA) shows free edge of disrupted tracheal wall (*white arrowhead*), paratracheal soft tissue gas (*asterisks*), and superficial laceration (*white arrows*). (*B*) Left lateral perspective CT three-dimensional (3D) surface shaded display (SSD) reconstruction shows focal tracheal mural defect (*black arrowheads*). (*C*) CT-3D SSD image shows left mandible fracture (*arrow*).

Although it may be caused by either a mucosal or transmural defect, it may also be unrelated to aerodigestive injury. In some instances, it may track from injuries in either the face (eg, fractures) or chest (eg, pneumomediastinum). Moreover, in the setting of penetrating trauma, it may be introduced by the penetrating object rather than resulting from transmucosal (see **Fig. 7**) or transmural injury[5,9] (**Fig. 8**). In addition, blunt laryngeal injuries, including those with significant mucosal injuries, may not be associated with soft tissue gas.[12]

In penetrating neck trauma, accurate assessment of wound tracts, including trajectory, is imperative. Wound tracts are usually delineated by soft tissue gas, hemorrhage, and possibly missile or fracture fragments[5,9] (see **Fig. 2**; **Fig. 9**). Structures along or within the tract are at risk of being injured, even if remote from the entry/exit wounds (see **Fig. 2**),[5,9,12] whereas injury may be excluded if the tract clearly spares these structures.[5,9] If a structure within the tract is not definitively injured, based on specific CT signs and/or clinical signs of injury, further work-up with other diagnostic tools (eg, endoscopy, esophagography) is necessary[5,8] (see **Fig. 9**).

At times, determination of the wound trajectory can be difficult, especially with trauma caused by

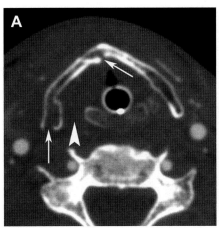
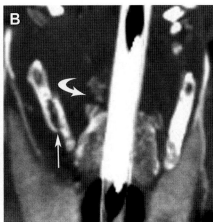

Fig. 5. A 36-year-old man struck in throat with a hockey puck. Axial (*A*) and coronal slab MIP (*B*) images from CTA show thyroid lamina (*straight arrows*) and arytenoid fractures (*curved arrow*) with cricoarytenoid joint disruption (*arrowhead*).

stabbings or low-velocity projectiles, as a result of the small diameter of the object and limited secondary cavitation around the tract.[5] Evaluation may also be complicated by comingling of multiple wounds or creation of secondary missile fragments (ie, bone, bullet) that form additional tracts with different trajectories.[5] Streak artifact from spinal hardware, bullet or shrapnel fragments, or metallic penetrating object remaining in situ (eg, knife) may obscure regions of interest, including injuries[5]; in this scenario, further evaluation by other diagnostic means is necessary to either diagnose or exclude an injury to structures within the tract.

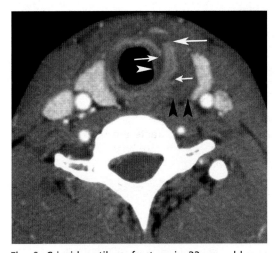

Fig. 6. Cricoid cartilage fracture in 22-year-old man following motor cycle crash (MCC). Axial CT shows comminuted cricoid cartilage (*arrows*), cricoid mucosal edema (*white arrowhead*), and paralaryngeal hematoma (*black arrowheads*) displacing the thyroid gland.

Computed tomography: diagnostic accuracy
Limited to penetrating injuries, CT has a sensitivity of 76% to 94.1%, specificity of 97% to 100%, and negative predictive value of 98.9%.[9,34,36] Direct CT findings of aerodigestive injury, mural defect (see Fig. 2; Fig. 10), and mucosal active bleeding are both 100% specific, but sensitivities are only 10.5% and 2.6%, respectively.[9] The direct CT signs of injury are important to recognize, but the accuracy of CT for diagnosing penetrating aerodigestive injuries hinges on identification of the deep soft tissue gas and specific wound trajectories. Madsen and colleagues[36] reported that the presence of soft tissue gas deep to the middle layer of the cervical fascia, fascia colli, and/or mediastinum is a sensitive but nonspecific sign of aerodigestive injury. Bodanapally and colleagues[9] reported that trajectory involving either the suprahyoid or the visceral deep neck spaces (Box 1) has a 97% sensitivity (Fig. 11) but only 55% specificity (see Fig. 9) for identifying an aerodigestive injury. Multiple investigators indicate CT negative for deep space extension of the tract virtually excludes penetrating aerodigestive injuries,[5,9,36] although Bodanapally and colleagues[9] reported false-negative scans for 3 of 6 esophageal injuries in their series. Therefore, it may be prudent to further evaluate patients with clinical signs and symptoms of an esophageal injury with endoscopy and/or esophagography.

CT may definitively show a blunt pharyngoesophageal injury[13,15] (see Fig. 8), but its accuracy for detecting blunt injuries has not been reported. Given the potentially deleterious consequences of a missed injury, when CT shows unexplained paraesophageal or parapharyngeal/retropharyngeal soft tissue emphysema (ie, unrelated to gas

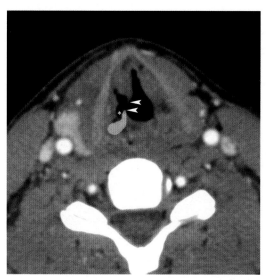

Fig. 7. A 16-year-old boy struck his neck on steering wheel in MVC. Axial CT shows mucosal defect (*arrowheads*) and submucosal gas (*asterisk*) adjacent to exposed cartilage of anteriorly subluxated arytenoid cartilage (*shaded yellow*).

tracking from other sites), further evaluation with endoscopy and/or esophagography should be considered.

Endoscopy

Endoscopy is an indispensable tool, complementary to diagnostic imaging, used in the assessment of aerodigestive injuries.[1,5,7–9,12,23,36] Endoscopy is used to:

- Exclude, diagnose, and/or thoroughly characterize laryngotracheal or pharyngoesophageal mucosal injuries[8,12,23]

- Evaluate for and differentiate between vocal cord dysfunction and cricoarytenoid joint injury[1,12]
- Evaluate for epiglottic injury[12]
- Diagnose or exclude injuries in patients with equivocal CT results[5,9,36]

In addition, in patients with laryngotracheal injuries, direct laryngoscopy may also be used to treat some injuries, including cricoarytenoid subluxation[37] and epiglottis avulsion.[12]

Esophagography

Used mainly in the setting of penetrating neck injuries, fluoroscopic esophagography (ie, pharyngoesophagography) plays a limited, but important, role in the diagnosis and characterization of acute pharyngoesophageal injuries (see **Fig. 8**). At most centers, the examination is typically biphasic: if an initial series of fluoroscopic-observed swallows of water-soluble contrast are negative, a single-contrast examination with thin barium contrast is performed.[5] In unconscious, intubated patients, in whom the endotracheal tube cuff protects the airway, the study can be performed by injecting contrast through an orogastric tube along the course of the esophagus.[8] However, in unconscious patients, the study may be difficult or impossible to perform.[5]

Even when successfully performed, the sensitivity of esophagography for showing pharyngoesophageal injuries is only 60% to 70%[8] with positive predictive value and specificity of 100%.[15] Esophagography may yield more false-negative results for detecting pharyngeal injuries relative to esophageal injuries, but it may also detect pharyngeal injuries missed by fiberoptic

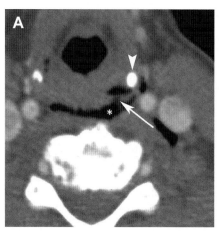

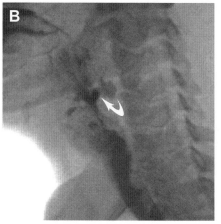

Fig. 8. (*A*) CTA shows full-thickness blunt pharyngeal injury (*straight arrow*) and retropharyngeal gas (*asterisk*), likely caused by perforation by the hyoid bone (*arrowhead*), secondary to MCC. (*B*) Esophagram better depicts size of mural defect (*curved arrow*), which was successfully treated nonoperatively.

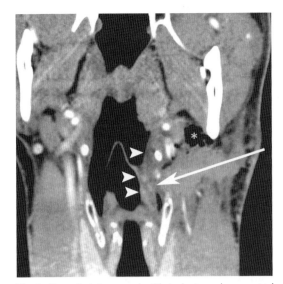

Fig. 9. Zone II stab wound with trajectory demarcated by hematoma (*white arrow*) extends to parapharyngeal region with adjacent pharyngeal mucosal thickening (*arrowheads*) and submucosal gas (*asterisk*), but no mucosal defect. Endoscopy and esophagography confirmed intact mucosa.

endoscopy.[15] In many centers, combination of endoscopy and esophagography is used, yielding a sensitivity of 100% for detecting injuries.[5,8]

Radiographs

The role of radiographs is limited in contemporary centers. They may localize bullet or shrapnel fragments, which may aid in estimating trajectory of the wound tract following penetrating trauma. In both blunt and penetrating trauma, they may be used to confirm the presence of clinically suspected soft tissue gas, which may indicate an

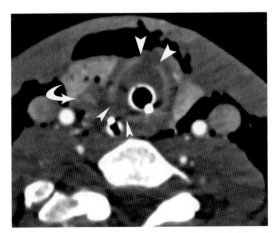

Fig. 10. Zone III GSW with anterior and posterolateral tracheal transmural injuries (*arrowheads*), as well as right thyroid lobe laceration (*curved arrow*).

Box 1
Deep spaces of the neck to assess for signs of penetrating aerodigestive injury

Suprahyoid Deep Space	Visceral Deep Space
Composed of multiple, smaller spaces	Central compartment lower neck, surrounding
Parapharyngeal spaces	Hypopharynx
Submandibular spaces	Larynx
Retropharyngeal space	Esophagus
Posterior third of sublingual space	Trachea

Data from Bodanapally UK, Shanmuganathan K, Dreizin D, et al. Penetrating aerodigestive injuries in the neck: a proposed CT-aided modified selective management algorithm. Eur Radiol 2016;26(7):2409–17.

---

aerodigestive injury.[20,38] Radiographs may also show signs of laryngotracheal separation.[38] However, any radiographic abnormality must be further assessed by some other diagnostic means.

Magnetic resonance imaging

Magnetic resonance (MR) imaging may be used to diagnose injuries to the laryngeal framework,[12,32,39] but it plays virtually no role in the acute evaluation of acute laryngeal injuries because of difficulties with patient monitoring; patient movement; and, in the setting of penetrating trauma, potentially ferromagnetic retained metallic foreign bodies.[5,7,12,32] To the author's knowledge, there are no peer-reviewed reports of the use of MR imaging to assess for acute pharyngoesophageal injuries in the medical literature.

LARYNGOTRACHEAL INJURIES
Laryngeal Injuries

Anatomic considerations
The larynx is a geometrically and mechanically complex organ, consisting of complicated cartilaginous framework, synovial joints, and multiple soft tissue structures.

The skeletal framework consists of multiple components composed of hyaline cartilage[12,32]:

- The tent-shaped thyroid cartilage, which has bilateral inferior and superior projections referred to as inferior and superior horns (cornua)
- The signet ring–shaped cricoid cartilage
- The paired, pyramidal arytenoid cartilages that anchor the vocal cords

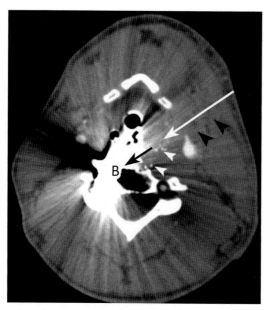

Fig. 11. CTA of zone II GSW shows wound tract (*white and black arrows*) demarcated by hemorrhage (*black arrowheads*) and bullet fragments (*white arrowheads*), in the parapharyngeal/retropharyngeal region, and bullet (B) with extensive streak artifact impacted in the spine. No pharyngeal defect was shown, but pharyngeal injury was inferred based on trajectory and confirmed by endoscopy.

As mentioned previously, the hyaline cartilage structures progressively mineralize and ossify with advancing age,[12,32] usually beginning in the second decade of life.[32] Heterogeneity of ossification is common and can periodically mimic a fracture,[12] especially in the thyroid cartilage.

Fibrocartilaginous components[12] of the skeletal framework include:

- The epiglottis, which protects the airway during swallowing, is attached to the thyroid cartilage by the thin, fibrous petiole
- Paired cuneiform and cuniculate cartilages at the tips of the arytenoid cartilages

Because they consist of fibrocartilage, the epiglottis, cuneiform cartilages, and cuniculate cartilages do not typically mineralize.[12] The cuneiform and cuniculate cartilages typically are not shown by routine imaging techniques.

There are 4 synovial joints, similar to others seen elsewhere in the bony skeleton, within the larynx.[12,32] Paired cricoarytenoid joints are at the superior, posterolateral cricoid cartilage and serve as the articulations between the cricoid and arytenoid cartilages.[12,32] The thyroid cartilage inferior horns laterally articulate with the cricoid cartilage via the paired cricothyroid joints,[12,32] which are in close proximity to the recurrent laryngeal nerves.[32]

The intrinsic soft tissue components of the larynx consist of mucosa, ligaments, and intrinsic muscles that may be impossible to definitively discriminate or project as discrete, identifiable structures (eg, true vocal cords).[12] Although it is difficult, and sometimes impossible, to exclude an injury with imaging, it is important to evaluate for discrete soft tissue injuries (eg, mucosal defect) or secondary signs of injury (eg, signs of vocal cord paralysis). Several extrinsic muscles and ligaments are also related to the larynx and its function, and, although either impossible to directly visualize with routine imaging or definitively discriminate from one another, associated injuries may be inferred in some instances.

Although, anatomically distinct from the larynx, the hyoid bone is both in very close proximity to and integrated with the function of the larynx.[12] Suspended between the suprahyoid muscles, infrahyoid (ie, strap) muscles, and stylohyoid ligaments, the hyoid bone does not directly articulate with either the larynx or another bone.[40] It is connected to the superior thyroid cartilage margins by the thyrohyoid ligament, which has areas of relative thickening referred to as ligaments.[12]

The triticeal cartilages are normal variants that are periodically visualized in the lateral thyrohyoid ligament, which extends between the superior horns of the thyroid cartilage and greater horns of the hyoid bone.[12] Triticeal cartilages are inconsistently visualized, and they are important only because they can mimic superior horn fractures.[12]

Injuries: general types
Although some injuries may be depicted or suggested by radiographs or MR imaging, most diagnosed with diagnostic imaging are done so with CT.

Fractures As with fractures diagnosed elsewhere in the skeleton, laryngeal fractures generally have the appearance of linear, partial-thickness, or full-thickness defects in the laryngeal cartilage.[12] When cartilage is heavily mineralized or ossified, fractures are typically complete (ie, full thickness) and, with increasing patient age and cartilaginous ossification, more frequently comminuted.[12] Because of its pliability, fractures through noncalcified cartilage may be incomplete (ie, greenstick or torus fractures).[12]

Dislocations and subluxations As with other synovial joints, cricoarytenoid and cricothyroid joint injuries may occur.[12,22,32,41–43] Types of injury include distraction, subluxation, and dislocation.

Mucosal injuries Mucosal injuries may be definitively diagnosed (see **Fig. 7**) or suggested (**Fig. 12**) with CT,[12,33] but they cannot be definitively excluded or fully characterized without endoscopy. Indirect CT signs of laryngeal injury have already been discussed in this article ("CT Image Interpretation: General Considerations").

Injuries: specific injuries

Thyroid cartilage fractures Thyroid cartilage fractures are typically vertical and either median (ie, through the apex) or paramedian through one or both of the laminae.[12,32,33] Horizontal fractures are typically superior and frequently result from strangulation or hanging[12] (**Box 2**).

Superior horn fractures may occur in isolation or with other fractures. They are frequently seen with strangulation or hanging[12,44] (see **Box 2**). Care must be taken not to confuse a normal variant triticeal cartilage for a displaced superior horn fragment; superior horn fracture fragments typically show a straight, defined margin that, when the cartilage is mineralized, is not corticated at the fracture site[12] (**Fig. 13**).

Inferior horn fractures frequently occur with cricoid cartilage fractures and cricothyroid joint injuries.[12]

Cricoid cartilage fractures Cricoid cartilage fractures most frequently occur with other laryngotracheal injuries.[12] However, isolated cricoid fractures have been reported as a result of strangulation[45] (see **Box 2**).

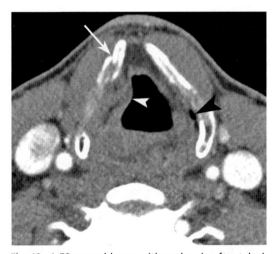

Fig. 12. A 59-year-old man with neck pain after television dropped onto his throat. Bubble of left submucosal gas (*black arrowhead*) caused by mucosal injury not shown by the CTA. Right submucosal hematoma (*white arrowhead*) caused by thyroid lamina fracture (*arrow*).

> **Box 2**
> **Laryngeal injuries associated with strangulation**
>
> Horizontal thyroid cartilage fractures
>
> Thyroid cartilage superior horn fractures
>
> Hyoid bone fractures
>
> Isolated cricoid cartilage fractures
>
> *Data from* Refs.[12,44,45]

Because it is a ring structure, cricoid fractures typically involve multiple sites[5,12] (see **Fig. 6**), which is important to identify because fragment depression may compromise the airway.

Mucosal tears occur with 50% of cricoid fractures.[12] Because the mucosa is normally tightly adherent to and indistinguishable from the cricoid cartilage, any submucosal density, submucosal gas, or mucosal thickening is always considered abnormal[32] (see **Fig. 6**) and should be considered a sign of a mucosal tear until proved otherwise by endoscopy. Cricoid mucosal tears may also contribute to airway compromise,[12] so it is important to recognize and report findings suspicious for cricoid cartilage mucosal injury.

Arytenoid cartilage fractures The arytenoid cartilages are the least commonly fractured of the laryngeal cartilages (see **Fig. 5**). Fifty percent of arytenoid fractures are bilateral, and they are frequently associated with thyroid cartilage and arytenoid cartilage fractures.[12]

Cricoarytenoid joint injuries The cricoarytenoid joints may subluxate or dislocate in any direction,[12,32] but anterior subluxations/dislocations are most common.[32] CT signs of cricoarytenoid joint injury include:

- Joint space widening (ie, distraction)[12] (**Fig. 14**)
- With anterior arytenoid subluxation/dislocation, anteromedial displacement of the arytenoid (see **Fig. 7**), anterior tipping of the arytenoid relative to the cricoid, inferior displacement of the ipsilateral vocal cord in relation to the uninjured side[32,41]
- With posterior subluxation/dislocation, superior position of the vocal cord in relation to the uninjured side[32,41]

Endoscopy is a vital part of the evaluation for cricoarytenoid joint injury, because it is required to definitively differentiate joint injury from vocal cord paralysis.[12,32] In addition, it may identify

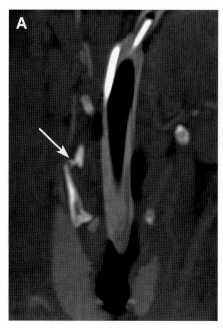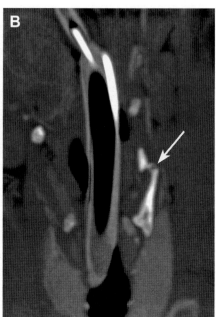

Fig. 13. (*A, B*) CTA oblique MPRs show bilateral medially displaced superior horn fractures (*arrows*).

one of the 36% of cricoarytenoid joint injuries that are not shown by CT.[32]

Cricothyroid joint injuries Cricothyroid joint injuries have been considered rare, but some investigators think they are underdiagnosed.[32] They typically occur with other laryngeal injuries, especially cricoid and inferior horn fractures.[12,32]

With CT, a cricothyroid joint injury should be suspected when there is asymmetric widening of the joint in relation to the uninjured joint[32] (**Fig. 15**). Images must be reconstructed in relation

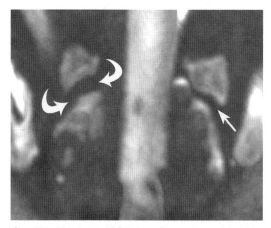

Fig. 14. Cricoarytenoid joint distraction caused by MCC. CT coronal slab MIP shows asymmetric widening (*curved arrows*) of the injured right cricoarytenoid joint relative to the normal left-sided joint (*arrow*).

to the true long axis of the trachea (ie, account for tilt or rotation of the neck), because off-axis reconstructions may mimic an injury and lead to a false-positive interpretation.[22,32]

Epiglottis injuries Epiglottis injuries are rare and may result from both blunt and penetrating trauma. Avulsions occur with disruption of the petiole, which connects the epiglottis and thyroid lamina.[12,39] Partial or full-thickness tears superior to and sparing the petiole may also occur[39] (**Fig. 16**).

Because the epiglottis usually is not calcified, injuries involving it can easily be missed by CT.[12,33] In addition, acute injuries may be masked by preepiglottic, epiglottic, and adjacent soft tissue swelling or hematomas.[12,39] Endoscopy is necessary for definitive diagnosis and potential repair.[12]

Hyoid bone fractures Because it is protected by the mandible and is a mobile structure without direct articulations, hyoid bone fractures are uncommon.[40] Isolated hyoid fractures occur but they most commonly occur in conjunction with mandible, thyroid cartilage, and cricoid cartilage fractures.[31,40] Hyoid fractures may also result in pharyngeal injuries caused by perforation by fracture fragments.[31] Hyoid fractures are frequently better appreciated with CT-3D reconstructed images[12] (**Fig. 17**).

Treatment is usually nonoperative,[31,40] with surgery reserved for patients with associated airway

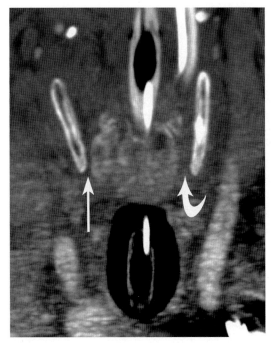

Fig. 15. A 49-year-old man with cricoarytenoid separation after being placed in a "scissors" chokehold. CTA coronal slab MIP shows widening of injured left cricoarytenoid joint (*curved arrow*) in relation to the normal joint (*straight arrow*).

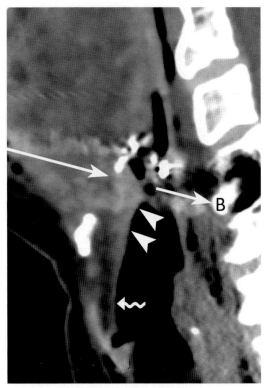

Fig. 16. Zone II GSW tract (*white arrows*) through pharynx with bullet embedded in C4 vertebral body (B). Injured distal epiglottis (*arrowheads*) is thickened and ill-defined in relation to normal proximal epiglottis (*wavy arrow*).

compromise, pharyngeal perforation that also requires surgery, or symptoms refractory to nonoperative management.[40]

Muscles The intrinsic muscles of the larynx are not clearly seen with CT and are easily masked by hemorrhage.[12] Extrinsic muscle (ie, suprahyoid and infrahyoid) and ligament (ie, thyrohyoid and stylohyoid) injuries are generally inferred by indirect signs of injury that include:

- Hematoma localized to given structure[12]
- Anterior tilting of the hyoid bone or hyoid bone anterior to thyroid cartilage, suggesting uninhibited action of the infrahyoid muscles caused by suprahyoid muscle disruption[12]
- Elevation of hyoid bone superior to level of C3 superior endplate, typically associated with complete laryngotracheal separation (**Fig. 18**), indicating uninhibited action of the suprahyoid muscles related to infrahyoid muscle disruption[12,38]

Laryngotracheal Junction and Tracheal Injuries

Injuries to the laryngotracheal junction or cervical trachea may result in either partial (see **Figs. 4** and **10**) or circumferential (see **Fig. 18**) mural disruption. Circumferential disruption

allows retraction of the elastic trachea into the lower neck or mediastinum[12] and is important to preoperatively differentiate from partial disruption.

Laryngotracheal separation

Laryngotracheal separation is a rare injury, usually caused by blunt trauma, that is usually fatal prior to the patient arrival at the hospital.[12,38] Injuries may be either partial or complete. Despite the dramatic nature of the injury, diagnosis is delayed in 40%.[12]

Blunt injuries are frequently caused by a clothesline mechanism,[12] and they usually occur at the cricotracheal junction,[12] cricothyroid membrane and cricothyroid joints,[43] or first tracheal ring.[12]

Because laryngotracheal separations are rare, the exact incidence of associated injuries is unknown, but they infrequently occur in isolation.[46] Typical associated injuries include:

- Complex cricoid cartilage fractures[12]
- Cervical esophageal injuries[43,46]
- Carotid artery injuries[46]

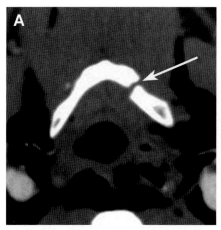
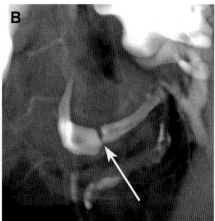

Fig. 17. CTA axial (*A*) and 3D volume-rendered (*B*) images show hyoid bone fracture (*arrows*) in 35-year-old after MCC.

Several imaging findings are associated with laryngotracheal separation and tracheal rupture:

- Direct visualization of the free edges of the defect[35] (see **Figs. 4** and **18**)

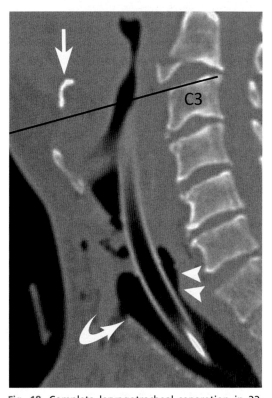

Fig. 18. Complete laryngotracheal separation in 22-year-old male motorcyclist caused by clothesline injury. Sagittal CTA image shows hyoid bone (*straight arrow*) cephalad to C3 superior endplate, endotracheal tube bulging beyond tracheal wall (*arrowheads*), and free edge of tracheal wall (*curved arrow*). Pharyngoesophageal junction was also found to be transected at surgery.

- Endotracheal tube retention cuff bulging through mural defect[12,35,46] (see **Fig. 18**)
- Endotracheal tube in false tract[38,46]
- Elevation of the hyoid bone superior to the C3 vertebral body superior endplate[38] (see **Fig. 18**), indicating complete laryngotracheal rupture or tracheal transection

Vocal Cord Paralysis or Paresis

In addition to intrinsic anatomic injury (eg, mucosal tear), both blunt and penetrating trauma may cause vocal cord dysfunction. Some cases of vocal cord dysfunction may be related to cricoarytenoid joint injury, but neurologic dysfunction characterized as either paralysis (ie, complete) or paresis (ie, partial) may occur.[32]

Vocal cord function relies on the integrity of the vagus nerves (CN X)[32] and their branches that serve the larynx, primarily through the recurrent laryngeal nerves, although the external branches of the superior laryngeal nerves account for motor function of the cricothyroid muscles. Consequently, vocal cord paralysis/paresis may result from an injury anywhere along the vagus nerve or its relevant branches.[32] Nerve injuries resulting in vocal cord dysfunction most frequently involve the recurrent laryngeal nerve in association with tracheal or laryngeal injury,[32] although proximal vagus nerve injury at the jugular foramen caused by skull base fracture or whiplash injury[47] does rarely occur.

Imaging findings

Several CT findings associated with vocal cord paralysis have been reported[32] (**Fig. 19**):

- Dilated ipsilateral piriform sinus
- Thickened medial aryepiglottic fold
- Dilated ipsilateral laryngeal ventricle

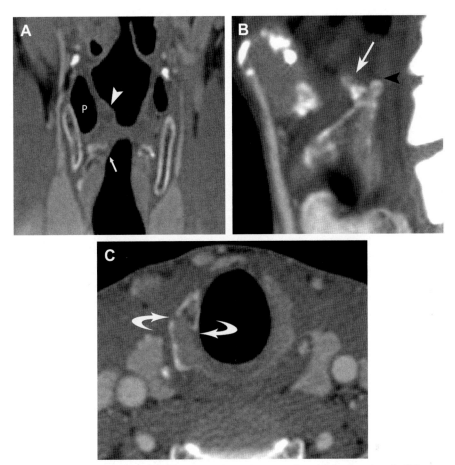

Fig. 19. A 41-year-old man with pain and dysphagia 2 days after assault to his face and neck. CTA coronal (*A*) and sagittal (*B*) MPRs show asymmetric right aryepiglottic fold thickening (*white arrowhead*), asymmetrically enlarged right piriform sinus, and slight medial rotation and anterior displacement of the right arytenoid cartilage (*straight arrows*) relative to the cricoid (*black arrowhead*). Axial image (*C*) shows subtle right-sided cricoid fracture (*curved arrows*) through small area of partial ossification. Endoscopy confirmed vocal cord paralysis, as well as loss of normal gag reflex.

- Anteromedial arytenoid rotation
- Ipsilateral true vocal cord fullness
- Dilated ipsilateral vallecula

Although findings of vocal cord paralysis can be identified in the setting of acute trauma, in the author's experience, the imaging diagnosis may be difficult because of hemorrhage, soft tissue swelling, and distortion of the normal laryngeal architecture. This difficulty reinforces the vital role played by endoscopy in fully characterizing laryngotracheal injuries,[12,32] including differentiating vocal cord paralysis/paresis from cricoarytenoid injury.

Laryngotracheal injury classification
The Schaefer-Fuhrman classification system is typically used to comprehensively grade or characterize laryngotracheal injuries (**Table 3**).[7,12,22]

Clinical examination, CT findings, and endoscopic findings are used to fully characterize an injury and assign it to the appropriate Schaefer-Fuhrman injury group.[7,12,37] Increasing group designation correlates with increasing severity of injury.[37]

Management
In many instances, treatment of laryngotracheal injuries may be nonoperative:

- Hyoid fractures[7]
- Laryngeal injury groups I or II[7,11,37]
- Tracheal injuries with small defect that has well-apposed, regular edges[7,20]

When diagnosed and treated early, Butler and colleagues[37] reported that patients with group I or II laryngeal injuries who were treated nonoperatively experienced long-term preservation of

Table 3	
Schaefer-Fuhrman laryngeal injury classification	
Group	**Injury Description**
0	Normal larynx
1	Minor endolaryngeal hematomas or lacerations without detectable fractures. No airway compromise
2	Moderately severe edema, hematomas, or lacerations without exposed cartilage or nondisplaced fractures. Partial airway compromise with varying degrees of severity
3	Massive laryngeal edema, large mucosal lacerations, exposed cartilage, displaced fractures, or vocal cord immobility. Airway compromised
4	Same as group 3 but with more severe anterior laryngeal disruption, unstable fractures, 2 or more fracture lines, or severe mucosal injuries
5	Complete laryngotracheal separation

Data from Refs.[7,12,22]

functional voice in 95% to 97%, normal deglutition in 99%, and normal airway function in 100%.

Surgery is generally reserved for group III to V laryngotracheal injuries.[11]

Pharyngoesophageal Injuries

Anatomic considerations
The location of the injury influences how it is treated. Specifically, because infra-arytenoid hypopharyngeal injuries are treated similar to esophageal injuries,[8,9] usually with surgery, every effort should be made to localize the site of the injury. Similarly, the size of the defect may determine whether the injury is treated surgically or nonoperatively,[9,18,20] so attempts should be made to determine the size of full-thickness defects.

Management
Many injuries, mostly pharyngeal, can be successfully treated nonoperatively by maintaining the patient nil per oral, using parenteral nutrition and IV antibiotics,[20] while closely monitoring the patient for signs of infection.

Injuries in which nonoperative treatment is typically successful include (see **Fig. 8**):

- Supra-arytenoid pharyngeal injuries[9]
- Small mural defects (<1.5–2 cm)[9,18,20]

Indications for surgical intervention include:

- Infra-arytenoid pharyngeal and esophageal transmural injuries[8,9]
- Large supra-arytenoid pharyngeal defect (>1.5–2 cm)[9,18,20]
- Supra-arytenoid laryngeal injury with extensive devascularized, necrotic tissue[9]

Successful nonoperative treatment of patients with esophageal injuries has been reported.[19] However, 22% to 39% of patients with infra-arytenoid pharyngeal or esophageal full-thickness mural injuries that are not surgically repaired develop deep soft tissue infections, which can spread to the mediastinum, causing mediastinitis and/or fistulas,[8] so surgical repair is the preferred option.

Regardless of whether treated nonoperatively or surgically, diagnosis of injury and initiation of treatment within 24 hours of injury improves patient outcomes.[8,48] In patients who require surgical repair, it has been reported that the time that treatment is initiated has a greater impact on outcome than the time of definitive surgical repair.[48] Therefore, regardless of treatment choice, it is incumbent on the radiologist to facilitate rapid diagnosis of pharyngoesophageal injury in order to promote good patient outcomes.

THYROID GLAND INJURIES
Diagnostic Work-up

In the nontrauma setting, ultrasonography is the preferred modality for imaging the thyroid gland. Although it is portable and can be performed in the trauma bay to assess the acutely injured patient while the patient is still undergoing initial assessment and resuscitation,[24] its use may be limited by a limited acoustic windows[25] caused by a cervical collar, hematoma, or soft tissue gas.

In the setting of acute neck trauma, IV-enhanced CT is the preferred diagnostic modality for imaging the thyroid gland, because it is unhindered by limited acoustic windows,[25] and it can be used to simultaneously assess for other, frequently associated injuries, such as laryngeal and carotid artery injuries.[24,25]

Ultrasonography and CT show comparable abnormalities[25,26,49]:

- Gland hematomas and contusions (**Figs. 20 and 21**)
- Lacerations (see **Fig. 21**)
- Paraglandular hematoma

CT scan may also show active bleeding into either the gland or an adjacent hematoma.[25]

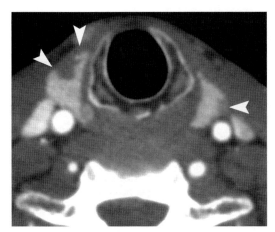

Fig. 20. CT of bilateral thyroid lobe contusions (*arrowheads*) caused by attempted strangulation.

Because of the close proximity of the recurrent laryngeal nerves, laryngoscopy has been recommended to assess for vocal cord dysfunction in patients with thyroid gland injuries.[24]

Injury Classification

A CT-based thyroid gland injury grading system was proposed by Heizmann and colleagues[25] (**Table 4**). Sonography could be used to obtain much of the information needed to grade injuries with this scheme, but it would be unable to identify laryngeal injuries.

Management

Heizmann and colleagues[25] recommended that thyroid gland injuries be managed as follows:

- Injury grades I/II and hemodynamically stable patient: observation and follow-up imaging
- Injury grades I/II, hemodynamically stable patient, and underlying disorder (eg, nodule): observation followed by elective surgery to address the underlying disorder
- Injury grades III/IV or any hemodynamically unstable patient: endotracheal intubation and emergency surgery

Recognizing that a patient may be hemodynamically stable but still show signs of airway compromise, Lemke and colleagues[26] advocated that any patient with progressive dyspnea or hoarseness should also undergo endotracheal intubation and immediate surgery.

Thyroid storm

Thyroid storm is a rare, extreme form of thyrotoxicosis, most frequently seen in patients with Graves disease, which is associated with mortality

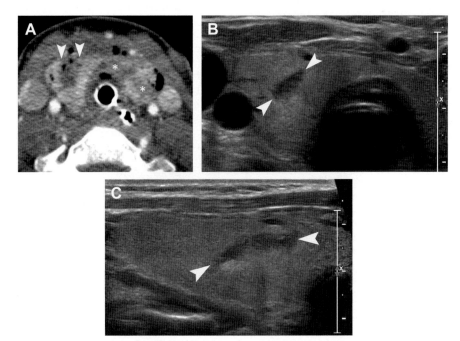

Fig. 21. (*A–C*) Blunt traumatic thyroid gland laceration in 34-year-old woman who jumped from a moving motor vehicle. Admission CT (*A*) shows right thyroid lobe laceration (*arrowheads*) containing air bubbles from an airway injury (not shown), as well as isthmus and left lobe ill-defined contusions (*asterisks*). Transverse (*B*) and longitudinal (*C*) gray-scale ultrasonography images obtained the next day show the linear, hypoechoic laceration (*arrowheads*).

Table 4
Computed tomography–based thyroid gland injury classification

Grade	Injury Description
I	Small lacerations, bleeding into nodule, subcapsular hematoma
II	Gland rupture either without or with paraglandular hematoma
III	Gland rupture with significant[a] neck hematoma and tracheal compression
IV	Gland rupture and neck hematoma associated with laryngeal, CCA/ICA injury, and/or internal jugular vein injury

Abbreviations: CCA, common carotid artery; ICA, internal carotid artery.
   [a] Significant is otherwise undefined.
   Data from Heizmann O, Schmid R, Oertli D. Blunt injury to the thyroid gland: proposed classification and treatment algorithm. J Trauma 2006;61(4):1012–5.

of 10% to 20%.[50] It manifests several clinical signs and symptoms (**Table 5**) that generally affect the cardiovascular, central nervous, and gastrointestinal systems.[50,51]

Typically, thyroid storm is initiated by a severe systemic insult (eg, sepsis, polytrauma, diabetic ketoacidosis) in either known[50] or unknown untreated[51] hyperthyroidism. However, it may also

Table 5
Clinical manifestations of thyroid storm

Systemic Dysfunction	Clinical Manifestations
Thermoregulatory	Fever
Cardiovascular	Tachycardia Atrial fibrillation Heart failure
CNS	Agitation Delirium Tremors Seizure Coma
GI	Nausea Vomiting Diarrhea Abdominal pain

Abbreviations: CNS, central nervous system; GI, gastrointestinal.
   Data from Carroll R, Matfin G. Endocrine and metabolic emergencies: thyroid storm. Ther Adv Endocrinol Metab 2010;1(3):139–45; and Delikoukos S, Mantzos F. Thyroid storm induced by blunt thyroid gland trauma. Am Surg 2007;73(12):1247–9.

result as a direct consequence of either direct blunt[51] or penetrating[52] trauma to a previously normal thyroid gland. Delikoukos and colleagues[51] hypothesized that thyroid storm related to direct glandular trauma occurs as a consequence of acinar rupture that results in the sudden release of thyroid hormones into the bloodstream.

The diagnosis of thyroid storm is clinical, but results for the necessary laboratory tests are usually unavailable in the acute setting,[51] and several of the manifestations (eg, abdominal pain, tachycardia, unconsciousness) are commonly encountered in acutely injured patients. Consequently, it is important for radiologists to correctly identify otherwise minor-appearing thyroid gland injuries, which may prompt clinicians to consider the diagnosis of trauma-induced thyroid storm in the appropriate context.

Shock thyroid

Shock thyroid is a CT manifestation of the hypoperfusion complex that is diagnosed when there is either clinically documented shock or diagnostic imaging that shows other signs of the hypoperfusion complex.[53] Shock thyroid may be seen in patients with both traumatic and nontraumatic causes of shock.[54] Because the thyroid region is not always included in scans performed to assess for the source of shock (eg, abdomen-pelvis CT for abdominal sepsis), it may be an underdiagnosed phenomenon.[54]

CT findings of shock thyroid are[53,54] (**Fig. 22**):

- Homogeneously low-density (4–10 Hounsfield units) paraglandular fluid that is usually more confluent anteriorly and may extend into the superior mediastinum
- Gland enlargement
- Heterogeneous thyroid enhancement

Importantly, there should be no focal thyroid lesion to suggest direct injury or preexisting abnormality.[53,54] CT scans of other regions may show additional signs of the hypoperfusion complex (see **Fig. 22**), including shock bowel, enlarged pancreas with peripancreatic edema, periportal edema, and/or decreased diameter of the inferior vena cava.

Three different pathophysiologic bases for shock thyroid have been proposed[53]:

- Third spacing of fluid secondary to IV fluid resuscitation
- Hypoperfusion of the gland that leads to cellular edema or death, resulting in fluid exudates
- Acute thyrotoxic response to hypovolemia

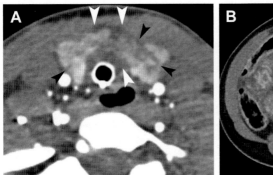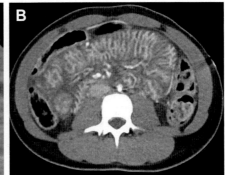

Fig. 22. Shock thyroid in 14-year-old boy who presented with severe hypotension following an MVC. Axial CT of neck (*A*) shows heterogeneous thyroid gland (*black arrowheads*) without focal abnormality and low-attenuation periglandular fluid (*white arrowheads*). Axial CT image of abdomen (*B*) shows hyperemic small bowel mucosa characteristic of shock bowel.

Regardless of the mechanism, euvolemia and return to normotension result in rapid return of normal appearance to the thyroid gland and adjacent tissue on follow-up imaging.[53,54] Consequently, it is important for radiologists to recognize and report shock thyroid as a manifestation of the hypoperfusion complex, rather than an injury or other abnormality warranting direct intervention.

SUMMARY

Neck visceral space trauma may result in several uncommon, but clinically important, injuries. Early diagnosis and treatment can improve outcomes but acute injuries are frequently missed by both clinicians and radiologists. To facilitate the best patient outcomes, it is incumbent on radiologists to understand the role of imaging in the work-up of both blunt and penetrating neck soft tissue trauma, recognize both the direct and indirect signs of injuries, and maintain a high index of suspicion in clinical settings in which neck visceral injuries are most likely to be to present.

REFERENCES

1. Soliman AM, Ahmad SM, Roy D. The role of aerodigestive tract endoscopy in penetrating neck trauma. Laryngoscope 2014;124(Suppl 7):S1–9.
2. Berkovitz B. Neck. In: Stranding S, editor. Gray's anatomy: the anatomical basis of clinical practice, 39th edition. Philadelphia: Elsevier Churchill Livingstone; 2005. p. 531, 560–1.
3. Stark DD, Moss AA, Gamsu G, et al. Magnetic resonance imaging of the neck. Part I: normal anatomy. Radiology 1984;150(2):447–54.
4. Berkovitz B. Surface anatomy of head and neck. In: Stranding S, editor. Gray's anatomy: the anatomical basis of clinical practice, 39th edition. Philadelphia: Elsevier Churchill Livingstone; 2005. p. 443.
5. Steenburg SD, Sliker CW, Shanmuganathan K, et al. Imaging evaluation of penetrating neck injuries. Radiographics 2010;30(4):869–86.
6. Khan S, Sliker C, Stein D, et al. Blunt external laryngeal injuries: factors that influence accurate prospective diagnosis with computed tomography. Radiological Society of North America 2016 Scientific Assembly and Annual Meeting. Chicago (IL), November 27–December 2, 2016. Available at: archive.rsna.org/2016/16014635.html. Accessed October 10, 2018.
7. Moonsamy P, Sachdeva UM, Morse CR. Management of laryngotracheal trauma. Ann Cardiothorac Surg 2018;7(2):210–6.
8. Demetriades D, Velmahos GG, Asensio JA. Cervical pharyngoesophageal and laryngotracheal injuries. World J Surg 2001;25(8):1044–8.
9. Bodanapally UK, Shanmuganathan K, Dreizin D, et al. Penetrating aerodigestive injuries in the neck: a proposed CT-aided modified selective management algorithm. Eur Radiol 2016;26(7):2409–17.
10. Nowicki JL, Stew B, Ooi E. Penetrating neck injuries: a guide to evaluation and management. Ann R Coll Surg Engl 2018;100(1):6–11.
11. Jalisi S, Zoccoli M. Management of laryngeal fractures–a 10-year experience. J Voice 2011;25(4):473–9.
12. Becker M, Leuchter I, Platon A, et al. Imaging of laryngeal trauma. Eur J Radiol 2014;83(1):142–54.
13. Misiak P, Jabłoński S, Terlecki A. Cervical esophageal rupture after blunt trauma resulting from a car accident. Kardiochir Torakochirurgia Pol 2016;13(3):262–4.
14. Niezgoda JA, McMenamin P, Graeber GM. Pharyngoesophageal perforation after blunt neck trauma. Ann Thorac Surg 1990;50(4):615–7.

15. Català J, Puig J, Muñoz JM, et al. Perforation of the pharynx caused by blunt external neck trauma. Eur Radiol 1998;8(1):137–40.

16. Hagr A, Kamal D, Tabah R. Pharyngeal perforation caused by blunt trauma to the neck. Can J Surg 2003;46(1):57–8.

17. Cross KJ, Koomalsingh KJ, Fahey TJ 3rd, et al. Hypopharyngeal rupture secondary to blunt trauma: presentation, evaluation, and management. J Trauma 2007;62(1):243–6.

18. Salemis NS, Georgiou C, Alogdianakis E, et al. Hypopharyngeal perforation because of blunt neck trauma. Emerg Radiol 2009;16(1):71–4.

19. Epstein MG, Costa SV, Carvalho FG, et al. Conservative treatment in isolated penetrating cervical esophageal injury: case report. Einstein (Sao Paulo) 2012; 10(4):505–7.

20. Goudy SL, Miller FB, Bumpous JM. Neck crepitance: evaluation and management of suspected upper aerodigestive tract injury. Laryngoscope 2002;112(5):791–5.

21. Nadig SK, Uppal S, Back GW, et al. Foreign body sensation in the throat due to displacement of the superior cornu of the thyroid cartilage: two cases and a literature review. J Laryngol Otol 2006; 120(7):608–9.

22. Robinson S, Juutilainen M, Suomalainen A, et al. Multidetector row computed tomography of the injured larynx after trauma. Semin Ultrasound CT MR 2009;30(3):188–94.

23. Schaefer SD. Management of acute blunt and penetrating external laryngeal trauma. Laryngoscope 2014;124(1):233–44.

24. Hara H, Hirose Y, Yamashita H. Thyroid gland rupture caused by blunt trauma to the neck. BMC Res Notes 2016;9:114.

25. Heizmann O, Schmid R, Oertli D. Blunt injury to the thyroid gland: proposed classification and treatment algorithm. J Trauma 2006;61(4): 1012–5.

26. Lemke J, Schreiber MN, Henne-Bruns D, et al. Thyroid gland hemorrhage after blunt neck trauma: case report and review of the literature. BMC Surg 2017;17(1):115.

27. Shanley CJ, Overbeck MC, Mazzara P, et al. Traumatic rupture of a cervical parathyroid adenoma. Surgery 1994;115(3):394–7.

28. Johnson NA, Tublin ME, Ogilvie JB. Parathyroid imaging: technique and role in the preoperative evaluation of primary hyperparathyroidism. AJR Am J Roentgenol 2007;188(6):1706–15.

29. Fahr ME, Thomas BW, Barker DE. Esophageal injury from cervical spine fracture in blunt trauma. Am Surg 2010;76(8):915–6.

30. Bodanapally UK, Sliker CW. Imaging of blunt and penetrating craniocervical arterial injuries. Semin Roentgenol 2016;51(3):152–64.

31. Chowdhury R, Crocco AG, El-Hakim H. An isolated hyoid fracture secondary to sport injury. A case report and review of literature. Int J Pediatr Otorhinolaryngol 2005;69(3):411–4.

32. Huang BY, Solle M, Weissler MC. Larynx: anatomic imaging for diagnosis and management. Otolaryngol Clin North Am 2012;45(6):1325–61.

33. Becker M, Duboé PO, Platon A, et al. MDCT in the assessment of laryngeal trauma: value of 2D multiplanar and 3D reconstructions. AJR Am J Roentgenol 2013;201(4):W639–47.

34. Conradie WJ, Gebremariam FA. Can computed tomography esophagography reliably diagnose traumatic penetrating upper digestive tract injuries? Clin Imaging 2015;39(6):1039–45.

35. Chen JD, Shanmuganathan K, Mirvis SE, et al. Using CT to diagnose tracheal rupture. AJR Am J Roentgenol 2001;176(5):1273–80.

36. Madsen AS, Oosthuizen G, Laing GL, et al. The role of computed tomography angiography in the detection of aerodigestive tract injury following penetrating neck injury. J Surg Res 2016;205(2):490–8.

37. Butler AP, Wood BP, O'Rourke AK, et al. Acute external laryngeal trauma: experience with 112 patients. Ann Otol Rhinol Laryngol 2005;114(5):361–8.

38. Tobias ME, Sack AD, Carter G, et al. Cricotracheal separation in blunt neck injury–the sign of hyoid bone elevation. A case report. S Afr J Surg 1989; 27(5):189–91.

39. Duda JJ Jr, Lewin JS, Eliachar I. MR evaluation of epiglottic disruption. AJNR Am J Neuroradiol 1996; 17(3):563–6.

40. Levine E, Taub PJ. Hyoid bone fractures. Mt Sinai J Med 2006;73(7):1015–8.

41. Alexander AE Jr, Lyons GD, Fazekas-May MA, et al. Utility of helical computed tomography in the study of arytenoid dislocation and arytenoid subluxation. Ann Otol Rhinol Laryngol 1997;106(12):1020–3.

42. Sataloff RT, Rao VM, Hawkshaw M, et al. Cricothyroid joint injury. J Voice 1998;12(1):112–6.

43. Bernat RA, Zimmerman JM, Keane WM, et al. Combined laryngotracheal separation and esophageal injury following blunt neck trauma. Facial Plast Surg 2005;21(3):187–90.

44. Charoonnate N, Narongchai P, Vongvaivet S. Fractures of the hyoid bone and thyroid cartilage in suicidal hanging. J Med Assoc Thai 2010;93(10):1211–6.

45. Oh JH, Min HS, Park TU, et al. Isolated cricoid fracture associated with blunt neck trauma. Emerg Med J 2007;24(7):505–6.

46. Reynolds JK, Dart BW 4th, Maxwell RA, et al. Tracheal transection with associated bilateral carotid and esophageal injuries after blunt neck trauma. Am Surg 2014;80(8):E232–3.

47. Helliwell M, Robertson JC, Todd GB, et al. Bilateral vocal cord paralysis due to whiplash injury. Br Med J (Clin Res Ed) 1984;288(6434):1876–7.

48. Makhani M, Midani D, Goldberg A, et al. Pathogenesis and outcomes of traumatic injuries of the esophagus. Dis Esophagus 2014;27(7):630–6.

49. Stunell H, O'Brien J, Benfayed W, et al. Thyroid gland rupture after blunt cervical trauma. J Ultrasound Med 2007;26(7):992.

50. Carroll R, Matfin G. Endocrine and metabolic emergencies: thyroid storm. Ther Adv Endocrinol Metab 2010;1(3):139–45.

51. Delikoukos S, Mantzos F. Thyroid storm induced by blunt thyroid gland trauma. Am Surg 2007;73(12):1247–9.

52. Delikoukos S, Mantzos F. Thyroid storm induced by trauma due to spear fishing-gun trident impaction in the neck. Emerg Med J 2007;24(5):355–6.

53. Brochert A, Rafoth JB. Shock thyroid: a new manifestation of the hypovolemic shock complex in trauma patients. J Comput Assist Tomogr 2006;30(2):310–2.

54. Han DH, Ha EJ, Sun JS, et al. Remarkable CT features of shock thyroid in traumatic and nontraumatic patients. Emerg Radiol 2017;24(3):319–24.

Imaging of Spine Trauma

Mark P. Bernstein, MD*, Matthew G. Young, DO, Alexander B. Baxter, MD

KEYWORDS

• Spinal injury • Spine fracture • Blunt trauma • CT

KEY POINTS

- The risk for cervical spine injury increases 6-fold in severely injured patients meeting trauma activation criteria. Liberal MDCT screening in these patients is advised.
- Clearing the cervical spine in the obtunded patient can be performed with a high quality negative CT alone according to 2 trauma associations.
- The AOSpine Classification provides a simple, comprehensive, and internationally recognized approach to understand and diagnose thoracolumbar spine injuries.

PART I: CERVICAL SPINE
Introduction

Every year in North America, approximately 3 million patients are evaluated for spinal injury, and 3% to 4% of blunt trauma patients presenting to the emergency department (ED) will have a cervical spine injury.[1,2] Failure to identify an unstable cervical spine injury can lead to devastating outcomes.

Both the National Emergency X-ray Utilization Study (NEXUS) and the Canadian C-Spine rule (CCR) criteria provide guidelines for imaging in suspected cervical spine injury. They have been validated in multiple studies,[3–8] and one or the other should be applied routinely in the ED. The authors use the NEXUS criteria, which they refer to as the 5 No's of NEXUS (Box 1) for its simplicity and because its application does not rely on mechanism of injury, a feature of the CCR that is often not readily available.

A note of caution: the risk for cervical spine injury increases more than 6-fold, and the sensitivity of NEXUS decreases substantially in severely injured patients meeting CDC trauma team activation criteria.[9,10] Liberal screening with multidetector computed tomography (MDCT) in these patients is advised.[10]

Clearing the Cervical Spine

In the alert asymptomatic patient who meets the NEXUS or CCR criteria, the cervical collar can be safely removed without imaging.[11,12] For all others, the standard of care imaging is MDCT.

The obtunded patient who is not examinable poses a difficult clinical situation. The Eastern Association for the Surgery of Trauma conditionally recommends cervical collar removal after a "negative high-quality C-spine CT scan result alone."[13] Although MR imaging had been advocated for these patients in the past, new literature has concluded MR imaging "had a lower health benefit and a higher cost compared with no follow-up after a normal CT finding in patients with obtunded blunt trauma to the cervical spine, a finding that does not support the use of MR imaging in this group of patients."[14]

The Western Trauma Association recently conducted a multi-institutional study with more than 10,000 patients to conclude "if the CT is adequate and negative, the collar may be removed with a low risk of clinically significant injury."[15] In this large study, there were 3 false-negative CTs (0.03%) that missed a clinically significant injury, but all had clinical examinations consistent with central cord syndrome. They state that MR imaging remains valuable only for "the patient who arrives with motor or sensory neurologic deficits or without witnessed movement of all extremities." At Bellevue Hospital in New York City, policy now exists to clear the obtunded patient with a negative cervical spine CT alone.

NYU Langone Health/Bellevue Hospital, 660 First Avenue, 3rd floor, New York, NY 10016, USA
* Corresponding author.
E-mail address: mark.bernstein@nyumc.org

Radiol Clin N Am 57 (2019) 767–785
https://doi.org/10.1016/j.rcl.2019.02.007
0033-8389/19/© 2019 Elsevier Inc. All rights reserved.

Classification

The cervical spine has long resisted a simple widely accepted classification system because of its unique and varied morphology from the C1 ring (atlas), to C2 with its dens (axis), to its articulation with the skull base. Consequently, many attempts at classification have instead focused on the "sub-axial" cervical spine from C3 through C7 vertebrae that share a more consistent morphology. What sets the subaxial cervical spine apart from the thor-acolumbar (TL) spine are its facet joints. Unlike the coronally oriented facets in the thoracic spine and the sagittally oriented facets in the lumbar spine, those in the subaxial cervical spine are oblique (in the coronal plane) and mobile. Consequently, the cervical facets play a much more critical role in injury morphology and stability. Moreover, many attempted classifications have suffered from poor interobserver agreement, largely in difficulty to classify facet involvement, and ability to compre-hensively dictate management. Thus, this article continues to describe these cervical spine injuries based on classic patterns of injury: flexion, exten-sion, and distraction.

Imaging

MDCT imaging of the cervical spine is performed with the cervical collar in place, and with the head lying directly on the CT table without a head holder or pillow to avoid flexion and to main-tain neutral positioning (**Fig. 1**A).

Image acquisition with thin-section algorithm produces high-quality multiplanar reformations (MPRs) to help identify the exact location and displacement of fractures and define the extent of any potential spinal canal, neuroforaminal, or vascular compromise. The authors recommend MPRs in all 3 planes no thicker than 2 mm, with ac-cess to source images as necessary.

An accurate clinical history that specifies any neurologic deficit and location of pain is essential for accurately interpreting subtle findings, particu-larly in the presence of degenerative disc disease.

In the setting of acute neurologic deficit, MR im-aging can provide useful information by identifying epidural hematoma, traumatic disc herniation, or spinal cord injury. However, the immediate clinical question in acute spine trauma is always, "Does the patient require surgical decompression?," and evaluation of canal and neuroforaminal patency is adequately accomplished by CT alone.

To avoid search pattern error, it is helpful to have a checklist in mind that will ensure that all impor-tant structures are examined:

Transaxial images

Assess the integrity and rotational alignment of each vertebra, the cervical soft tissues, and spinal canal diameter. There should be an intact osseous ring at each level surrounding the spinal cord, and normal facet articulations no wider than 2 mm (**Fig. 1**B, C).

Midline sagittal images

Evaluate the anterior spinal line, posterior spinal line, and spinolaminar line. Each should be smooth and continuous. The interspinous distances should be uniform. The basion-dens interval (BDI) should be less than 9.5 mm, and the atlantodental interval should be less than 3 mm in adults. Prever-tebral fat stripe should lie just anterior to the verte-bral bodies in the midline (**Fig. 1**D).

Parasagittal images

The bilateral atlanto-occipital articulations (referred to as the atlanto-occipital intervals [AOIs]) should be congruent and no wider than 1.4 mm. All facets should be fully covered, parallel, and no wider than 2 mm (**Fig. 1**E).

Coronal images

The occipital condyles (OC), C1 and C2, should be aligned and intact (**Fig. 1**F). The combined dis-tance between dens and the lateral masses of C1 should total less than 7 mm.

Keep in mind that at imaging, any osseous displacement or malalignment that existed at the moment of impact may be reduced by recoil and mus-cle spasm and subsequently immobilized with a hard collar potentially masking signs of instability. Close attention to subtle malalignment between vertebral bodies or facet joints can reveal the abnormality.

A visual familiarity with the range of cervical spine fractures and injuries is invaluable. This re-view describes several characteristic cervical spine injuries, their mechanisms, variants, imaging hallmarks, and pitfalls.

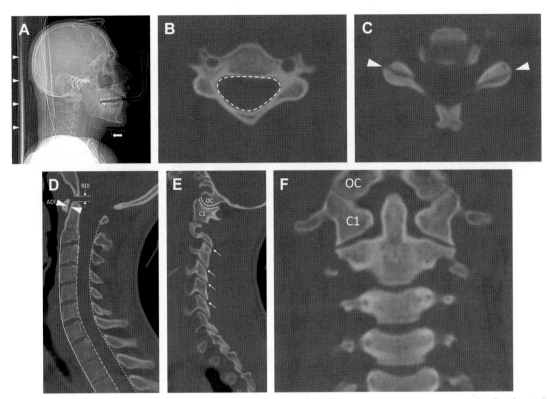

Fig. 1. Normal cervical spine imaging. (A) CT acquisition is performed with the patient in a cervical collar (arrow) with the head flat on the CT table (arrowheads) in neutral position. (B) Transaxial CT image through the vertebral ring with intact bone surrounding the spinal canal (dashed ring). (C) Transaxial CT image through the level of the facets with normal uniform appearance (arrowheads). (D) Midsagittal CT image outlining the anterior vertebral body line (solid line), posterior vertebral body line (larger dashed line), and spinolaminar line (smaller dashed line). The normal BDI measures <9.5 mm, and the normal atlantodental interval is <3 mm in adults (arrowheads). (E) Parasagittal reformation demonstrates the normal AOI between the OC and the lateral mass of C1. The AOI is congruent and less than 1.4 mm wide. Arrows point to parallel normal facet joints. (F) Coronal reformation through the upper cervical spine shows the normal relationship between the OC and the lateral masses of C1.

Atlanto-Occipital Dissociation

Relevant mechanism, anatomy, cause

Atlanto-occipital dissociation (AOD) includes atlanto-occipital dislocation, distraction, and subluxation. Although atlanto-occipital dislocation is often lethal and associated with striking imaging findings, AOD and subluxation may be survivable, and imaging signs can be subtle and easily overlooked. These craniocervical junction injuries are severe and unstable and typically result from high-energy trauma. Distraction, often combined with flexion or extension, causes craniocervical ligament disruption. AOD is invariably accompanied by severe neurologic deficits, typically with concomitant multisystem injuries.

Imaging findings

On MDCT, the normal BDI should be less than 9.5 mm (Fig. 2A). In AOD injuries, the BDI is increased and may be associated with avulsion fractures of the basion, tip of the dens, or OC. On parasagittal reformations, the AOIs are wider than 1.4 mm or subluxed (Fig. 2B). Subarachnoid

hemorrhage at the foramen magnum is common (Fig. 2C).

MR imaging typically reveals prevertebral soft tissue edema, ligamentous disruption, spinal cord injury, and epidural hematoma.

CT angiography, MR angiography, or conventional angiography should be performed to evaluate for cervical vascular dissection or occlusion.

Atlas Injuries: Jefferson Fracture and Unstable Variants

Relevant mechanism, anatomy, cause

The first cervical vertebra (C1, atlas) is a simple bony ring that articulates with the OC and supports the cranium. Its unique shape allows for great range of motion. The transverse ligament holds the dens in place immediately behind the anterior arch of C1; its integrity is the key determinant of atlanto-axial stability.

Jefferson fractures result from an axial load in which force is transmitted through the OC to the

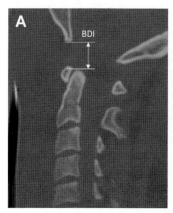
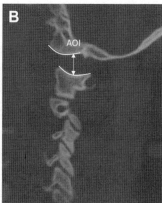
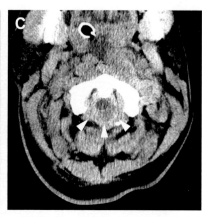

Fig. 2. Atlanto-occipital distraction. (*A*) Midsagittal CT reformation shows an increased BDI. (*B*) Parasagittal CT image shows severe widening and lack of congruence of the AOI. (*C*) Transaxial CT image through the craniocervical junction demonstrates extensive hemorrhage within the spinal canal surrounding the spinal cord (*arrowheads*).

lateral masses of C1 that disrupt the ring-shaped vertebra in one of several common patterns.

Imaging findings

The classic Jefferson fracture is a 4-part C1 burst fracture, with 2 anterior and 2 posterior arch fractures (**Fig. 3**A). This injury is a decompressive injury with radial displacement of the fracture fragments and widening of the spinal canal. As an isolated injury, the classic Jefferson burst is both mechanically and neurologically stable.

Atypical Jefferson fractures are unstable fractures produced by asymmetric axial loading and result in 2 or 3 fractures of the C1 ring (**Fig. 3**B). The transverse ligament is invariably disrupted, permitting C1-2 subluxation and widening of the atlanto-dental interval.

Combined lateral displacement of fracture fragments on either side of the dens ≥7 mm is diagnostic of transverse ligament injury and instability. This measurement, known as the rule of Spence, can be made on transaxial or coronal

MPRs but is only applicable in the presence of a fracture. Another sign of instability is avulsion of the C1 tubercle; this is the insertion site of the transverse ligament. MR imaging evaluates the transverse ligament directly and is highly sensitive for the diagnosis of transverse ligament rupture.

Subaxial Cervical Spine (C3-C7)

Hyperflexion injuries

Relevant mechanism, anatomy, cause Subaxial hyperflexion injuries represent a spectrum from hyperflexion sprain, to anterior subluxation, to bilateral interfacetal dislocation to the flexion teardrop fracture (**Fig. 4**). These injury patterns reflect increasingly severe ligamentous disruptions from the posterior-most supraspinous ligament, progressing anteriorly to the interspinous ligaments, facet capsular ligaments, and ligamentum flavum. This group of ligaments is collectively referred to as the posterior ligament complex, or posterior ligamentous complex (PLC).

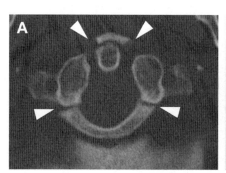
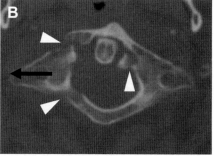

Fig. 3. C1 (atlas) fractures. (*A*) Transaxial CT image of a Jefferson fracture characterized by 2 anterior and 2 posterior arch fractures (*arrowheads*). There is no significant C1-C2 subluxation. (*B*) Jefferson variant fracture with right-sided fractures of the anterior and posterior arches and left tubercle (*arrowheads*). Note the lateral subluxation of the right lateral mass fracture fragment (*arrow*) indicative of instability.

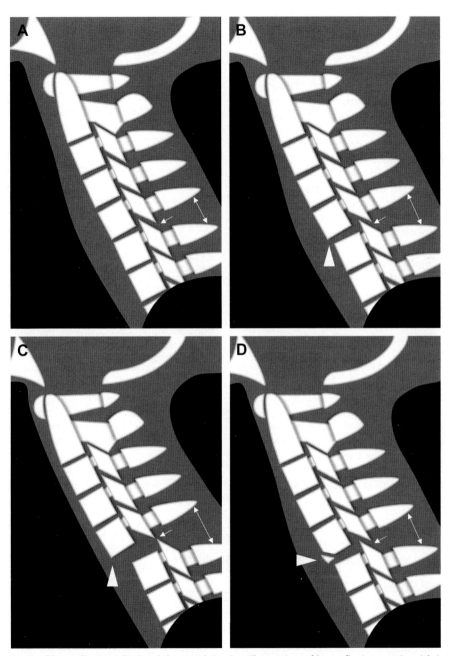

Fig. 4. Spectrum of hyperflexion injuries. (*A*) Lateral C-spine illustration of hyperflexion sprain with interspinous widening (*doubleheaded arrow*) and facet widening (*arrow*). (*B*) Lateral C-spine illustration of anterior subluxation characterized by interspinous widening (*doubleheaded arrow*), facet malalignment (*arrow*), and vertebral subluxation (*arrowhead*). (*C*) Lateral C-spine illustration of bilateral facet dislocation characterized by interspinous widening (*doubleheaded arrow*), facet dislocation (*arrow*), and approximately 50% anterior translation of the upper vertebral segment (*arrowhead*). (*D*) Lateral C-spine illustration of a flexion teardrop fracture. This results from hyperflexion followed by an axial load that breaks off the teardrop fragment (*arrowhead*). The hallmarks of hyperflexion are seen with interspinous widening (*doubleheaded arrow*) and facet widening and malalignment (*arrow*). Patients with flexion teardrop fractures typically present with anterior cord syndrome.

Disruption of the PLC alone does not lead to spinal instability. The mildest of these injuries, the hyperflexion sprain, is limited to PLC injury and is mechanically stable. Anterior subluxation indicates disruption of the posterior longitudinal ligament (PLL) in addition to the PLC and is unstable.

The radiologic evaluation of hyperflexion sprain and anterior subluxation can be challenging, and missed injury can lead to significant morbidity, including pain, kyphosis, delayed vertebral dislocation, and neurologic deficit. Because imaging signs are subtle and their significance as evidence of occult ligamentous instability may not be appreciated, particular care is necessary in evaluating the patient with near normal imaging and persistent pain or any neurologic impairment.

Imaging findings Imaging features of progressively severe hyperflexion injuries are outlined in Table 1.

Pitfalls Cervical straightening or reversal of the normal lordosis may occur from muscle spasm and should be distinguished from true anterior subluxation. Close attention to facet alignment on sagittal CT and posterior disc spacing is most helpful in this regard (Fig. 5).

Degenerative changes may be confused with traumatic subluxation. Degenerated facet joints are most commonly narrowed, with thinning of the bony facet from long-term wear. In contrast, facet joints in cases of traumatic subluxation are abnormally widened.

If CT findings are equivocal, MR imaging can detect edema of the cervical ligaments and soft tissues.

Hyperextension injuries

Relevant mechanism, anatomy, cause Hyperextension injuries include the hyperextension teardrop fracture and the highly unstable hyperextension-dislocation. They are ligamentous and osseous disruptions that progress from anterior to posterior (in contrast to hyperflexion injuries). The anterior longitudinal ligament (ALL) and anterior annulus fibrosus are disrupted in mild injuries with progressive extension through the posterior disc annulus, PLL, ligamentum flavum, and facet joint capsules in more severe cases. Hyperextension-dislocation commonly results in a central cord syndrome, characterized by weakness in the upper extremities and to a lesser extent in the lower extremities.

Hyperextension injuries account for 25% of cervical spine injuries and result from direct frontal impact or through a whiplash effect. They may be associated with frontal hematomas or facial bone fractures, particularly in the elderly.

Imaging Findings

The hyperextension teardrop fracture typically involves the upper cervical spine (C2 or C3) and is characterized by a teardrop fragment at the anterior-inferior corner of the vertebral body (Fig. 6A). In contrast to the flexion teardrop fracture, the hyperextension teardrop fracture plane is vertical rather than horizontal and reflects osseous avulsion from the ALL. Hyperextension teardrop fractures are mechanically stable.

Table 1
Hallmarks of hyperflexion injuries from posterior to anterior

Hallmarks of Hyperflexion Injuries	
Interspinous widening	Supraspinous + interspinous ligament disruption
Uncovered, widened, perched, or jumped facets	PLC disruption
Widened posterior disc space	PLC + PLL disruption
Focal kyphosis	PLC + PLL disruption
Anterior subluxation	PLC + PLL + ALL disruption
Teardrop fracture	PLC + PLL + ALL disruption + axial load

The severity of the injury increases as the injury progresses anteriorly (down the list).

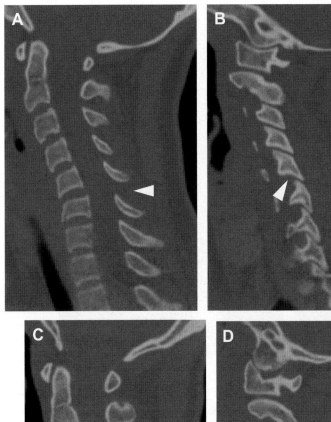

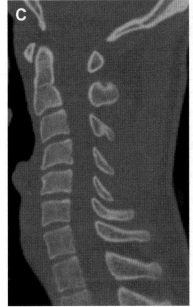

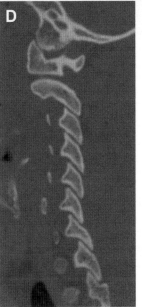

Fig. 5. Hyperflexion sprain compared with muscle spasm. (*A*) Midsagittal CT image of hyperflexion sprain with focal kyphosis at C5-C6 and interspinous widening (*arrowhead*). (*B*) Parasagittal CT image shows uncovering of the C6 facet (*arrowhead*) in hyperflexion sprain. (*C*) Midsagittal CT image in muscle spasm shows reversal the normal cervical lordosis without focal kyphosis. Close attention to the parasagittal CT images (*D*) shows normal facet alignment and is therefore reassuring that this is not an injury.

Although hyperextension-dislocation injuries are severe and unstable, imaging signs are often subtle. As in hyperflexion injuries, severe soft tissue disruption and displacement occur at the moment of trauma but may not be evident on later imaging because recoil, muscular spasm, and cervical collar immobilization in a cervical collar can lead to a near-normal spine examination. Hyperextension injuries usually involve the lower cervical spine. Signs on sagittal CT include subtle anterior intervertebral disc space widening, anterior vertebral avulsion fragments, and facet malalignment (**Fig. 6**B). MR imaging reveals the extent of ligamentous disruption, soft tissue edema, disc herniation, and spinal cord injury.

Fused Spine Hyperextension Injury

Relevant mechanism, anatomy, cause
Ankylosing spondylitis (AS) and diffuse idiopathic skeletal hyperostosis (DISH) are conditions characterized by intervertebral bony bridging and

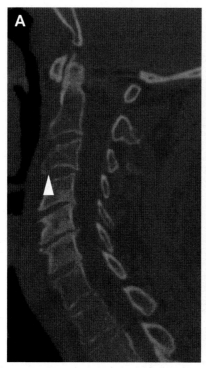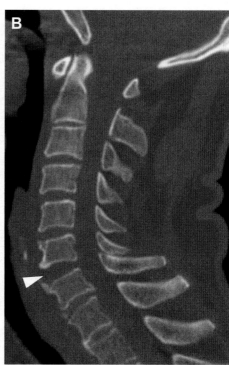

Fig. 6. Hyperextension injuries. (*A*) Midsagittal CT image shows a small hyperextension teardrop fragment (*arrowhead*), a mechanically stable injury. (*B*) Midsagittal CT image shows anterior disc space widening at C6-C7 (*arrowhead*) from a hyperextension fracture-dislocation injury. Although the injury looks subtle and not very dramatic, the ALL, PLL, and ligamentum flavum are all injured. Recoil and muscle spasm reduce the dislocation, which is subsequently immobilized in a cervical collar. Typically, these patients present with a central cord syndrome, and further assessment with MR imaging is indicated.

poor underlying bone quality. The rigid, fused spine in patients with AS and DISH is susceptible to fracture with even mild hyperextension.

Many patients with fused-spine hyperextension fractures have associated spinal cord injury with profound neurologic deficits at presentation. Others may be neurologically asymptomatic, but if a fracture is present and not detected, the possibility of delayed neurologic injury increases significantly. Because up to 25% of patients with a fused-spine fracture will have additional, noncontiguous, fractures, the entire spine should always be imaged when a single fracture is detected.

Imaging findings

A high index of suspicion should be maintained with trauma patients who have rigid spines because unstable hyperextension fractures may be occult. The occult nature of these injuries is due to both frequent spontaneous reduction and underlying osteoporosis, particularly in those with advanced disease.

Because fractures in fused spine patients are often horizontal, findings on axial images may be subtle or undetectable. Sagittal CT reformations best reveal these fractures, which involve the

vertebral body, the fused disc space, or both, and can cross all ossified ligaments from anterior to posterior (**Fig. 7**).

PART II: THORACOLUMBAR SPINE
Introduction

TL spine fractures are found in up to 18% of trauma patients and are often associated with transient or permanent neurologic deficits. Noncontiguous vertebral injuries are present in about 20% of cases. Missed fractures are associated with a higher incidence of neurologic injury.

Many classification systems have been proposed over the past half century, including the 2-column model by Holdsworth (1970),[16] the 3-column model by Denis (1983),[17] the AO/Magerl classification (1994),[18] and the Thoracolumbar Injury Classification and Severity Score (TLICS; 2005).[19] TLICS was designed to incorporate fracture morphology, status of the PLC, neurologic status, and clinical factors relevant for therapeutic decision making and prognosis. One of the major practical limitations of TLICS is the reliance on MR imaging for assessment of PLC integrity, an imaging modality that may not be readily available at all trauma centers.

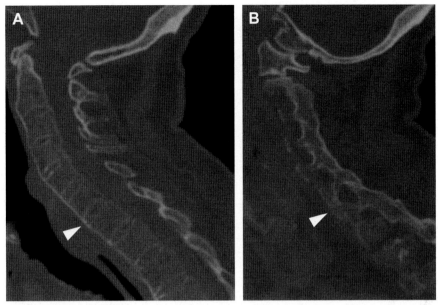

Fig. 7. Fused spine hyperextension fracture. (*A*) Midsagittal CT image in a patient with AS reveals a subtle hairline fracture across the fused disc space at C6-C7 (*arrowhead*). (*B*) Parasagittal CT image shows the hairline fracture extending across the spine (*arrowhead*). A high index of suspicion is necessary in patients with rigid spine disease to identify these fractures.

The AOSpine Thoracolumbar Spine Injury Classification System[20] was introduced in 2013 as a simple, comprehensive, and internationally accepted descriptive approach to TL injuries. In addition, it does not rely on MR imaging for primary classification.

Imaging

MDCT imaging of the TL spine is the primary initial imaging study for TL trauma and should be performed if any of the following are present:

1. Back pain or midline tenderness
2. Local signs of TL injury
3. Abnormal neurologic signs
4. Cervical spine fracture
5. Glasgow Coma Score (GCS) less than 15
6. Major distracting injury
7. Alcohol or drug intoxication[21]

In polytrauma patients, MPRs of the TL spine from the thorax-abdomen-pelvis scans may be used. The authors recommend MPRs in all 3 planes be no thicker than 2 mm, with access to source images as necessary.

MR imaging is useful for evaluating patients after a TL fracture has been found on a screening MDCT. MR imaging is especially useful for evaluating spinal cord injury, spinal cord or cauda equina compression, and ligamentous injury.

Interpretation

To avoid observational error, it is helpful to have a checklist in mind that will ensure that all important structures are evaluated (**Table 2**) Corresponding CT anatomy and alignment are outlined in **Fig. 8**. Conditions to bear in mind include acute fracture, epidural hematoma, paraspinous hematoma, and contributing conditions, such as fused vertebrae, AS, and DISH.

Anatomy

Functional segments

The TL spine consists of 3 functional segments: thoracic spine (T1-10), TL junction (T11-L2), and lumbar spine (L2-L5).

The thoracic functional segment is characterized by a mild kyphotic curvature, coronal orientation of the facet joints, and a narrow spinal canal. Because the first through 10th ribs connect the thoracic spine to the sternum, the thoracic spine is the most rigid portion of the axial skeleton. Flexion and extension of the thoracic spine are limited by the coronal orientation of the facet joints (**Fig. 9**). The dominant motion of the thoracic spine is lateral flexion in the coronal plane.

The TL junction (T11-L2) is a transitional segment that connects the relatively inflexible thoracic spine to the mobile lumbar spine. Vertebral injuries tend to occur in transitional areas where stress is concentrated, that is, craniocervical junction (occiput-C2), cervicothoracic

Table 2			
Computed tomographic checklist for evaluating the thoracolumbar spine			
Midline Sagittal	**Parasagittal**	**Coronal**	**Transaxial**
Anterior vertebral line	Facets	Lateral vertebral lines	Vertebral bodies
Posterior vertebral line	Articular processes	Spinous processes	Pedicles
Spinolaminar line	Pedicles	Transverse processes	Laminae
Interspinous distances	Pars interarticularis		Facets
Vertebral body			Spinous processes
Spinous processes			Spinal canal volume and
Perivertebral soft tissues			diameter
			Prevertebral soft tissues
? Vertebral fracture	? Facet widening	? Interpedicular	? Vertebral fracture
? Vertebral height loss		widening	? Vertebral height loss
? Retropulsed fragment		? Interspinous widening	? Retropulsed fragment
? Epidural hematoma			? Epidural hematoma

junction (C7-T1), and TL junction (T11-L2). In fact, almost 60% of thoracic and lumbar spine fractures occur from T11-L2.[18] Facets in this region are intermediate in orientation (see **Fig. 9**), compared with the coronally oriented thoracic facet joints and the sagittally oriented lumbar facet joints.

The lumbar functional segment (L3-5) is characterized by a lordotic curvature, sagittal orientation of the facet joints (see **Fig. 9**), larger intervertebral discs, and a larger spinal canal. The sagittal orientation of the facet joints allows flexion and extension but limits lateral bending and rotation.

Spinal segment and ligamentous connections

Two adjacent TL vertebrae and their interconnecting ligamentous structures constitute a spinal segment. The vertebrae are connected and stabilized by the ALL, intervertebral disc, PLL, ligamentum flavum, facet capsules, interspinous ligaments, supraspinous ligament, and intertransverse ligaments (**Fig. 10**).

The ALL runs continuously along the anterior spinal column from the skull base to the sacrum. It is a strong ligament, firmly attached to the anterior vertebral bodies, that primarily limits hyperextension. The PLL runs from the skull base to the sacrum and is firmly attached to the posterior margins of the vertebral bodies/endplates and posterior disc annulus. The PLL prevents hyperflexion and reinforces the intervertebral disc.

Posterior ligamentous complex

The PLC plays a key role in stabilizing the TL spine and is composed of the ligamentum flavum, interspinous ligament, articular facet capsules, and supraspinous ligament (see **Fig. 10**). The ligamentum flavum connects adjacent laminae at the posterior aspect of the spinal canal. Because of its high composition of elastin, the ligamentum flavum assists in returning the spine to an upright position after flexion. The interspinous ligament connects the spinous processes from C1-S1. The supraspinous ligament is a strong cordlike ligament that connects the tips of the spinous processes from C7 to the sacrum. These ligaments function to limit hyperflexion. The facet capsules surround the facet joints and help keep the spine in line during motion. Because of the poor healing potential of the PLC, injury of this structure often requires surgical intervention to prevent late deformity.

Tension band concept

The osseous and ligamentous structures that prevent distraction, hyperextension, and hyperflexion of the TL spine are considered tension bands. The anterior tension band limits hyperextension and is formed by the ALL and anterior disc annulus. The posterior tension band limits hyperflexion and is formed by the posterior bony arch and the PLC. When either tension band is disrupted, the other acts as a hinge, preventing gross displacement. If both tension bands are disrupted, there may be gross displacement at the injured segment.

STABILITY

Fracture stability is an important concept that surgeons apply in determining whether surgical or nonoperative treatment is most appropriate. Determination of stability remains controversial, and more than a dozen classification systems have been proposed for evaluating TL injuries. To date, no single globally accepted classification system for spinal instability has been developed.

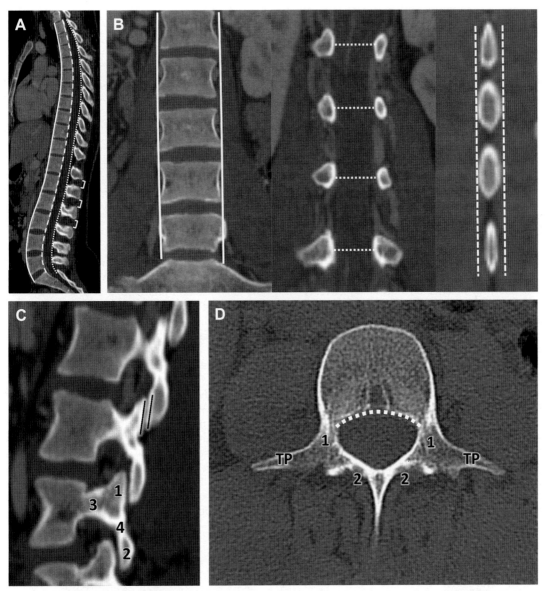

Fig. 8. TL-spine anatomy. (*A*) Midline sagittal images of the TL spine. The anterior vertebral line (*solid line*), posterior vertebral line (*dashed line*), and spinolaminar line (*dotted line*) should be smooth and continuous, without step-offs. The interspinous distances should be uniform (*brackets*). (*B*) Coronal images of the TL spine. The lateral vertebral lines (*solid line*) should be smooth, without step-offs. The interpedicular distances should be uniform (*dotted line*). The spinous processes should be aligned (*dashed lines*). (*C*) Parasagittal images. All facets should be fully covered and parallel (*black lines*). The superior (1) and inferior (2) articular processes of the facets, pedicles (3), and pars interarticularis (4) should be intact. (*D*) Transaxial images. The posterior vertebral body (*dashed line*), laminae (1), and pedicles (2) should form an intact ring at each level. The transverse processes should be intact (TP).

A commonly cited, comprehensive definition of stability was proposed by White and Panjabi[22] in 1980 as "the ability of the spine under physiologic loads to limit patterns of displacement so as not to damage or irritate the spinal cord and nerve roots and, in addition, so as to prevent incapacitating deformity or pain due to structural changes."

AO Spine Thoracolumbar Spine Injury Classification System

Developed in 2013, the AOSpine Thoracolumbar Spine Injury Classification System describes 3 morphologic types of injuries to the TL spine, compression injuries (type A), tension band injuries

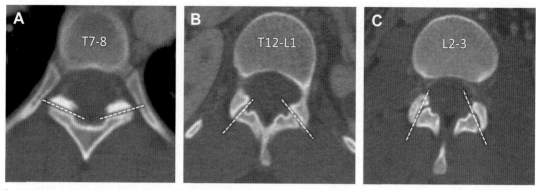

Fig. 9. Representative orientations of the facet joints on transaxial CT (*dashed lines*). (*A*) Coronal orientation of the thoracic facet joints limit flexion and extension. (*B*) Intermediate orientation of the TL junction facet joints. (*C*) Sagittal orientation of the lumbar facet joints limits lateral bending.

(type B), and displacement/translational injuries (type C) (**Table 3**).[20] Each successive injury type and subtype indicate an ascending severity of injury. As a simple yet comprehensive, internationally accepted, pathway to describe these injuries, this part focuses on this classification system to describe TL spine injuries.

In 2016, Kepler and colleagues[23] applied AOSpine criteria to create the Thoracolumbar AOSpine Injury Score (TL AOSIS) (**Table 4**). The score is based on 3 basic parameters: morphologic classification of the fracture, neurologic status, and clinical modifiers. A trial of nonoperative treatment is indicated for patients with a score less than 4. Patients with scores greater than 5 should undergo early surgical intervention. Scores of 4 or 5 should be individualized based on surgeon and patient variables.

Type A (compression) injuries
A0 injuries are isolated nonstructural fractures of the spinous or transverse processes (**Fig. 11**). Although A0 fractures are usually not associated with spinal instability, transverse process avulsions indicated high-energy trauma and may be associated with significant visceral injury.

A1 injuries include wedge compression fractures (**Fig. 12**A, B) and single endplate impaction fractures (**Fig. 12**C). Wedge compression fractures involve the anterior vertebral body wall (anterior column) and a single endplate. A1 fractures always spare the posterior vertebral body wall.

A2 injuries include split or pincer-type fractures that involve both superior and inferior endplates (**Fig. 13**). If the fracture involves the posterior vertebral body wall, it should be considered a burst subtype fracture (A3 or A4).

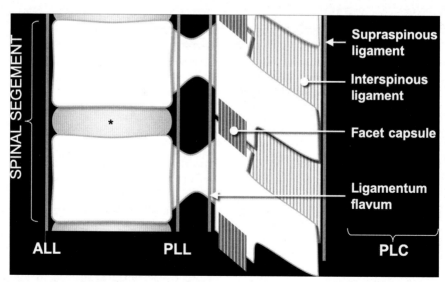

Fig. 10. Spinal segment and ligamentous connections. The vertebrae are connected by an ALL, intervertebral disc (*asterisk*), PLL, and PLC.

Table 3
AOSpine thoracolumbar spine injury classification system and thoracolumbar AOSpine Injury Score

AOSpine Thoracolumbar Spine Injury Classification System	Thoracolumbar AOSpine Injury Score Points
Type A: Compression fractures	
A0: Minimal injuries such as transverse process fractures	0
A1: Wedge compression	1
A2: Pincer compression injury	2
A3: Incomplete burst fracture	3
A4: Complete burst fracture	4
Type B: Tension band injuries	
B1: Osseous disruption of the tension band	5
B2: Posterior tension band injury	6
B3: Anterior tension band injury	7
Type C: Displacement/translational injuries	8

Table 4
The thoracolumbar AOSpine Injury Score neurologic status and modifiers

Subgroup	Description	Thoracolumbar AOSpine Injury Score Points
Neurologic status		
N0	No neurologic injury	0
N1	Resolved temporary injury	1
N2	Injury to a nerve root	2
N3	Incomplete cord or cauda equina injury	4
N4	Complete spinal cord injury	4
Nx	A reliable neurologic examination cannot be obtained	3
Patient-specific modifiers		
M1	Ambiguity in the integrity of the PLC	1
M2	Patient-specific concerns that will affect the treatment algorithm (ie, AS, severe burst)	0

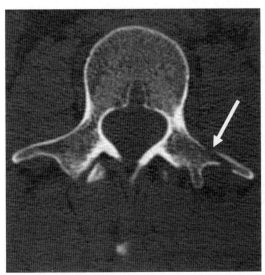

Fig. 11. A0 injury, nonstructural fractures. Transaxial CT shows a mildly displaced fracture of the left transverse process of L2 (*arrow*).

A3 injuries (incomplete burst fractures) involve both the anterior and the posterior vertebral body walls and a single endplate (**Fig. 14**). These fractures represent injuries of the anterior and middle columns of Denis, sparing the posterior tension band. For all burst fractures (A3 and A4), it is important to describe the amount of osseous retropulsion, spinal canal narrowing, and the degree of kyphotic angulation.

A4 injuries (complete burst fractures) involve the anterior and posterior vertebral body walls and both endplates (**Fig. 15**). Split fractures involving the posterior vertebral wall are included in this group. In both A3 and A4 injuries, a vertically oriented lamina fracture may occur and does not necessarily indicate failure of the posterior tension band. Transverse fractures through the posterior arch indicate disruption of the posterior tension band and should be classified as a type B injury.

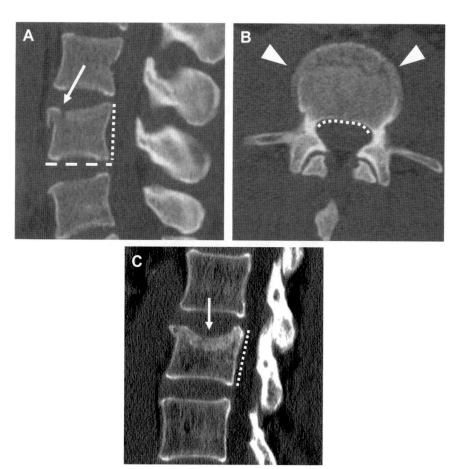

Fig. 12. A1 injury, compression fracture. (A) Sagittal CT reformat shows a superior wedge compression fracture of L2 involving the superior endplate and anterior vertebral body wall (*arrow*). Note the intact posterior vertebral body wall (*dotted line*) and inferior endplate (*dashed line*). (B) Transaxial CT shows the fracture involving the anterior vertebral body and anterior cortex (*arrowheads*), sparing the posterior vertebral body wall (*dotted line*). (C) Sagittal CT reformats show a mildly depressed superior endplate impaction fracture of a lumbar vertebral body (*arrow*), sparing the posterior vertebral body wall (*dotted line*).

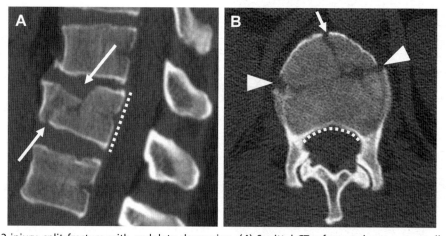

Fig. 13. A2 injury, split fracture with endplate depression. (A) Sagittal CT reformat shows a coronally oriented fracture involving the superior and inferior endplates with mild superior endplate depression (*arrows*). Note the intact posterior vertebral body wall (*dotted line*). (B) Transaxial CT shows the coronal orientation of the fracture (*arrowheads*) with a component that involves the anterior vertebral body wall (*arrow*). Note the intact posterior vertebral body (*dotted line*).

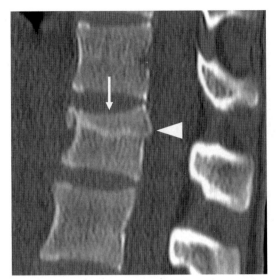

Fig. 14. A3 injury, incomplete burst fracture. Sagittal CT reformat shows a mildly retropulsed fracture of the posterior vertebral body wall (*arrowhead*). The fracture only involves the superior endplate (*arrow*), which distinguishes this from a subtype A4 injury.

Type B (tension band) injuries

Type B injuries disrupt either the anterior or the posterior tension band, but not both. The intact tension band acts as a hinge and prevents dislocation at the injured level. Imaging clues of a posterior tension band injury include transverse posterior arch fractures, interspinous widening, and facet joint distraction.

B1 injuries (monosegmental transosseous tension band disruption/bony Chance fractures) involve a single vertebral body level sparing the disc space (**Fig. 16**). B1 injuries are due to hyperflexion with a fulcrum of rotation anterior to the vertebral body (ie, lap belt) typically at the TL junction. On CT imaging, B1 fractures are characterized by a horizontally oriented posterior arch fracture that often extends into the vertebral body. Pedicles, transverse processes, laminae, and spinous process may be involved. If the vertebral body fracture involves the intervertebral disc space, the fracture is classified as a B2 injury (Chance variant).

B2 injuries (posterior tension band disruption/Chance variant fractures) are bony and ligamentous tension band injuries. These injuries are often associated with vertebral body compression (subtype A3 or A4) injuries (**Fig. 17**).

B3 injuries (anterior tension band disruption) result from hyperextension with disruption of the anterior tension band, including the ALL. The PLC remains intact and prevents gross displacement of the posterior elements. Hyperextension injuries are uncommon in the general spine trauma population[23] and are often associated with a

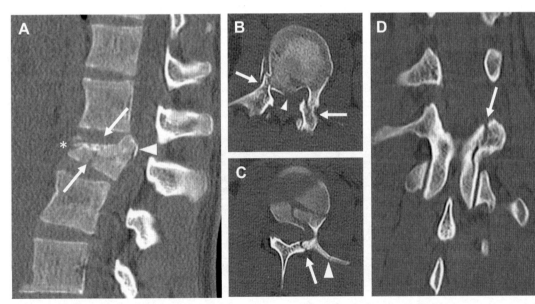

Fig. 15. A4 injury, complete burst fracture. (*A*) Sagittal CT reformat shows fractures of both the anterior and the posterior vertebral body walls with osseous retropulsion (*arrowhead*). The fracture involves both the superior and inferior endplates (*arrows*). There is mild kyphotic angulation (*asterisk*) without interspinous widening. (*B*) Transaxial CT shows fracture involvement of the posterior vertebral body wall (*arrowhead*) and bilateral pedicles (*arrows*). (*C*) Transaxial CT shows a nondisplaced vertically oriented fracture of the left pedicle (*arrow*) and a nondisplaced fracture of the left transverse process (*arrowhead*). (*D*) Coronal CT reformat shows a vertically oriented nondisplaced fracture of the left lamina (*arrow*).

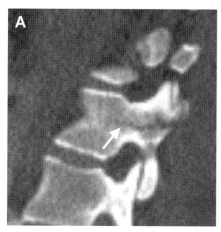
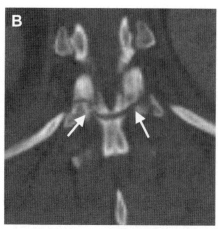

Fig. 16. B1 injury, transosseous tension band disruption/Chance fracture. (A) Sagittal CT reformat shows a horizontally oriented fracture through the vertebral body extending into the pedicle (arrow), sparing the adjacent disc space. (B) Coronal CT reformat shows propagation of the horizontally oriented fracture into the bilateral pedicles and base of the spinous process (arrows).

fused/ankylosed spine (AS or DISH). In patients with these conditions, B3 injuries may occur with trivial trauma, such as a fall from sitting or a low-speed motor vehicle accident.[23] On CT imaging, B3 injuries are characterized by a transverse fracture that involves both anterior and middle columns. The fracture may primarily involve the fused disc space and appear as anterior distraction (Fig. 18). B3 injuries typically require surgical stabilization.

Type C (displacement/translational injuries)
These injuries involve failure of both the anterior and the posterior tension bands (osseous and ligamentous), allowing for displacement beyond the physiologic range of the injured segment

(Fig. 19). Type C injuries may be displaced in any plane and include rotational injuries. These fractures always require surgical stabilization unless contraindicated.

Diagnostic Algorithm for Coding the Morphologic Injury Patterns

A systematic approach is needed while evaluating TL injuries in order to relay pertinent information to surgeons (Fig. 20). Each injured vertebra or spinal segment should be classified.

The first question to ask is: Is there translation or vertical displacement with separation? If yes, the injury should be classified as a type C (displacement/translation) injury. If not, the second question to ask is whether there could be a tension band

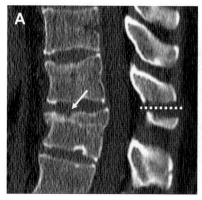
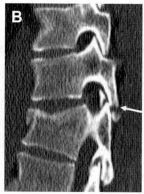
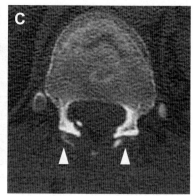

Fig. 17. B2 injury, posterior tension band disruption. (A) Sagittal CT reformat shows a horizontally oriented fracture of the T10 spinous process (dotted line), indicative of posterior tension band disruption. Anteriorly, there is a compression type fracture of the vertebral body (arrow). (B) Parasagittal CT reformat shows fractured and distracted T10-11 facets (arrow). (C) Transaxial CT shows bilateral "naked" T11 superior articulating facets (arrowheads).

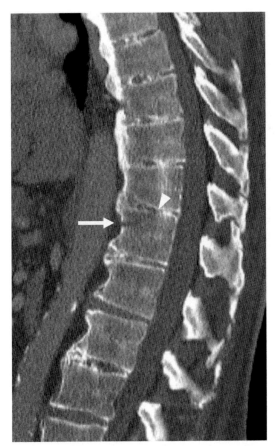

Fig. 18. B3 injury, anterior tension band disruption/distraction hyperextension injury. Sagittal CT reformat shows flowing anterior vertebral ossification compatible with DISH. There is a minimally displaced fracture involving the anterior T12 vertebral body wall (*arrow*) extending into the ossified T11-12 disc space (*arrowhead*). Note that there is no gross displacement at the injured segment due to the intact posterior hinge.

injury involving the anterior ligamentous complex or PLC. If a PLC injury is present and limited to 1 bony segment, a subtype B1 (classic Chance fracture) is diagnosed. If more than 1 vertebral segment is involved, it is a B2 (Chance variant fracture). If there is anterior distraction indicating a hyperextension injury (often in the setting of an ankylosed spine), it is a B3.

If the injury is neither a dislocation nor tension band injury, and a vertebral fracture is present, it is a type A injury. If the posterior vertebral body wall and both endplates are involved, it is an A4 (complete burst) fracture. If the posterior vertebral wall and only 1 endplate are involved, it is an A3 (incomplete burst) fracture. If the fracture involves both endplates but spares the posterior vertebral body wall, it is an A2 (pincer/split) fracture. If only a single endplate is fractured and the posterior vertebral body wall is normal, it is an A1 (wedge/impaction) fracture. Isolated nonstructural fractures that spare the vertebral body (transverse or spinous process fractures) are designated A0.

PITFALLS AND FRACTURE MIMICS

Several developmental variants may mimic fractures. Limbus vertebrae are identified by a small corticated triangular osseous fragment at the anterosuperior or anteroinferior corner of the vertebral body. Unfused ossicles, round, corticated ossific densities at the sites of secondary ossification centers, are typically seen at the tips of the facet articular processes or spinous processes. Mild wedging of both superior and inferior endplates of a TL junction vertebra without underlying fracture line is considered physiologic.

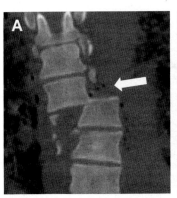
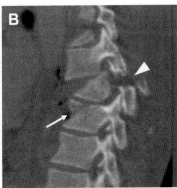
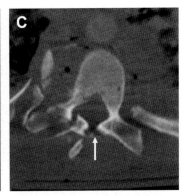

Fig. 19. C injury, displacement/dislocation injury. (*A*) Coronal CT reformat shows total disruption of the spinal column with right lateral displacement of T7 relative to T8 (*large arrow*). These findings are indicative of disruption of the anterior and posterior tension bands. (*B*) Parasagittal CT reformat shows a subtype A1 compression fracture of the T8 vertebral body (*arrow*) as well as distracted fractures of the posterior arch and facets (*arrowhead*). (*C*) Transaxial CT shows the rotational component of the type C injury as well as the comminuted fracture of the posterior arch of T8 (*arrow*).

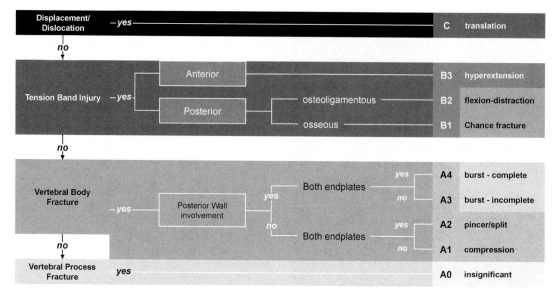

Fig. 20. AOSpine TL classification system.

REFERENCES

1. Milby AH, Halpern CH, Guo W, et al. Prevalence of cervical spinal injury in trauma. Neurosurg Focus 2008;25(5):E10.
2. Hasler RM, Exadaktylos AK, Bouamra O, et al. Epidemiology and predictors of cervical spine injury in adult major trauma patients. J Trauma Inj Infect Crit Care 2012;72(4):975–81.
3. Stiell IG, Clement CM, McKnight RD, et al. The Canadian C-spine rule versus the NEXUS low-risk criteria in patients with trauma. N Engl J Med 2003;349(26):2510–8.
4. Coffey F, Hewitt S, Stiell I, et al. Validation of the Canadian c-spine rule in the UK emergency department setting. Emerg Med J 2011;28(10):873–6.
5. Griffith B, Kelly M, Vallee P, et al. Screening cervical spine CT in the emergency department, phase 2: a prospective assessment of use. AJNR Am J Neuroradiol 2013;34(4):899–903.
6. Paxton M, Heal CF, Drobetz H. Adherence to Canadian C-spine rule in a regional hospital: a retrospective study of 406 cases. J Med Imaging Radiat Oncol 2012;56(5):514–8.
7. Duane TM, Young A, Mayglothling J, et al. CT for all or selective approach? Who really needs a cervical spine CT after blunt trauma. J Trauma Acute Care Surg 2013;74(4):1098–101.
8. Duane TM, Wilson SP, Mayglothling J, et al. Canadian cervical spine rule compared with computed tomography: a prospective analysis. J Trauma Inj Infect Crit Care 2011;71(2):352–7.
9. Sasser SM, Hunt RC, Faul M, et al, Centers for Disease Control and Prevention (CDC). Guidelines for field triage of injured patients: recommendations of the National Expert Panel on Field Triage, 2011. MMWR Recomm Rep 2012;61(RR-1):1–20.
10. Duane TM, Young AJ, Vanguri P, et al. Defining the cervical spine clearance algorithm: a single-institution prospective study of more than 9,000 patients. J Trauma Acute Care Surg 2016;81(3):541–7.
11. Hoffman JR, Mower WR, Wolfson AB, et al. Validity of a set of clinical criteria to rule out injury to the cervical spine in patients with blunt trauma. National Emergency X-Radiography Utilization Study Group. N Engl J Med 2000;343:94–9.
12. Stiell IG, Wells GA, Vandemheen KL, et al. The Canadian C-spine rule for radiography in alert and stable trauma patients. JAMA 2001;286:1841–8.
13. Patel MB, Humble SS, Cullinane DC, et al. Cervical spine collar clearance in the obtunded adult blunt trauma patient: a systematic review and practice management guideline from the Eastern Association for the Surgery of Trauma. J Trauma 2015;78(2):430–41.
14. Wu X, Malhotra A, Geng B, et al. Cost-effectiveness of magnetic resonance imaging in cervical clearance of obtunded blunt trauma after a normal computed tomographic finding. JAMA Surg 2018;153(7):625–32.
15. Inaba K, Byerly S, Bush LD, et al. Cervical spinal clearance: a prospective Western Trauma Association Multi-institutional Trial. J Trauma Acute Care Surg 2016;81(6):1122–30.
16. Holdsworth F. Fractures, dislocations, and fracture-dislocations of the spine. J Bone Joint Surg Am 1970;52(8):1534–51.
17. Denis F. The three column spine and its significance in the classification of acute thoracolumbar spinal injuries. Spine (Phila Pa 1976) 1983;8(8):817–31.

18. Magerl F, Aebi M, Gertzbein SD, et al. A comprehensive classification of thoracic and lumbar injuries. Eur Spine J 1994;3:184–201.

19. Vaccaro AR, Lehman RA Jr, Hurlbert RJ, et al. A new classification of thoracolumbar injuries: the importance of injury morphology, the integrity of the posterior ligamentous complex, and neurologic status. Spine (Phila Pa 1976) 2005;30(20):2325–33.

20. Vaccaro AR, Oner C, Kepler CK, et al, AOSpine Spinal Cord Injury & Trauma Knowledge Forum. AOSpine thoracolumbar spine injury classification system: fracture description, neurological status, and key modifiers. Spine (Phila Pa 1976) 2013;38(23):2028–37.

21. American College of Radiology ACR appropriateness criteria clinical condition: suspected spine trauma. Available at: https://acsearch.acr.org/docs/69359/Narrative/. Accessed October 21, 2018.

22. White AA, Panjabi MM. Clinical biomechanics of the spine. 2nd edition. Philadelphia: Lippincott; 1990. p. 30–342.

23. Kepler CK, Vaccaro AR, Schroeder GD, et al. The thoracolumbar AOSpine injury score. Global Spine J 2016;6(4):329–34.

Imaging of Cardiovascular Thoracic Emergencies
Acute Aortic Syndrome and Pulmonary Embolism

Gene Kim, MD, Hristina Natcheva, MD*

KEYWORDS

- Aortic dissection • Intramural hematoma • Pulmonary embolism • Pulmonary angiography
- Aortic aneurysm

KEY POINTS

- Cardiovascular injuries represent the second most common cause of death among trauma victims in the United States, with motor vehicle collisions accounting for more than 80% of all blunt thoracic trauma.
- Acute aortic syndrome refers to the triad of aortic pathology, which includes aortic dissection, intramural hematoma, and penetrating atherosclerotic ulcer. Aortic dissection represents the majority of acute aortic syndrome cases.
- Venous thromboembolism/pulmonary embolism should be an important clinical consideration in the symptomatic trauma patient due to its high morbidity and mortality in the recovery period. CT pulmonary angiography is the preferred first-line diagnostic imaging modality for the detection of pulmonary emboli thanks to its high sensitivity, specificity, wide availability, and speed of acquisition.

INTRODUCTION

Cardiovascular injuries represent the second most common cause of death among trauma victims in the United States.[1] Given the nonspecific nature and variable severity of symptoms, such as chest pain and shortness of breath, as well as confounding and overlapping clinical presentations in the setting of additional injuries, diagnosis of cardiovascular injuries can be challenging. Therefore, understanding the classification and pathophysiology of cardiovascular trauma is essential for timely diagnosis and treatment.

PATHOPHYSIOLOGY

Considering the mechanism of injury of trauma victims, motor vehicle collisions account for more than 80% of all blunt thoracic injury followed by crush injuries at 5% (eg, fall from heights). Kinetic energy is transmitted through the chest wall via direct impact, with compression of the heart between the anterior spinal elements and the chest wall, with a change in the inertia of the organs as well the blood pool. Additionally, rapid deceleration with velocities of less than 20 miles per hour have been reported in cases of cardiac injury. Cardiovascular injury may be present in cases of blunt thoracic trauma without visible sequelae of injury to the chest wall. Furthermore, abdominal trauma may cause upward displacement of solid abdominal viscera, which also may result in cardiac injury.[2] External forces, such as atmospheric changes surrounding the victim (ie, explosion), also may lead to cardiovascular trauma. The

Disclosure Statement: The authors have no financial interests to disclose.
Department of Radiology, Boston Medical Center, Boston University School of Medicine, 820 Harrison Avenue, FGH Building, Radiology Administration, Boston, MA 02118, USA
* Corresponding author.
E-mail address: Hristina.Natcheva@bmc.org

different mechanisms of injury with variable severity can lead to a spectrum of cardiovascular injuries involving the heart, pericardium, coronary vasculature, and great vessels and cause nonimaging complications, such as arrhythmias.[1]

ACUTE AORTIC SYNDROME

Although not limited to a singular entity, acute aortic syndrome (AAS) typically refers to the triad of aortic pathology, which includes aortic dissection (AD), intramural hematoma (IMH), and penetrating atherosclerotic ulcer (PAU). These entities should be viewed as different points on a spectrum and may occur in isolation or concurrently because they all originate from injury of the intimomedial layer of the aorta. The shared pathophysiology and their indistinguishable signs and symptoms, which include acute, abrupt onset of severe chest and/or back pain, require rapid and accurate diagnosis and classification, because there are differences in clinical management and prognosis.

Aortic Dissection

With an incidence of 2.6 to 3.6 cases per 100,000 persons annually, AD represents a majority of AAS cases.[3] AD is defined as a tear in the intimal layer of the aorta, with formation of an intimomedial dissection flap and a false lumen. As blood enters the media, a double-barreled aorta is formed with 2 distinct lumens. The true lumen is lined by the intimal layer whereas the false lumen is the blood contained within the separated medial layer. If the pressure differential results in higher pressures within the false lumen, the true lumen may be compressed or even effaced, leading to end-organ ischemia due to occlusion of branch vessels. The direction and degree of circumferential involvement of the AD are variable, which leads to differences in classification.

The 2 most widely used anatomic classifications of AD are based on the location and degree of involvement of the aorta and its branches and include the Stanford and DeBakey classifications (**Fig. 1**). The Stanford classification is used more widely due to its simplicity and correlation with clinical management. It also is used to characterize the location of IMH and PAUs. Stanford type A AD involves the ascending aorta and may extend to the distal aortic arch or descending aorta. It typically is treated as a surgical emergency (**Figs. 2–4**). Stanford type B AD involves the aorta distal to the brachiocephalic arteries and usually is managed medically (**Figs. 5–7**).[4]

The complications of acute AD are varied but usually stem from compromised or abnormal perfusion

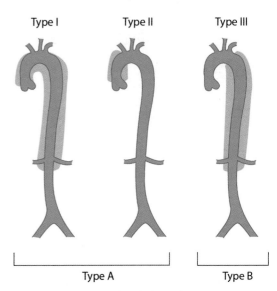

DeBakey Classification

Type I   Type II   Type III

Type A   Type B

Stanford Classification

Fig. 1. Stanford and DeBakey classification of ADs. AD involving the ascending and descending aorta (Stanford Type A, DeBakey type I, left), ascending aorta (Stanford Type A, DeBakey type II, middle), and descending aorta (Stanford Type B, DeBakey type III, right).

of the aortic branch vessels and involvement of the aortic valve or pericardium.[5] For example, if the coronary arteries are involved, patients may present with myocardial ischemia or infarction; if the aortic valve is involved, patients may present with aortic insufficiency and resultant acute congestive heart failure. There also is concern for cerebral ischemia and mesenteric ischemia if the dissection involves the brachiocephalic vessels and the abdominal visceral vessels, respectively. Other feared complications of AD, in particular Stanford type A, include hemopericardium and pericardial tamponade as well as rupture of the dissection. Considering the potential high mortality and morbidity of these varied complications, a timely and accurate diagnosis of AD is essential.

Multidetector CT angiography currently is the modality of choice for diagnosis of AAS given its rapid acquisition and wide availability as well as postprocessing capabilities, which can be useful for both detailed assessment and preoperative planning.[6] CT angiography provides excellent visualization of the false lumen, which is contained within the aortic medial layer and separated from the true lumen by the intimal flap.[7] The standard CT protocol involves a noncontrast series covering the entire aorta and extending into the iliac arteries, followed by an arterial-phase contrast-

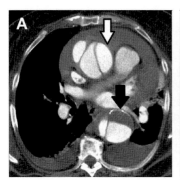
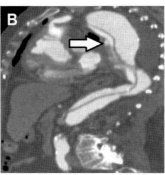

Fig. 2. (*A*) Axial arterial phase image demonstrates Stanford type A AD involving the ascending and descending aorta. The true lumen (*white arrow*) is hyperdense and mildly compressed by the false lumen, which is less densely opacified. Note the small bilateral pleural effusions and moderate-sized pericardial effusion. Thrombus is seen in the false lumen within the descending aorta (*black arrow*). (*B*) Sagittal reconstruction demonstrates the dissection flap (*white arrow*) extending into the abdominal aorta.

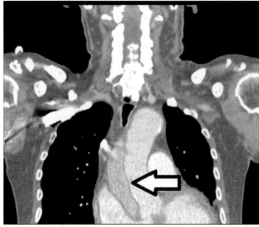

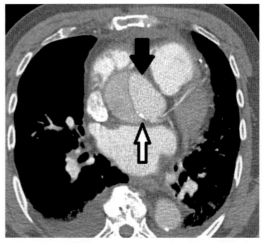

Fig. 3. Coronal arterial phase image demonstrates a Stanford type A dissection involving the proximal ascending aorta sparing the brachiocephalic vessels (*white arrow*).

Fig. 4. Axial contrast-enhanced image demonstrates Stanford type A dissection (*black arrow*) limited to the ascending aorta. The true lumen is hyperdense relative to the false lumen. Intimal calcifications (*white arrow*) confirm the location of the true lumen. Note the left coronary artery is supplied by the true lumen, and there are bilateral pleural effusions.

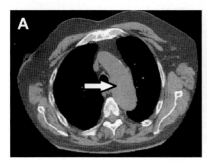
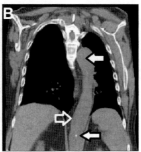

Fig. 5. (*A*) Axial noncontrast image demonstrates Stanford type B dissection with a faintly hyperattenuating intimal flap (*white arrow*) extending from the distal aortic arch to the proximal abdominal aorta. (*B*) Coronal noncontrast image demonstrates the true lumen (*white outlined arrow*) with intimal calcifications along the right-aspect of the intimal flap (*white arrows*).

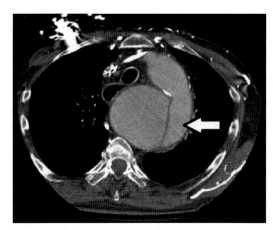

Fig. 6. Axial contrast-enhanced image shows Stanford type B dissection with a large aneurysm of the proximal descending aorta and hyperdense true lumen (*white arrow*).

enhanced scan with a standard 25-second postinjection delay at a rate of 4 mL/s to 5 mL/s.[6] ECG-gated imaging also may be used to reduce the motion artifact associated with cardiac movement and pulsatile motion of the proximal aorta. The non–contrast-enhanced series aides in identifying hyperdense IMH and a thrombosed false lumen as well as displaced intimal calcifications.

Intramural Hematoma

IMH is the second most common entity in the triad of AAS, comprising approximately 6% to 20% of cases. Characteristic imaging findings include a hyperdense crescentic collection or eccentric thickening of the aortic wall.[6,8] Historically, IMH has been considered a distinct entity from AD, suspected to result from rupture of the vasa vasorum within the intimomedial layer and the formation of an aortic wall hematoma while the intima

remains intact. Advancements in CT imaging, however, as well as corroboration with surgical pathology variably confirm the coexistence of IMH and intimal flap in some cases.[9,10] Therefore, IMH and AD more accurately are thought of as entities on the spectrum of AAS rather than separate disease processes. As with AD, CT angiography is the preferred modality for detection of IMH, with a protocol including nonenhanced and arterial-enhanced series through the entire aorta and iliac arteries.

Like AD, IMH is categorized using the Stanford classification based on location within the aorta, which has important prognostic implications. Stanford type A IMHs typically require surgical management given the increased risk of aneurysm formation, progression to type AD, pericardial/pleural effusions, and aortic rupture.[6] Stanford type B IMHs generally can be managed medically or with delayed planned surgical intervention (**Figs. 8–9**).

Apart from classification, assessment of the maximum aortic diameter also imparts prognostic value. An IMH with a concurrent aortic aneurysm has an increased risk for negative outcomes, including progression to AD, incomplete resolution, rupture, and death.[11,12] Some literature suggests there is an increase in adverse events when the maximum aortic diameter is greater than 48 mm to 55 mm for Stanford type A IMHs.[10,12] For Stanford type B IMHs, the suggested cutoff for maximum aortic diameter is reported to be 40 mm.[13,14] In addition to the maximum diameter of the aorta, the thickness of the IMH itself is an important imaging characteristic. Increased IMH thickness of greater than 10 mm measured in the axial plane perpendicular to the longitudinal axis to the aortic lumen increases the risk of adverse outcomes, including

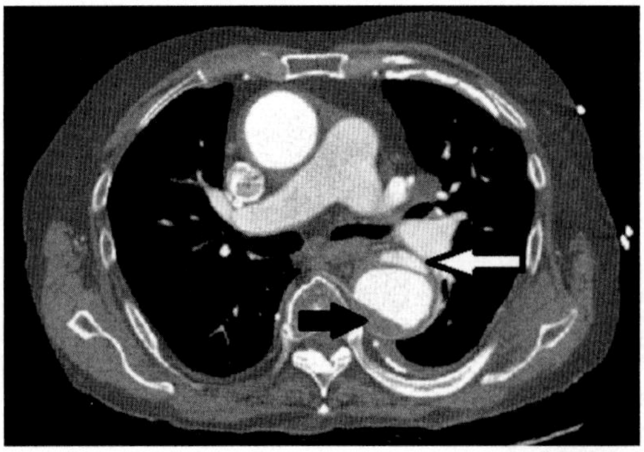

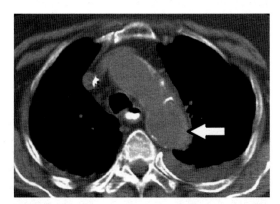

Fig. 7. Axial arterial-phase image demonstrates Stanford type B dissection with a compressed true lumen (*white arrow*). There is partial thrombosis of the false lumen (*black arrow*). Note the trace right pleural effusion with pleural calcifications.

Fig. 8. Axial noncontrast image demonstrates a crescentic hyperdense IMH in the distal aortic arch ([*white arrow*] Stanford type B IMH). There is a right pleural effusion and oral contrast within the esophagus.

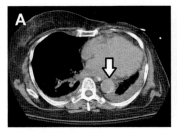
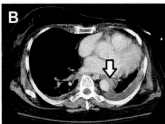

Fig. 9. (*A*) Axial noncontrast image demonstrates a hyperdense Stanford type B IMH in the descending aorta without a visible intimal flap (*white arrow*). (*B*) Axial arterial phase image demonstrates narrowing of the aortic lumen by the IMH (*white arrow*). Note the small right pleural effusion.

AD, progression of extent of the hematoma, and incomplete resorption.[10–12,15]

The last important consideration when evaluating the extent or severity of disease includes evaluation for focal contrast enhancement within the IMH. This important imaging finding can manifest in 2 ways—ulcer-like projections (ULPs) and intramural blood pools—and is likely to occur with thick IMHs.[16] A ULP is characterized by a focal outpouching of contrast visibly communicating with the aortic lumen via a broad neck greater than 3 mm; intramural blood pools are defined as focal contrast enhancement with an imperceptible communication to the aortic lumen or a neck less than 3 mm.[15,16] There is increased adverse outcome risk with larger size and depth of ULPs, with the literature suggesting a threshold of approximately 10 mm to 20 mm in diameter and 5 mm to 10 mm in depth as well as increased poor prognosis and risk of adverse events, including AD, aneurysm, or rupture when the ULP involves the ascending aorta or aortic arch.[9,11,13]

Penetrating Atherosclerotic Ulcer

PAUs comprise approximately 2% to 7% of AAS cases, occurring less commonly than AD and IMH.[17–19] PAUs are defined as a disruption of the internal elastic lamina, with varying degrees of extension through the layers of the aorta. Depending on the degree of extension, PAUs may lead to IMH, pseudoaneurysm formation, and transmural rupture if they extend through the adventitia. As the name implies, PAUs are strongly associated with atherosclerotic disease and, therefore,

commonly found in the descending aorta (>90%) and in elderly patients.[6,20] There is increased mortality associated with PAUs involving the ascending aorta and aortic arch, with a risk of aortic rupture of approximately 33% to 40%.[21,22] Comparatively, ULPs typically are not associated with atherosclerotic plaques and occur mainly in the ascending aorta and aortic arch.[15,23]

PULMONARY EMBOLISM

As a significant cause of morbidity and mortality in the recovery of posttraumatic patients, venous thromboembolisms (VTEs) should be an important clinical consideration in the symptomatic trauma patient.[24] The Virchow triad, consisting of venous stasis, endothelial damage, and hypercoagulability, was established more than a century ago as the pathophysiologic basis of thromboembolism.[25] VTEs are believed to occur most commonly 5 days to 7 days after trauma due to immobility promoting venous stasis and clot formation. Approximately 25% of pulmonary emboli (PE), however, occur during the first 4 days after clinical presentation and a minority can be seen within several hours posttrauma.[26–28]

As with other posttraumatic thoracic pathology, patients can develop nonspecific signs and symptoms, such as tachypnea, tachycardia, and dyspnea, which may be attributed to etiologies other than PE. In combination with the variable timing of formation of PEs and difficulty in attributing signs and symptoms, astute clinical suspicion leading to diagnosis and clinical management is critical.

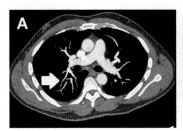
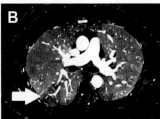

Fig. 10. (*A*) Axial CTPA image demonstrates occlusive PE within a subsegmental artery of the right lower lobe (*white arrow*). (*B*) Axial iodine distribution map image at the same level, demonstrates matching wedge-shaped perfusion abnormality (*white arrow*).

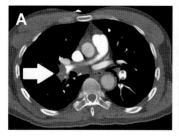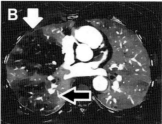

Fig. 11. (*A*) Axial CTPA image demonstrates occlusive PE (*white arrow*) within the distal right main pulmonary artery. (*B*) Axial iodine distribution map image demonstrates large geographic areas of hypoperfusion within the right upper/middle lobe (*white arrow*) and lower lobe (*black arrow*).

With its high sensitivity and high specificity rates, ranging from 83% to 100% and 89% to 96%, respectively, as well as its speed of acquisition and wide availability, CT pulmonary angiography (CTPA) is the preferred first-line diagnostic imaging modality for the detection of PE.[29,30] Moreover, CTPA, can provide anatomic and physiologic clues that may lead to important ancillary information, such as an estimate of right ventricular function. Standard protocol revolves around the goal of maximizing contrast opacification of the pulmonary arterial circulation. The dose of contrast is typically patient-specific based on renal function and body habitus. Either contrast timing using a test bolus or bolus tracking in a region of interest centered within the main pulmonary artery can be used for appropriate timing to achieve maximal pulmonary arterial opacification.

Acute Pulmonary Embolism

Acute PEs can be occlusive or nonocclusive. Occlusion is characterized by a concave or rounded intraluminal defect, with contrast opacifying the pulmonary artery proximal to the obstruction. There also may be enlargement of the involved pulmonary artery due to impaction of the embolus by pulsatile flow.[31,32] Nonocclusive defects may be centrally or eccentrically located within the

lumen of the pulmonary artery or may form acute angles with the arterial wall.[32] Contrast should be seen partially opacifying the involved vessel and its distal branches.

Sequelae of occlusive PE include pulmonary infarcts, which typically appear as peripheral wedge-shaped lung parenchymal opacities (**Figs. 10 and 11**).[33] New dual energy and spectral CT technology allows visualization of hypo-perfused lung using iodine distribution maps. In addition, there may be findings indicating right ventricular strain or dysfunction, including increased right ventricular cavity diameter in relation to the left ventricular cavity diameter (right ventricular:left venticular ratio), flattening or leftward deviation of the interventricular septum, and reflux of contrast into the inferior vena cava and hepatic veins (**Fig. 12**).[34]

Chronic Pulmonary Embolism

Chronic PEs also can present with complete vessel obstruction or may be partially occlusive defects with several differentiating features. Complete obstruction usually presents as a filling defect with a convex margin relative to contrast

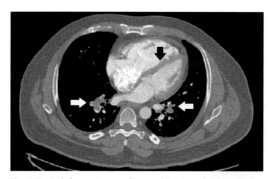

Fig. 12. Axial contrast enhanced image demonstrates multiple occlusive PE within segmental pulmonary arteries of the lower lobes (*white arrows*) as well as flattening of the interventricular septum (*black arrow*) and right ventricular enlargement, consistent with right heart strain.

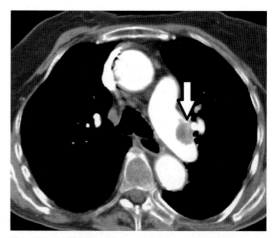

Fig. 13. Axial CTPA image demonstrates a nonocclusive convex defect (*white arrow*) along the wall of the left main pulmonary artery suggestive of a chronic PE.

within the vessel (**Fig. 13**). The pulmonary artery distal to the obstruction may be narrowed in caliber due to contraction or atresia.[31] There is variable appearance of nonocclusive chronic PEs, which may present as crescent-shaped filling defects with obtuse angles in relation to the arterial wall, web-like or flap-like opacities characterized by a network of thin linear filling defects of varying complexity within a contrast opacified pulmonary artery, and abrupt vessel narrowing due to recanalization.[31,32] Additional findings of chronic PE include anatomic changes related to pulmonary hypertension, such as enlargement of the main pulmonary artery greater than 33 mm in diameter.[35]

SUMMARY

Cardiovascular injuries represent the second most common cause of death among trauma victims in the United States. Their sometimes vague and overlapping symptoms could present a diagnostic challenge to even the most astute of clinicians. Moreover, delays in diagnosis may result in catastrophic outcomes. Computed tomoangiography with its wide availability and rapid acquisition plays an important role in the timely diagnosis and management of cardiovascular pathology, including AAS and PE, and, therefore, is the imaging modality of choice in the emergency setting. Knowledge of the imaging characteristics and nuances of these pathologic entities is essential for every radiologist.

REFERENCES

1. El-Chami MF, Nicholson W, Helmy T. Blunt cardiac trauma. J Emerg Med 2008;35(2):127–33.
2. Tenzer MLMD. The spectrum of myocardial contusion: a review. J Trauma 1985;25(7):620–7.
3. Tsai TT, Nienaber CA, Eagle KA. Acute aortic syndromes [review]. Circulation 2005;112(24):3802–13.
4. Hagan PG, Nienaber CA, Isselbacher EM, et al. The International Registry of Acute Aortic Dissection (IRAD): new insights into an old disease. JAMA 2000;283(7):897–903.
5. Mészáros I, Mórocz J, Szlávi J, et al. Epidemiology and clinicopathology of aortic dissection. Chest 2000;117(5):1271–8.
6. Nienaber CA. The role of imaging in acute aortic syndromes. Eur Heart J Cardiovasc Imaging 2013; 14(1):15–23.
7. Ueda T, Chin A, Petrovitch I, et al. A pictorial review of acute aortic syndrome: discriminating and overlapping features as revealed by ECG-gated multidetector-row CT angiography. Insights Imaging 2012; 3(6):561–71.
8. Harris KM, Braverman AC, Eagle KA, et al. Acute aortic intramural hematoma: an analysis from the International Registry of Acute Aortic Dissection. Circulation 2012;126(11 Suppl 1):S91–6.
9. Kitai T, Kaji S, Yamamuro A, et al. Detection of intimal defect by 64-row multidetector computed tomography in patients with acute aortic intramural hematoma. Circulation 2011. Available at: https://www.ahajournals.org/doi/full/10.1161/CIRCULATIONAHA.111.037416. Accessed September 4, 2018.
10. Sawaki S, Hirate Y, Ashida S, et al. Clinical outcomes of medical treatment of acute type a intramural hematoma. Asian Cardiovasc Thorac Ann 2010;18(4): 354–9.
11. Lee YK, Seo JB, Jang YM, et al. Acute and chronic complications of aortic intramural hematoma on follow-up computed tomography: incidence and predictor analysis. J Comput Assist Tomogr 2007; 31(3):435–40.
12. Song J-K, Yim JH, Ahn J-M, et al. Outcomes of patients with acute type a aortic intramural hematoma. Circulation 2009. Available at: https://www.ahajournals.org/doi/full/10.1161/CIRCULATIONAHA.109.879783. Accessed September 5, 2018.
13. Sueyoshi E, Imada T, Sakamoto I, et al. Analysis of predictive factors for progression of type B aortic intramural hematoma with computed tomography. J Vasc Surg 2002;35(6):1179–83.
14. Sueyoshi E, Sakamoto I, Uetani M, et al. CT analysis of the growth rate of aortic diameter affected by acute type B intramural hematoma. AJR Am J Roentgenol 2006;186(6 Suppl 2):S414–20.
15. Wu M-T, Wang Y-C, Huang Y-L, et al. Intramural blood pools accompanying aortic intramural hematoma: CT appearance and natural course. Radiology 2011;258(3):705–13.
16. Park K-H, Lim C, Choi JH, et al. Prevalence of aortic intimal defect in surgically treated acute type a intramural hematoma. Ann Thorac Surg 2008;86(5): 1494–500.
17. Corvera JS. Acute aortic syndrome. Ann Cardiothorac Surg 2016;5(3):188–93.
18. Eggebrecht H, Plicht B, Kahlert P, et al. Intramural hematoma and penetrating ulcers: indications to endovascular treatment. Eur J Vasc Endovasc Surg 2009;38(6):659–65.
19. Nathan DP, Boonn W, Lai E, et al. Presentation, complications, and natural history of penetrating atherosclerotic ulcer disease. J Vasc Surg 2012;55(1): 10–5.
20. Litmanovich D, Bankier AA, Cantin L, et al. CT and MRI in diseases of the aorta. AJR Am J Roentgenol 2009;193(4):928–40.
21. Coady MA, Rizzo JA, Hammond GL, et al. Penetrating ulcer of the thoracic aorta: what is it? How do we recognize it? How do we manage it? J Vasc Surg 1998;27(6):1006–16.

22. Tittle SL, Lynch RJ, Cole PE, et al. Midterm follow-up of penetrating ulcer and intramural hematoma of the aorta. J Thorac Cardiovasc Surg 2002;123(6):1051–9.

23. Sueyoshi E, Matsuoka Y, Sakamoto I, et al. Fate of intramural hematoma of the aorta: CT evaluation [Miscellaneous Article]. J Comput Assist Tomogr 1997;21(6):931–8.

24. Geerts WH, Code KI, Jay RM, et al. A prospective study of venous thromboembolism after major trauma. N Engl J Med 1994;331(24):1601–6.

25. Rogers FB, Osler TM, Shackford SR. Immediate pulmonary embolism after trauma: case report. J Trauma 2000;48(1):146–8.

26. Menaker J, Stein DMM, Scalea TM. Incidence of early pulmonary embolism after injury. J Trauma 2007;63(3):620–4.

27. Menaker J, Stein DMM, Scalea TM. Pulmonary embolism after injury: more common than we think? J Trauma 2009;67(6):1244–9.

28. O'malley KFMD, Ross SEMD. Pulmonary embolism in major trauma patients. J Trauma 1990;30(6): 748–50.

29. Qanadli SD, Hajjam ME, Mesurolle B, et al. Pulmonary embolism detection: prospective evaluation of dual-section helical ct versus selective pulmonary arteriography in 157 patients. Radiology 2000; 217(2):447–55.

30. Stein PD, Fowler SE, Goodman LR, et al. Multidetector computed tomography for acute pulmonary embolism. N Engl J Med 2006. https://doi.org/10.1056/NEJMoa052367.

31. Wittram C, Kalra MK, Maher MM, et al. Acute and chronic pulmonary emboli: angiography–CT correlation. Am J Roentgenol 2006;186(6_supplement_2): S421–9.

32. Wittram C, Maher MM, Yoo AJ, et al. CT angiography of pulmonary embolism: diagnostic criteria and causes of misdiagnosis. Radiographics 2004;24(5): 1219–38.

33. Coche EE, Müller NL, Kim KI, et al. Acute pulmonary embolism: ancillary findings at spiral CT. Radiology 1998;207(3):753–8.

34. Contractor S, Maldjian PD, Sharma VK, et al. Role of helical CT in detecting right ventricular dysfunction secondary to acute pulmonary embolism. J Comput Assist Tomogr 2002;26(4):587–91.

35. Edwards PD, Bull RK, Coulden R. CT measurement of main pulmonary artery diameter. Br J Radiol 1998; 71(850):1018–20.

Imaging of Cardiac Trauma

Yuhao Wu, MD[a,b], Sadia R. Qamar, MBBS[b], Nicolas Murray, MD, FRCPC[b],
Savvas Nicolaou, MD, FRCPC[b,*]

KEYWORDS

- Multidetector computed tomography (MDCT) • Cardiac trauma • Pericardial/myocardial injury
- Coronary artery injury • Ascending aortic injury • Pulmonary trunk injury
- Emergency and trauma radiology

KEY POINTS

- Cardiac trauma can present in up to 76% of patients following trauma to the chest and is associated with high mortality rates. Early diagnosis and treatment are essential to reduce deaths from cardiac trauma.
- Multidetector computed tomography is considered the gold-standard diagnostic imaging in diagnosing and characterizing cardiac trauma, and should be used in all patients presenting with abnormal electrocardiogram or Troponin I levels following chest trauma.
- The spectrum of cardiac injuries ranges from pericardial contusion to coronary artery injuries. It is imperative for emergency and trauma radiologists to become familiar with the different injury patterns of cardiac trauma.

INTRODUCTION

Cardiac trauma, which can present in up to 76% of patients following chest trauma, is the second most common cause of death in trauma after central nervous system injuries.[1] There are approximately 900,000 reported cases of cardiac trauma in the United States every year.[1] The most common cause of cardiac trauma is motor vehicle accidents (83%), followed by crush injuries (5.7%) and bicycle accidents (2.9%).[2] Because traumatic cardiac injuries often have high mortality rates, it is essential to have a high degree of suspicion for cardiac injuries in all patients presenting after trauma to the chest. Diagnostic imaging plays a critical role in the diagnosis and evaluation of cardiac trauma so that early intervention can be initiated to reduce the mortality of these patients.

In this review article, we present the clinical features of cardiac trauma and discuss the role of diagnostic imaging. We also showcase the spectrum of pathologic imaging findings, with a focus on the use of multidetector computed tomography (MDCT), which has become the gold standard for imaging cardiac trauma.

ETIOLOGY AND PATHOPHYSIOLOGY OF CARDIAC TRAUMA

Cardiac trauma can be broadly categorized into blunt and penetrating cardiac trauma. Blunt trauma to the chest results in the compression of the heart between the sternum and the posterior spine in compression injuries, or anterior translation of the heart against the sternum in deceleration injuries.[3,4] In most cases, this result in pericardial and myocardial contusion. Blunt injuries with greater impact may lead to damage to the cardiac free wall, interventricular septum, the tensor apparatus, and cusps of the cardiac valves,

Disclosure Statement: The University of British Columbia Master Research Agreement with Siemens AG. However, there was no commercial funding received for this study.
[a] Faculty of Medicine, University of British Columbia, 317 - 2194 Health Sciences Mall, Vancouver V6T 1Z3, Canada; [b] Emergency and Trauma Radiology, Vancouver General Hospital, 950 West 10th Avenue, Vancouver V5Z 1M9, Canada
* Corresponding author. Emergency and Trauma Radiology, Vancouver General Hospital, 950 West 10th Avenue, Vancouver, British Columbia V5Z 1M9, Canada.
E-mail address: savvas.nicolaou@vch.ca

Radiol Clin N Am 57 (2019) 795–808
https://doi.org/10.1016/j.rcl.2019.02.006

as well as the coronary arteries.[4] Because of its anterior position, the right ventricle is the most susceptible cardiac chamber in pericardial and myocardial contusions. However, the mitral and aortic valves are more commonly injured than the tricuspid and pulmonic valves due to the relatively higher mural pressures in the left heart chambers.[4]

Penetrating cardiac trauma includes stab wounds, which commonly result in ventricular involvement, and projectile injuries, which often results in hemodynamic instability.[3] It is a highly fatal pattern of injury, with previously reported mortality of up to 94% in patients before reaching the hospital.[5] Recent advances in prehospital care and rapid transportation have significantly reduced prehospital mortality.[4] Nevertheless, the mortality of penetrating trauma remains high, with gunshot wounds being more fatal than stab wounds.[6]

CLINICAL MANIFESTATIONS

The signs and symptoms of cardiac trauma are often nonspecific, and clinical presentation may range from being asymptomatic to being in cardiogenic shock. Chest pain in the presence of sternal, clavicular, or rib injuries increases the suspicion for cardiac trauma.[1] Other commonly associated injuries include pneumothorax (which occurs in 39% of the patients), hemothorax (31%), and lung contusions (13%).[4] On physical examination, bruising is seen in approximately 30% of the patients, and new murmurs or pericardial rubs may indicate intrinsic cardiac involvement.[1]

According to the Eastern Association for the Surgery of Trauma guidelines, all patients with suspected blunt cardiac trauma should receive an electrocardiogram (ECG) and Troponin I level. Troponin I, instead of creatine kinase–muscle/blood (CK-MB), should be used because CK-MB is neither sensitive nor specific for cardiac injury.[7] Cardiac injury can be ruled out only if patients have both normal ECG and Troponin I levels.[8] The most common abnormal findings on ECG are ST segment changes ≥1 mm (seen on 41% of the abnormal ECGs), T-wave inversions (31%), and right bundle branch block (15%).[9]

ROLE OF DIAGNOSTIC IMAGING IN CARDIAC TRAUMA

Medical imaging plays a crucial role in the diagnosis and characterization of cardiac trauma in patients with abnormal ECG and/or Troponin I levels, and helps to the guide the management of these patients.

Radiography

Chest radiograph is often the initial imaging modality obtained at most North American emergency departments and trauma centers following acute chest trauma. Signs suggestive of cardiac trauma include skeletal fractures (sternal, clavicular, or rib fractures), hemothorax (shown in **Fig. 1**), pericardial fluid, pneumopericardium, and widened mediastinum. However, chest radiograph has a low sensitivity and specificity for cardiac injuries because of its inability to delineate overlying anatomic structures and patients' poor inspiratory effort in the setting of severe chest pain or decreased consciousness. For this reason, cross-sectional imaging is required for assessing the anatomic and hemodynamic details of the heart.[10]

Echocardiogram

Before the advent of multidetector computed tomography (MDCT), echocardiogram was widely used as the cross-sectional imaging modality for assessing for cardiac trauma.[11] The most common findings include regional wall hypokinesis/akinesis, right ventricular dilation, pericardial effusion, and aortic injuries.[9] It also can detect associated injuries such as ventricular septal rupture and valvular injuries, as well as complications including development of intracardiac thrombi.[4] It remains as the imaging modality of choice for diagnosis of cardiac tamponade, which manifests as abnormal ventricular dimension changes during inspiration,

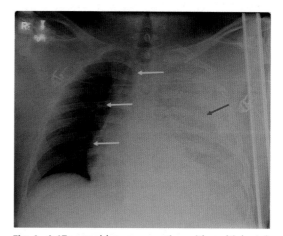

Fig. 1. A 17-year-old man presenting with multiple stab wounds following an altercation. On clinical assessment, there was a large laceration (3 cm) just below and to the left of the nipple. He had decreased air entry. Chest radiograph shows complete opacification of the left hemithorax (*red arrow*) with deviation of the mediastinal structures to the right (*green arrows*). He was taken to the operating room and underwent anterolateral thoracotomy, which showed a left ventricular stab wound that was subsequently repaired.

ventricular diastolic collapse, right atrial compression, dilated inferior vena cava, and swinging heart within the pericardium.[12,13] **Fig. 2** demonstrates an example of CT and trans-thoracic echocardiogram that show features of cardiac tamponade.

However, echocardiogram has several limitations. Trans-thoracic echocardiogram (TTE) can produce suboptimal images in patients with obesity, subcutaneous emphysema, mechanical ventilation, or chest tube insertion.[14] For this reason, trans-esophageal echocardiogram (TEE) is preferred over TTE because of its higher diagnostic accuracy, but it is semi-invasive and may be contraindicated in patients with hypotension, cervical spine trauma, or tracheal and esophageal structural abnormalities.[13] In addition, TEE cannot delineate the distal ascending aorta and proximal descending aorta due to obscuration by the airways.[14]

Computed Tomography

The American College of Radiology recommends MDCT as the gold-standard diagnostic imaging test for all thoracic trauma and states that it should be used in patients presenting with high-impact trauma, abnormal chest radiograph findings, altered mental status, distracting injuries, or suspected thoracic injuries. CT angiography (CTA), in combination with chest radiography, should be routinely used in suspected aortic injuries, given its high sensitivity and noninvasive nature (compared with pulmonary aortography).[10] In addition, the development of ECG-gated cardiac MDCT has allowed the heart to be captured during diastole so that high-resolution images of the heart, great vessels, and coronary arteries can be generated in a noninvasive fashion with minimal motion artifacts.[13,15]

At the authors' institution (Vancouver General Hospital, Vancouver, Canada), prospective systolic-triggered ECG synchronized cardiac-gated coronary CTA is performed with second generation 128-slice dual-source CT scanners. **Table 1** shows the MDCT protocol and **Fig. 3** describes the clinical algorithm for patients

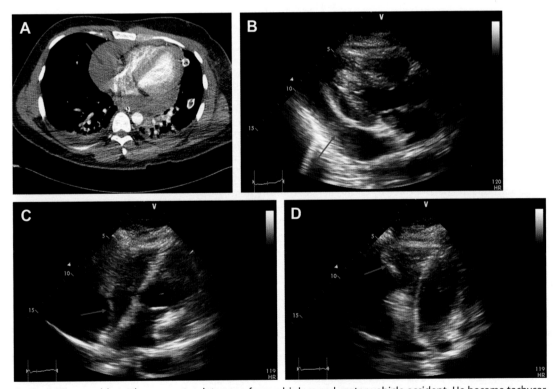

Fig. 2. A 33-year-old gentleman post polytrauma from a high-speed motor vehicle accident. He became tachycardiac and hypotensive on presentation. Over the course of the few minutes, he then proceeded to become bradycardiac and eventually progressed to pulseless electrical activity. He was resuscitated with 30 minutes of cardiopulmonary resuscitation. Contrast-enhanced CT (*A*) shows that there is a large pericardial effusion (*red arrow*) with mass effect on the contour of the heart and narrowing of the right atrium (*orange arrow*). The follow-up echocardiogram confirmed the presence of a large pericardial effusion (*red arrow, B*) with right atrial collapse (*red arrow, C*), and diastolic right ventricular collapse (*red arrow, D*). This is indicative of pericardial tamponade. He received aggressive fluid resuscitation and emergent pericardial drainage.

Table 1
Multidetector computed tomography protocol for imaging traumatic cardiac injuries at Vancouver General Hospital

Technique	Prospective ECG-Gated Cardiac CT
Tube potential	100 kV for BMI <30 120 kV for BMI >30
Tube current	300–500 mA with ECG tube current modulation
Scan direction	Cranial to caudal
Scan volume	Heart to diaphragm (14–16 cm)
Size	0.5–0.6 mm reconstruction with 40% overlap, 512 × 512 matrix, FOV 25 cm
Detector collimation	128 × 0.6 mm
Cardiac phase reconstruction	Relative triggering 30%–40% of RR interval, or Absolute triggering 250 ms after R wave
Contrast bolus tracking	An automated bolus-tracking algorithm is used to monitor the attenuation within the ascending aorta; CT scanning is automatically triggered when vessel enhancement reaches 100 Hounsfield units after contrast injection
IV contrast injection	50–80 mL Optiray contrast, followed by 50 mL 30% contrast/70% saline mixture, and finally 30 mL of saline
IV contrast injection rate	5 mL/s
Heart rate	Baseline
Beta-blocker	May be utilized
Nitroglycerine	May be utilized

Abbreviations: BMI, body mass index; CT, computed tomography; ECG, electrocardiogram; FOV, field of view; IV, intravenous.

Dose-reduction can be achieved by (1) use of prospective ECG-gated technique with narrow window acquisition, ECG tube current modulation and limited pulse windows; (2) utilization of BMI-based tube voltage reduction; (3) automated kV reduction tool based on tomogram attenuation profile; (4) adaptive collimation limiting helical over spiral scanning; (5) deploying iterative reconstructive techniques to reduce noise and ultimately reduce dose.

The quality of the cardiac CT can be optimized by achieving (1) heart rate <65 beats per minute by administering beta-blocker (metoprolol 5–20 mg IV or 50–100 mg orally) 1 hour before the CT; lowering the heart rate widens diastole and decreases beat to beat variability; (2) coronary arterial dilatation for optimal visualization can be achieved by administering 0.4 to 0.8 mg SL nitroglycerine 5 minutes before contrast injection; (3) reconstruction algorithms to reduce beam-hardening artifacts due to iodine mimicking ischemia; (4) edge enhancing reconstruction algorithms usage to reduce noise due to extensive coronary calcifications or coronary stents.

presenting with suspected cardiac trauma at our institution.

Recent advances in dual-energy CT (DECT), which uses 2 distinct energy levels to differentiate materials that have similar attenuation values on conventional CT, may be valuable in detecting blunt cardiac trauma. DECT can be used to generate perfusion mapping of the heart, as shown in **Fig. 4**, by quantifying the amount of iodine based on the attenuation characteristics of iodine when it is penetrated by 2 X-ray spectra at different energy levels. Based on this principle, iodine maps can be generated to assess for the luminal patency of coronary arteries and myocardial function and perfusion at greater accuracy than single-energy CT.[16,17] Although not routinely used in clinical practice, DECT has great potential in the future of cardiac trauma imaging.

MR Imaging

MR Imaging is not indicated in the setting of acute cardiac trauma because of its long acquisition time, but may be used to detect posttraumatic complications. Delayed enhancement MR Imaging, which involves the injection of gadolinium agents followed by T1-weighted pulse sequence 10 to 30 minutes later, can demonstrate areas of post-traumatic myocardial infarction (MI) and distinguish between viable and nonviable myocardium.[18]

SPECTRUM OF FINDINGS IN CARDIAC TRAUMA
Pericardial Contusion/Rupture/Cardiac Luxation

The pericardial space lies between the visceral and parietal layers of the pericardium and may

MANAGEMENT ALGORITHM FOR BLUNT CARDIAC AND THORACIC TRAUMA

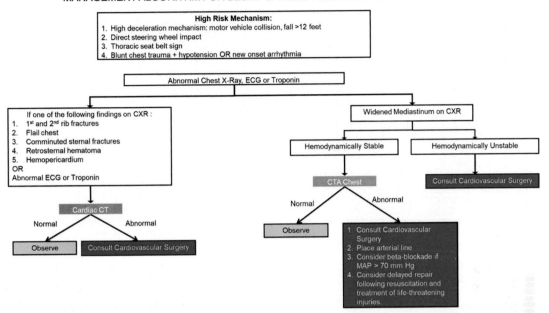

Fig. 3. The clinical algorithm for management of blunt cardiac and thoracic trauma at Vancouver General Hospital. CXR, chest radiograph. (*Courtesy of* Vancouver General Hospital, Vancouver, British Columbia, Canada; with permission.)

normally contain up to 50 mL of serous fluid that facilitates movement of the heart within the pericardium. Pericardial injuries range from small pericardial contusions (shown in **Fig. 5**) to large contusions that result in pericardial tamponade (shown in **Fig. 6**) by forming clots to seal the fibrous pericardium and prevent hemorrhagic extravasation into the thoracic cavity. Pericardial tears, however, can extend across the entire pericardium and result in pericardial rupture (shown in **Fig. 7**). They account for 0.5% of all patients with blunt trauma, but is a highly fatal finding, with mortality rates of 25%.[19]

The most lethal complication of pericardial injury is cardiac luxation (shown in **Fig. 8**), which is associated with right-sided pericardial tears. It occurs when the heart becomes dislocated into the right hemithorax and torsed along the axis made by the inferior vena cava and the great vessels. This can result in arrhythmias and hypotension causing hemodynamic collapse. Tears along the diaphragmatic surface of the pericardium may result in either cardiac herniation into the abdomen or the herniation of abdominal contents into the pericardium (shown in **Fig. 9**).[20]

On chest radiograph, the presence of air within the pericardium (ie, pneumopericardium) is suggestive of underlying pericardial injury. Cardiac

luxation and herniation can manifest in the displacement of the cardiac silhouette, an unusually shaped cardiac contour, as well as the presence of colonic contents within the pericardium.[20]

CT provides higher spatial resolution, and can help differentiate pneumopericardium from pneumomediastinum and pneumothorax. Focal pericardial defect is a direct indication of pericardial injury and can be seen as dimpling or discontinuity within the pericardium. Cardiac herniation manifests in altered cardiac axis, presence of air within the empty pericardium ("empty pericardial sac sign"), and altered cardiac contour ("collar sign"). In contrast to radiographs, CT provides excellent resolution of pericardial effusions. The combination of hemorrhagic fluid within the pericardium, distended central veins (inferior vena cava, superior vena cava, hepatic and renal veins), and displaced cardiac chamber contour are all suggestive of cardiac tamponade.[20]

Myocardial/Ventricular Contusion/Rupture

Myocardial contusion occurs after the myocardium impacts against the sternum or the vertebrae, or from shearing forces within the thorax. It occurs in 10% to 75% of all blunt cardiac traumas and is associated with deceleration

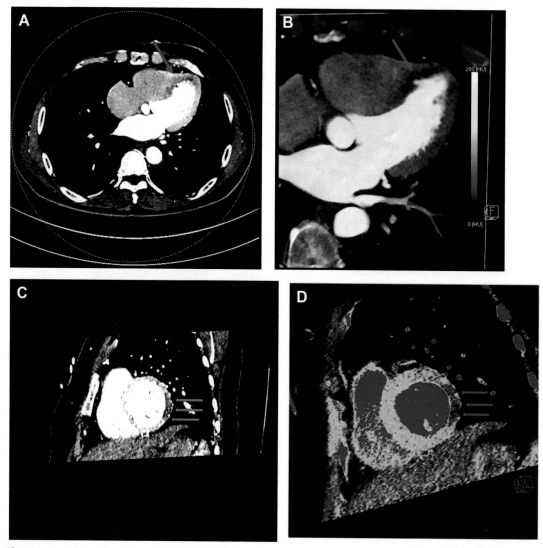

Fig. 4. Conventional CT (*A*) and DECT (*B*) showing decreased iodine uptake in the septal wall suggesting decreased perfusion to the area (*red arrows*). Conventional CT (*C*) and DECT (*D*) in another patient shows a perfusion defect in the left ventricular free wall (*blue and red arrows*, respectively).

injuries where the body is moving at more than 20 miles per hour.[13,21] There is a large variance in reported incidence because definitive diagnosis can be made only by seeing myocardial necrosis on histologic samples, which can be attained only at the time of autopsy.[21] On histology, there are patchy areas of necrosis and hemorrhage, which eventually heal by myocardial fibrosis and scarring. In contrast to MI, in which there is gradual transition between infarcted tissue and normal tissue on histology, myocardial contusion results in a distinct boundary between normal and contused tissue.[21]

The right ventricle is particularly susceptible to myocardial contusion because of its anterior and

retrosternal location. Although MDCT may be nonspecific for myocardial contusion, it is more useful for detecting associated mediastinal, pulmonary, and aortic injuries.[22] **Fig. 10** shows a case of myocardial contusion with associated pulmonary injuries.

Myocardial rupture is a rare, but often-fatal injury with a reported incidence of 0.16% to 2% among all trauma patients.[23] It can result from direct compression of the heart and increased intrathoracic pressure, or may be a delayed complication of myocardial contusion.[24] The disruption and rupture of myocardium leads to pericardial effusion and tamponade, and also can cause conduction abnormalities and result in

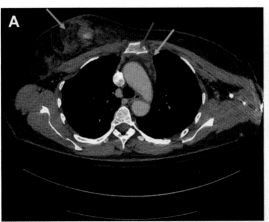

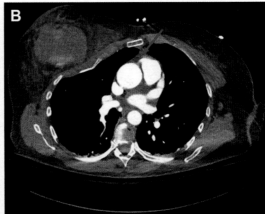

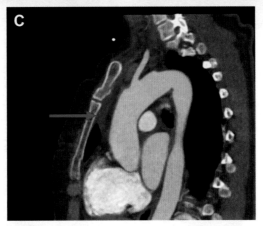

Fig. 5. A 61-year-old woman brought to hospital after polytrauma following motor vehicle collision. (*A*) A CT angiogram of the chest showed a comminuted fracture of the sternal manubrium (*red arrow*) with associated mediastinal hematoma (*green arrow*). There is also active bleeding from a branch of the right internal mammary artery, manifesting in breast hematoma (*orange arrow*). (*B, C*) The mediastinal hematoma (*red arrows*) extends to the origins of the aorta and the pulmonary trunk. This pattern of injury is suspicious for cardiac contusion.

arrhythmias. Early diagnosis is crucial for guiding prompt surgical management of myocardial rupture. MDCT may show focal myocardial disruption/discontinuity, communication between cardiac chambers and the pericardial space, or active contrast extravasation into the surrounding space.[25] This is shown in **Fig. 11**.

Traumatic Septal Defect

Ventricular septal defects (VSDs) are the most common type of traumatic septal defects, with a reported incidence between 1% and 5% following cardiac trauma.[26] Early VSDs occur within 48 hours from the initial trauma and result either from mechanical compression of the heart

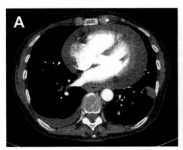

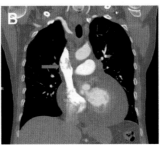

Fig. 6. MDCT showing signs of cardiac tamponade, which includes (*A*) inversion of the right atrial wall (*dashed blue curve*), and (*B*) distention of the superior vena cava (*blue arrow*), both of which are signs of increased intracardiac pressure.

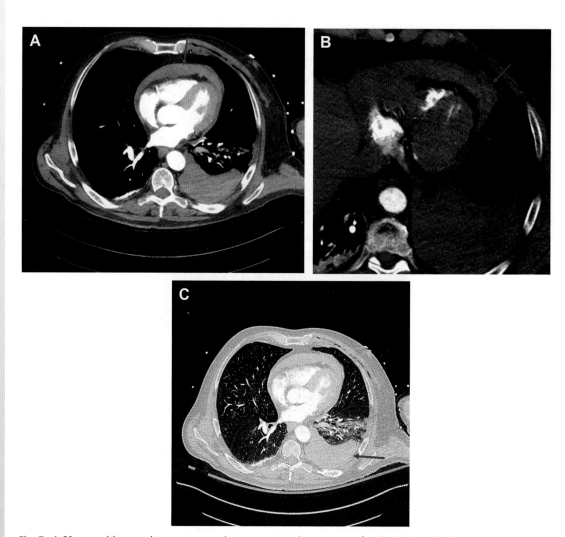

Fig. 7. A 60-year-old man who presents to the emergency department after being impaled by a spike. ECG-gated arterial-phase CT with cardiac reformats was performed. (*A*) There is a moderate-sized hemorrhagic pericardial effusion (*red arrow*) (average attenuation = 66 Hounsfield units). (*B*) There is also a small volume of blood (*red arrow*) lying outside the pericardial surface in keep with penetrating pericardial injury and pericardial tear. (*C*) In the lung window, there is also an associated left lower lobe laceration (*green arrow*) with moderate-sized left hemothorax (*red arrow*, average attenuation = 72 Hounsfield units). An emergent sternotomy was performed with evacuation of hemopericardium and hemothorax. The pericardial tear was repaired, and the patient recovered well with no complications.

or from penetrating injuries. The ventricles are most vulnerable to compression during late diastole after the atrial kick, when the they are filled with blood and all the valves are closed. Late VSDs occur as delayed complications from inflammatory response, which leads to disruption of microvascular flow, causing liquefactive infarction and septal rupture. Early VSDs are often larger and more severe septal defects that require emergent surgery and are associated with higher mortality. By contrast, late VSD rarely requires emergent surgery and has more favorable prognoses.[27] Traumatic atrial septal defects (ASDs)

and combined ASDs and VSDs are less common, although they have been reported in case studies.[28,29]

Valve Injuries

Valve injuries after cardiac trauma are rarely reported in the literature. Aortic and mitral valves are the most commonly involved valves because of the higher intramural pressure in the left heart. They are injured when there is increased intracardiac pressure across a closed competent valve. The aortic valve is most vulnerable during

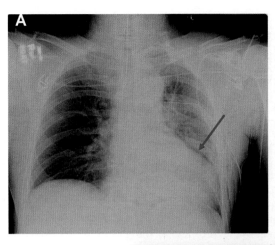

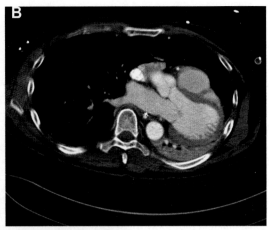

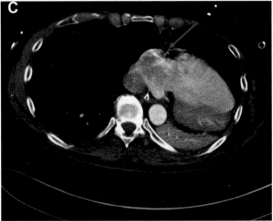

Fig. 8. A 59-year-old man involved in motor vehicle accident after rolling over while traveling at 100 km/h. (*A*) Chest radiograph shows a left-deviated cardiac shadow with pneumopericardium (*red arrow*). (*B*) ECG-gated cardiac CT performed showed that the cardiac apex is posterolaterally displaced to the left. (*C*) There is dimpling and indentation along the right atrioventricular wall with herniation of pericardial fat (*red arrow*). These findings are suspicious for pericardial rupture with cardiac luxation. This patient subsequently underwent bovine patch repair of the pericardial rupture.

early diastole when a traumatic force can generate high pressure gradients across the aortic valve, resulting in the tear of one of the aortic valve cusps (most commonly the noncoronary cusp). The mitral valve is most easily injured during late diastole and early systole when the

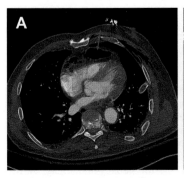

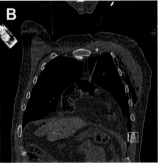

Fig. 9. An 84-year-old gentleman who was a restrained driver in a motor vehicle crash in which he was T-boned from the driver's side. Axial (*A*) and coronal (*B*) reformats of contrast-enhanced CT of the chest, which was performed as part of the whole-body CT, showed that the colon and omental fat (*red arrows*) extends superiorly from the abdomen into the pericardial sac adjacent to the heart, causing significant mass effect on the right heart. This is concerning for traumatic rupture of the central tendon of the diaphragm. He proceeded to the operating room, where the transverse colon and omentum was pulled down from the chest and the diaphragmatic hernia was repaired.

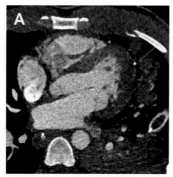
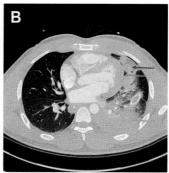

Fig. 10. A 29-year-old man presenting with thoracoabdominal gunshot wound and hemorrhagic shock. ECG-gated spiral CT coronary angiogram was performed with functional imaging. (A) There was a bullet fragment (*red arrow*) adjacent to the left ventricular side wall at the mid-cardiac level outside the myocardium. On functional imaging (not shown), there is marked hypokinesis at this level consistent with myocardial contusion. (B) There is also small residual left pneumothorax with extensive pulmonary contusions (*red arrow*), hemothorax (*green arrow*), and pneumatocele formation (*orange arrow*) suggestive of pulmonary laceration.

inciting force impacts on the fully loaded ventricle and stretches the mitral apparatus. The most common mitral valve injury is the rupture of papillary muscles, followed by chordae tendineae and leaflet injury.[30]

Coronary Artery Injuries

Coronary artery injuries account for approximately 2% of all blunt cardiac trauma and range from intimal tears to complete coronary artery rupture. MI can result from coronary artery intimal tears or vasospasm, disruption of atherosclerotic plaques, and epicardial hematoma.[31] The left anterior descending (LAD) artery is the most commonly injured artery due to its anterior location in the heart. In a literature review of 77 patients with MI following blunt cardiac trauma, Christensen and colleagues[32] found that the LAD artery injury occurred in 71% of patients, followed by the right coronary artery (19.0%), the left main coronary artery (6.4%), and the left circumflex artery (3.2%). Fig. 12 shows a case of traumatic occlusion of the left circumflex artery. The prognosis of

traumatic MI is generally favorable (with a mortality rate of 6.5%), as most patients are younger than 45 and have only single-vessel involvement.

Compared with traumatic MI, coronary artery rupture results from higher-energy traumatic forces and can often have fatal consequences, as it leads to sudden development of hemopericardium and cardiac tamponade. It can occur from laceration by an adjacent rib, from shearing forces during cranio-caudal deceleration, or from chest compression during held inspiration (ie, Compression-Valsalva injury), which leads to sudden increases in the intramural pressure within the coronary arteries. Coronary artery rupture tends to occur in elderly patients with underlying atherosclerosis, as the disease remodels the coronary vessels into rigid tubes that are more prone to rupture. The accumulation of blood in the pericardium leads to the development of cardiac tamponade, resulting in hemodynamic shock. Despite its grim prognosis, Abu-Hmeidan and colleagues[31] found that there is often a sufficient time-window (ranging from 2 to 56 hours) between initial injury to death, which provides adequate time for

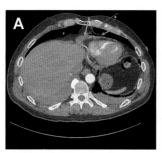
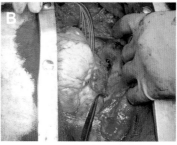

Fig. 11. A 49-year-old man who presented to the hospital after suffering 3 stab wounds to the chest. (A) On arterial-phase CT chest, there are anterior chest wall stab tracts (*red arrows*) that pass the entire chest wall to the pleural space. There is a moderate-volume hemopericardium (*green arrow*) with an internal air-fluid level (*orange arrow*). This was suspicious for penetrating injury of the right ventricular myocardium. (B) He was taken to the operating room, where it was found that there was a full-thickness laceration of the right atrium. He subsequently underwent repair of the right atrium.

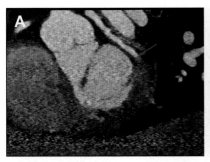
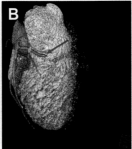

Fig. 12. A 34-year old man who suffered blunt chest trauma after falling from a snowboard. He had persistent chest pain refractory to morphine, and his troponin was elevated at 1.35. ECG-gated CT (*A*) and post-processed 3-dimensional model of the heart (*B*) show the left circumflex artery abrupt cutoff (*red arrows*), in keeping with traumatic occlusion. He was treated with aspiration thrombectomy and drug-eluting stent placed in the left circumflex artery. He was discharged with dual-antiplatelet therapy for 1 year and aspirin for life.

patients to undergo appropriate operative management.

Because of its noninvasive nature, rapid acquisition times, and high spatial and temporal resolution, ECG-gated MDCT is often used as the first-line modality for imaging of coronary tears, dissection, and thrombosis. These patients can be further assessed using coronary angiography or intracoronary ultrasound to guide proper management.[33]

Injuries to the Great Vessels

Injuries to the aortic root and ascending aorta account for approximately 5% of all thoracic aorta injuries. Azizzadeh and colleagues[34] categorized traumatic aortic injuries into 4 grades based on severity: (1) grade 1: intimal tear/minimal aortic injury; (2) grade 2: intramural hematoma; (3) grade 3: aortic pseudoaneurysms; and (4) grade 4: free rupture. Patients with grade 1 injuries can be managed medically, but those with higher-grade injuries require operative

interventions with either open repair or endovascular graft repair. MDCT has recently replaced conventional aortography for detecting ascending aortic injuries, and has a negative predictive value approaching 100%.[35] **Figs. 13** and **14** show grade 1 and grade 2 injuries of the ascending aorta, respectively.

Injuries to the pulmonary artery are extremely rare in patients presenting with thoracic trauma. In a series of 585 autopsies conducted after blunt trauma, only 4 had injury to the main pulmonary artery.[36] They are, however, fatal injuries with survival rates of less than 30%.[37] Thus, it is important to be vigilant for pulmonary artery injuries, which can occur from deceleration, fall from a height, or from imprints from the steering wheel. Patients can present in various ways: (1) massive hemothorax from injury to the hilar structures; (2) contained hemorrhage leading to aneurysm formation; (3) delayed onset of large pleural effusion; and (4) pericardial tamponade.[38] Chest radiograph may show widened

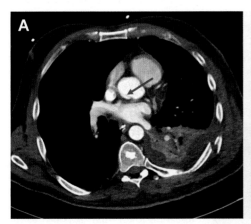
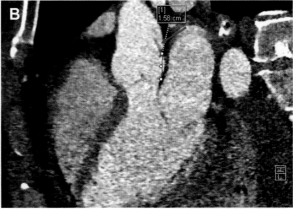

Fig. 13. Axial (*A*) and Sagittal (*B*) reformats of ECG-gated CT images obtained following intravenous contrast shows that there is a short flap arising in the noncoronary cusp of the aortic valve (*red arrows*), (approximately 16 mm distal to the aortic annulus) in the proximal ascending aorta. This was deemed to be not requiring operative intervention and the patient remained stable over the remainder course of hospitalization.

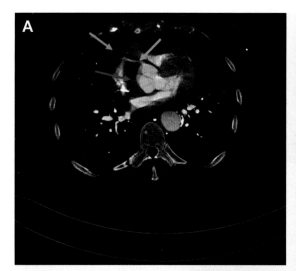

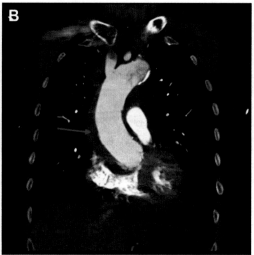

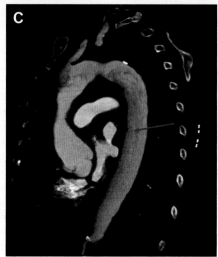

Fig. 14. Axial (*A*), coronal (*B*), and sagittal (*C*) images of a 65-year-old woman who received intravenous contrast-enhanced trauma protocol of the chest, abdomen, and pelvis. There is a crescent-shaped intramural hematoma (*red arrows*) arising from the aortic root along the ascending aorta, as well as an area of contrast extravasation (*green arrow*) at the junction of the ascending and proximal transverse aorta. In addition, there is a component of hemopericardium (*orange arrow*), and mixing of blood within the aorta (*purple arrow*).

mediastinum, first rib fracture, scapular fracture, or hemopneumothorax.[37] MDCT may demonstrate active contrast extravasation from the pulmonary artery and allows for surgical planning before thoracotomy. **Fig. 15** shows an example of pulmonary artery injury.

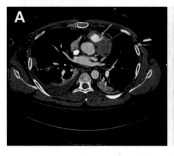

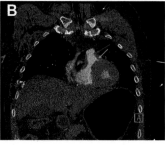

Fig. 15. Axial (*A*) and coronal (*B*) images of pulmonary artery injury following motor vehicle accident. There is soft tissue thickening representing contained hematoma (*red arrows*) surrounding the pulmonary trunk with irregular contrast pooling (*green arrows*) that appears to be continuous with the main pulmonary trunk, suggestive of pulmonary artery injury.

SUMMARY

Traumatic cardiac trauma is the second most common cause of trauma-related deaths. Clinicians should have a high index suspicion for cardiac injuries following chest trauma. Diagnostic imaging plays a crucial role in directing the early diagnosis and management of cardiac trauma. In the past few decades, MDCT has evolved to become the gold-standard imaging modality because of its rapid acquisition, high resolution, and noninvasive nature. To accurately diagnose and characterize the extent of cardiac injuries, radiologists need to understand the mechanism of cardiac trauma and become familiar with the common injury patterns.

REFERENCES

1. El-Chami MF, Nicholson W, Helmy T. Blunt cardiac trauma. J Emerg Med 2008;35(2):127–33.
2. van Wijngaarden MH, Karmy-Jones R, Talwar MK, et al. Blunt cardiac injury: a 10 year institutional review. Injury 1997;28(1):51–5.
3. Navid F, Gleason TG. Great vessel and cardiac trauma: diagnostic and management strategies. Semin Thorac Cardiovasc Surg 2008;20(1):31–8.
4. Restrepo CS, Gutierrez FR, Marmol-Velez JA, et al. Imaging patients with cardiac trauma. Radiographics 2012;32(3):633–49.
5. Campbell NC, Thomson SR, Muckart DJ, et al. Review of 1198 cases of penetrating cardiac trauma. Br J Surg 1997;84(12):1737–40.
6. Mina MJ, Jhunjhunwala R, Gelbard RB, et al. Factors affecting mortality after penetrating cardiac injuries: 10-year experience at urban level I trauma center. Am J Surg 2017;213(6):1109–15.
7. Bertinchant JP, Polge A, Mohty D, et al. Evaluation of incidence, clinical significance, and prognostic value of circulating cardiac troponin I and T elevation in hemodynamically stable patients with suspected myocardial contusion after blunt chest trauma. J Trauma 2000;48(5):924–31.
8. Clancy K, Velopulos C, Bilaniuk JW, et al. Screening for blunt cardiac injury: an Eastern Association for the Surgery of Trauma practice management guideline. J Trauma Acute Care Surg 2012;73(5 Suppl 4):S301–6.
9. García-Fernández MA, López-Pérez JM, Pérez-Castellano N, et al. Role of transesophageal echocardiography in the assessment of patients with blunt chest trauma: correlation of echocardiographic findings with the electrocardiogram and creatine kinase monoclonal antibody measurements. Am Heart J 1998;135(3):476–81.
10. Chung JH, Cox CW, Mohammed TL, et al. ACR appropriateness criteria blunt chest trauma. J Am Coll Radiol 2014;11(4):345–51.
11. Vignon P, Boncoeur MP, François B, et al. Comparison of multiplane transesophageal echocardiography and contrast-enhanced helical CT in the diagnosis of blunt traumatic cardiovascular injuries. Anesthesiology 2001;94(4):615–22 [discussion: 615A].
12. Fowler NO. Cardiac tamponade. A clinical or an echocardiographic diagnosis? Circulation 1993; 87(5):1738–41.
13. Co SJ, Yong-Hing CJ, Galea-Soler S, et al. Role of imaging in penetrating and blunt traumatic injury to the heart. Radiographics 2011;31(4):E101–15.
14. Chirillo F, Totis O, Cavarzerani A, et al. Usefulness of transthoracic and transoesophageal echocardiography in recognition and management of cardiovascular injuries after blunt chest trauma. Heart 1996; 75(3):301–6.
15. Malbranque G, Serfaty JM, Himbert D, et al. Myocardial infarction after blunt chest trauma: usefulness of cardiac ECG-gated CT and MRI for positive and aetiologic diagnosis. Emerg Radiol 2011; 18(3):271–4.
16. Schwarz F, Ruzsics B, Schoepf UJ, et al. Dual-energy CT of the heart—principles and protocols. Eur J Radiol 2008;68(3):423–33.
17. Sade R, Kantarci M, Ogul H, et al. The feasibility of dual-energy computed tomography in cardiac contusion imaging for mildest blunt cardiac injury. J Comput Assist Tomogr 2017;41(3):354–9.
18. Vogel-Claussen J, Rochitte CE, Wu KC, et al. Delayed enhancement MR imaging: utility in myocardial assessment. Radiographics 2006;26(3): 795–810.
19. Chughtai T, Chiavaras MM, Sharkey P, et al. Pericardial rupture with cardiac herniation. Can J Surg 2008;51(5):E101–2.
20. Adams A, Fotiadis N, Chin JY, et al. A pictorial review of traumatic pericardial injuries. Insights Imaging 2012;3(4):307–11.
21. Bansal MK, Maraj S, Chewaproug D, et al. Myocardial contusion injury: redefining the diagnostic algorithm. Emerg Med J 2005;22(7):465–9.
22. Baxi AJ, Restrepo C, Mumbower A, et al. Cardiac injuries: a review of multidetector computed tomography findings. Trauma Mon 2015;20(4):e19086.
23. Nan YY, Lu MS, Liu KS, et al. Blunt traumatic cardiac rupture: therapeutic options and outcomes. Injury 2009;40(9):938–45.
24. Pevec WC, Udekwu AO, Peitzman AB. Blunt rupture of the myocardium. Ann Thorac Surg 1989;48(1): 139–42.
25. Golshani B, Dong P, Evans S. Traumatic cardiac injury: ventricular perforation caught on CT. Case Rep Radiol 2016;2016:9696107.
26. Olsovsky MR, Topaz O, DiSciascio G, et al. Acute traumatic ventricular septal rupture. Am Heart J 1996;131(5):1039–41.

27. Ryan L, Skinner DL, Rodseth RN. Ventricular septal defect following blunt chest trauma. J Emerg Trauma Shock 2012;5(2):184–7.

28. Ortiz Y, Waldman AJ, Bott JN, et al. Blunt chest trauma resulting in both atrial and ventricular septal defects. Echocardiography 2015;32(3):592–4.

29. Menaker J, Tesoriero RB, Hyder M, et al. Traumatic atrial septal defect and papillary muscle rupture requiring mitral valve replacement after blunt injury. J Trauma 2009;67(5):1126.

30. Kan CD, Yang YJ. Traumatic aortic and mitral valve injury following blunt chest injury with a variable clinical course. Heart 2005;91(5):568–70.

31. Abu-Hmeidan JH, Arrowaili AI, Yousef RS, et al. Coronary artery rupture in blunt thoracic trauma: a case report and review of literature. J Cardiothorac Surg 2016;11(1):119.

32. Christensen MD, Nielsen PE, Sleight P. Prior blunt chest trauma may be a cause of single vessel coronary disease; hypothesis and review. Int J Cardiol 2006;108(1):1–5.

33. Torres-Ayala SC, Maldonado J, Bolton JS, et al. Coronary computed tomography angiography of spontaneous coronary artery dissection: a case report and review of the literature. Am J Case Rep 2015; 16:130–5.

34. Azizzadeh A, Keyhani K, Miller CC, et al. Blunt traumatic aortic injury: initial experience with endovascular repair. J Vasc Surg 2009;49(6):1403–8.

35. Sun X, Hong J, Lowery R, et al. Ascending aortic injuries following blunt trauma. J Card Surg 2013; 28(6):749–55.

36. Mattox KL. Approaches to trauma involving the major vessels of the thorax. Surg Clin North Am 1989; 69(1):77–91.

37. Daon E, Gorton ME. Traumatic disruption of the innominate and right pulmonary arteries: case report. J Trauma 1997;43(4):701–2.

38. Ambrose G, Barrett LO, Angus GL, et al. Main pulmonary artery laceration after blunt trauma: accurate preoperative diagnosis. Ann Thorac Surg 2000;70(3):955–7.

Imaging of Traumatic Shoulder Girdle Injuries

Nicholas M. Beckmann, MD*, Latifa Sanhaji, MD, Naga R. Chinapuvvula, MD,
O. Clark West, MD

KEYWORDS

- Trauma • Shoulder • Classification • Glenohumeral • Acromioclavicular • Sternoclavicular
- Humerus • Scapula

KEY POINTS

- Traumatic shoulder girdle injuries are a common injury encountered in the emergency center.
- It is vital that the appropriate radiographic positioning is performed when evaluating for suspected injury of the shoulder girdle, because shoulder girdle injuries can be easily missed on imaging.
- Upright radiographs should also be performed whenever possible to avoid misdiagnosis or under-diagnosis of injury to the shoulder.
- Advanced imaging using computed tomography or magnetic resonance imaging is usually not required to assess shoulder girdle injuries.
- However, a low threshold should be held for performing advanced imaging when there is suspected scapula injury, shoulder instability, or injury to the medial clavicle.

INTRODUCTION

The shoulder girdle is the musculoskeletal architecture that connects the arm to the thorax and is defined as the scapula, clavicle, and supporting soft tissues. Traumatic shoulder girdle injuries are one of the most common injuries seen in trauma patients presenting to emergency centers. Like many types of traumatic injury, shoulder girdle trauma has a bimodal age and gender distribution, with shoulder girdle injuries occurring most frequently in young men and elderly women.[1] The spectrum of shoulder girdle injuries is broad, ranging from mild soft tissue contusions that can be managed conservatively to complex combined fracture and soft tissue injuries, resulting in dissociation of the upper extremity from the thorax that may require emergent surgical stabilization and treatment of concomitant neurovascular injuries.

Shoulder girdle injuries can be difficult to diagnose on clinical examination due to the intimate relationship between the shoulder and thorax, which can result in posttraumatic deformity of the shoulder girdle being masked by normal thoracic soft tissue contours. Imaging plays a vital role in both identification and characterization of traumatic shoulder girdle injuries. However, identification of shoulder girdle injuries on imaging can be challenging as well. The complex osteology of the shoulder as well as supine positioning for imaging can result in the misdiagnosis of shoulder girdle injuries and underappreciation of the extent of injury.

In this article, the authors review the epidemiology, mechanism, classification, and imaging evaluation of the most important traumatic injuries of the shoulder girdle to identify in patients presenting to the emergency center. For this review, the imaging evaluation is focused on the radiographic and computerized tomographic (CT) appearance of injuries, because these are the 2 predominate imaging modalities used in the emergency center to assess shoulder girdle injuries.

Department of Diagnostic and Interventional Imaging, McGovern Medical School, The University of Texas Health Science Center at Houston, 6431 Fannin Street, 2.130B, Houston, TX 77030, USA
* Correspondong author.
E-mail address: Nicholas.M.Beckmann@uth.tmc.edu

Radiol Clin N Am 57 (2019) 809–822
https://doi.org/10.1016/j.rcl.2019.02.013
0033-8389/19/© 2019 Elsevier Inc. All rights reserved.

Although not a focus of the review, the role of magnetic resonance imaging (MR imaging) in evaluating associated injuries is also discussed.

DISCUSSION
Osseous Anatomy

The clavicle is a long bone that serves as a bridge between the sternum and scapula (**Fig. 1**A). In order to accommodate the wide range of motion about the shoulder, the clavicle has precarious bony support at its articulations, relying mainly on soft tissues to maintain alignment. The medial two-thirds of the clavicle are tubular, with the medial end of the clavicle considered the head of the clavicle. Along the undersurface of the clavicle head is the attachment site of the costoclavicular ligament. This attachment site may be visualized as either a raised (called the costal tubercle) or depressed (called the rhomboid fossa) region along the inferior clavicle surface. The lateral third of the clavicle is more bladelike in appearance and contains the conoid tubercle along the undersurface of the clavicle, which is the insertion site of the conoid band of the coracoclavicular ligament.

The clavicle articulates with the manubrium medially at the sternoclavicular joint and the scapula laterally at the acromioclavicular (AC) joint. Most of the stability of both of these joints is derived from strong intrinsic and extrinsic ligaments. Most of the stability of the sternoclavicular joint is created by strong anterior and posterior sternoclavicular capsule ligaments with the costoclavicular ligament, interclavicular ligament, and articular disc providing minor support. The 2 main stabilizers of the AC joint are the superior and inferior acromioclavicular capsule ligaments and the coracoclavicular ligament, which spans from the coracoid process of the scapula to the undersurface of the lateral clavicle. The coracoclavicular ligament is composed of 2 bands: the conoid band that attaches to the conoid tubercle of the clavicle and the trapezoid band that attaches lateral to the conoid tubercle.

The scapula is a triangle-shaped bone composed of a body, glenoid, and 2 processes (**Fig. 1**B). The main triangle portion of the scapula is the body that has 3 borders: superior, medial, and lateral. The scapula body tapers laterally to form the glenoid, which articulates with the humeral head at the glenohumeral joint. The glenoid neck forms the cylinder of bone bridging the glenoid articular surface with the scapula body. The 2 processes of the scapula, the acromion and coracoid, are involved in the articulation between the scapula and clavicle as well as serve as attachment sites for several muscles.

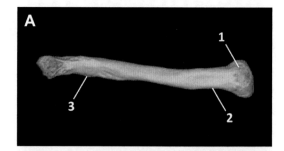

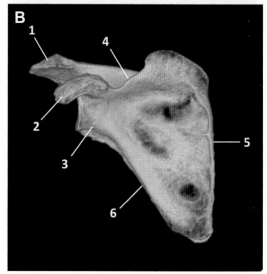

Fig. 1. Osseous anatomy of the clavicle and scapula. (*A*) Frontal view of the clavicle: (1) clavicle head, (2) costal tubercle, (3) conoid tubercle. (*B*) Frontal view of the scapula: (1) acromion process, (2) coracoid process, (3) gelnoid neck, (4) superior border, (5) medial border, (6) lateral border.

Sternoclavicular Joint Injury

Sternoclavicular joint injuries are rare traumatic injuries of the shoulder girdle. Sternoclavicular joint injuries comprise 1% to 3% of all shoulder girdle injuries, with a reported annual incidence of only approximately 3 cases per 100,000 people.[2,3] Because of their rarity, the demographics of sternoclavicular injuries are difficult to determine. Like most traumatic injuries, there is a predilection for sternoclavicular joint injuries to occur in men, with a reported man to woman ratio of 1.3 to 2.0:1.[3,4] Most sternoclavicular joint injuries are seen in young to middle-aged adults. The average reported age at the time of injury is 29 to 40 years.[3,4]

Anterior sternoclavicular joint dislocations are more common than posterior dislocations, although, exactly how much more frequent is a debated question. Anterior sternoclavicular joint dislocations have been reported as being from

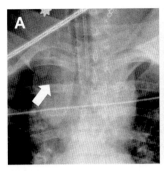
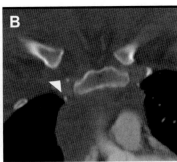

Fig. 2. Anterior sternoclavicular dislocation. (*A*) Coned AP chest radiograph centered at the sternoclavicular joints shows widening of the right sternoclavicular joint (*arrow*). (*B*) Widening is better appreciated on coronal CT image of the chest (*arrowhead*).

1.5 to 9 times more common than posterior dislocations.[2–4] Anterior dislocations most commonly occur from an indirect force caused by a blow to the lateral aspect of the shoulder, and patients will typically present with pain and palpable lump over the sternoclavicular joint. Posterior dislocations are the result of either direct impact to the sternoclavicular joint driving the clavicle posterior or an indirect blow to the posterolateral shoulder. A subtle depression of the skin surface can be seen in posterior dislocations; however, this depression may be masked by soft tissue swelling, making posterior dislocations difficult to diagnosis on physical examination. Posterior dislocations have a significantly higher rate of complications than anterior dislocations, because the posteriorly displaced clavicle can compress the airway, esophagus, or neurovascular structures in the upper mediastinum. Almost one-third of patients with posterior sternoclavicular dislocation report dyspnea and/or dysphagia at presentation, and approximately 15% will have evidence of vascular compression.[5]

Sternoclavicular joint dislocations can be impossible to diagnosis on standard shoulder radiographs and easily missed on clavicle radiographs. A typical clavicle series is composed of 2 images: a standard anteroposterior (AP) view and an AP view with 15° to 30° of cephalic angulation. Malalignment of the sternoclavicular joint is best appreciated on the cephalic angulated view where an anterior dislocation will appear as superior displacement of the medial clavicle relative to the sternoclavicular joint and posterior dislocation will appear as inferior displacement. An anterior oblique view centered on the sternoclavicular joint and with the patient rotated 20° to 30° away from the x-ray tube may also be helpful in identifying malalignment of the sternoclavicular joint when the joint is not well seen on clavicle radiographs. A low threshold should be maintained for obtaining cross-sectional imaging with either CT or MR imaging to assess alignment because of the difficulty

in visualizing the sternoclavicular joint on radiographs (**Fig. 2**). CT with contrast is also recommended for all patients with posterior dislocation identified on radiographs to evaluate the relationship of the clavicle with the airway and mediastinal vascular structures (**Fig. 3**).

The medial clavicle physis is one of the last physes in the body to fuse, typically not fusing until 22 to 25 years of age.[6] Approximately half of adolescents and young adults with an unfused medial clavicle physis presenting with sternoclavicular joint injury will have a fracture through the physis instead of a pure sternoclavicular dislocation.[7] Fracture through the physis can be difficult to reduce, increasing the likelihood that the patient will require open reduction.[7] These physeal fractures can be indistinguishable from a true sternoclavicular dislocation on radiographs and CT when the epiphysis lacks mineralization (**Fig. 4A**).

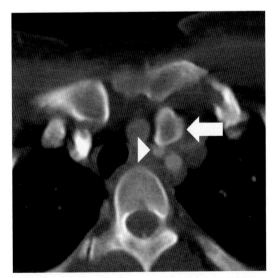

Fig. 3. Posterior sternoclavicular dislocation. Axial CT image of the chest shows posterior displacement of the clavicle head (*arrow*), abutting the left common carotid artery (*arrowhead*).

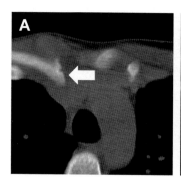
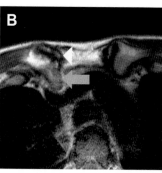

Fig. 4. Sternoclavicular transphyseal fracture-dislocation. (*A*) Axial CT image of chest shows posterior displacement of clavicle head in a 20-year-old man with unossified medial clavicle epiphysis (*white arrow*). (*B*) Axial T2-weighted MR image showing posterior displaced metaphyseal component of clavicle head (*gray arrow*) with epiphyseal component of the clavicle head displaced anteriorly, interposed between the metaphysis of the clavicle head and the sternum (*white arrowhead*).

MR imaging has been shown to effectively demonstrate the displaced epiphyseal fragment of these transphyseal fractures and may be a useful for preoperative planning in patients under the age of 25 years presenting with sternoclavicular joint injury (**Fig. 4B**).[8]

Clavicle Fracture

Clavicle fractures are a fairly common injury, comprising slightly less than 5% of fractures.[9] Most clavicle fractures are the result of a direct blow, either during a fall or high-energy trauma such as a motor vehicle collision. The clavicle can be divided into medial, middle, and lateral thirds, and clavicle fractures are often categorized by which third of the clavicle is involved by the fracture. The middle third of the clavicle is defined as the shaft of the clavicle medial to the conoid tubercle and lateral to the costal tubercle. Fractures through the medial and lateral thirds follow a unimodal distribution in men and women where these fractures are seen most frequently in young men and older women. In distinction, fractures through the middle third of the clavicle have a bimodal age distribution in men where incidence of the fracture peaks in young adults and again in the elderly. Middle third fractures have a unimodal age distribution in women with peak incidence in older women.[9] The decision whether to surgically treat a clavicle fracture is very complex and depends on many factors, including the clavicle fracture pattern, patient functional status, comorbidities, and associated soft tissue and bony injuries. For the purposes of this discussion, the authors focus on the imaging characteristics of the fracture that help guide surgical treatment.

Fractures through the middle third of the clavicle are the most common type of clavicle fractures, comprising 65% to 76% of all cases.[10,11] The more displaced the midclavicle fracture, the more likely surgical fixation will be performed with fractures displaced by more than 1 shaft width, more than 2 cm shortening, or with a "z-shaped" fracture pattern usually requiring fixation (**Fig. 5A**). Midclavicular fractures may also visibly tent the skin on radiographs (**Fig. 5B**). When tenting of the skin is identified, it is important that radiologist alerts the clinician, because these fractures require urgent reduction to avoid soft tissue compromise.

Fractures through the lateral third of the clavicle comprise 22% to 30% of clavicle fractures. Fractures through the distal clavicle can involve the

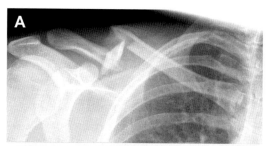
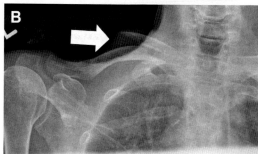

Fig. 5. Middle third clavicle fractures. (*A*) AP view of the clavicle demonstrating the z-shaped, or "zed", fracture pattern of the midclavicle. The z-shaped fracture pattern is a displaced segmental fracture of the clavicle with inferior displacement of the distal fragment and vertical orientation of the segmental fragment producing a characteristic "z-shaped" appearance. (*B*) AP oblique view of the clavicle demonstrating superior displacement of a midclavicle fracture causing tenting of the skin surface (*arrow*).

acromioclavicular joint or coracoclavicular attachment and, therefore, functionally behave as an acromioclavicular separation. The most important characteristics to describe when evaluating these fractures are displacement, comminution, involvement of the acromioclavicular joint, and location relative to the coracoclavicular ligament insertion. The conoid tubercle can be useful as a reference point for the medial margin of the coracoclavicular ligament, with the coracoclavicular ligament extending approximately 1.5 cm lateral to the conoid tubercle (Fig. 6).[12]

Fractures through the medial third of the clavicle are the least common fracture pattern, comprising just 2% to 5% of clavicle fractures. Similar to sternoclavicular joint injuries, medial clavicle fractures can be easily missed on radiographs (Fig. 7). Close inspection of the medial clavicle should be performed on all radiograph examinations of the shoulder and clavicle. Medial clavicle fractures can be categorized similar to sternoclavicular joint injuries as being either anteriorly or posteriorly displaced. Anteriorly displaced fractures are more common and are usually treated nonoperatively. Posteriorly displaced fractures run the same risk of vascular and airway compromise as posterior sternoclavicular dislocation and will typically undergo surgical fixation.

Most clavicle fractures are diagnosed on either routine shoulder or clavicle radiographs. Dedicated clavicle radiographs can be useful in assessing AP displacement of the fracture, which is not easily appreciated on routine shoulder radiographs. It is vital that imaging is performed with the patient upright because supine imaging can underestimate the degree of fracture displacement or mask an associated acromioclavicular separation. CT is rarely needed in assessment of fractures involving the middle and lateral thirds of the clavicle but can be very useful in both the diagnosis and preoperative planning of medial clavicle fractures. There is little utility in MR imaging for the assessment of clavicle fractures.

Acromioclavicular Separation

Any injury to the stabilizing ligaments of the AC joint is termed an "AC separation," even if actual separation of the AC joint does not occur. Most AC separations are the result of direct impact, usually from a fall onto the shoulder. AC joint injuries are one of the most common traumatic soft tissue injuries. The estimated incidence of AC joint injury, including both AC joint contusions and separations, is 45 cases per 100,000 people, and the estimated annual incidence of AC separations alone is 14 cases per 100,000 people.[1,13] The incidence of AC separation varies considerably depending on age and gender. The incidence of AC separations in men peaks in the third decade of life when men have approximately 10 times the incidence of AC separation as women. After the third decade, the incidence of AC separation in men steadily declines until the seventh decade in life when men only have a slightly higher incidence of AC separation compared with women. The incidence of AC separation in women remains relatively steady during the first 5 decades of life followed by a

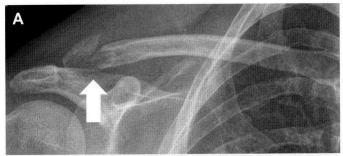

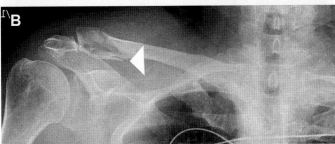

Fig. 6. Distal third clavicle fractures. (*A*) Coned AP radiograph of the clavicle demonstrating mildly displaced distal clavicle fracture distal to the coracoclavicular ligament insertion on the clavicle (*arrow*). (*B*) AP radiograph of the clavicle demonstrating comminuted distal clavicle fracture that extends to involve the conoid tubercle indicating involvement of the coracoclavicular insertion on the clavicle (*arrowhead*).

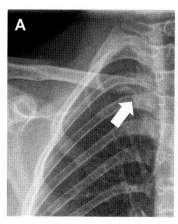
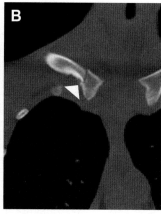

Fig. 7. Medial third clavicle fracture. (*A*) Coned AP view of the clavicle shows subtle fracture through the medial clavicle just medial to the rhomboid fossa (*arrow*). (*B*) Coronal chest CT better demonstrates the mildly displaced medial clavicle fracture (*arrowhead*).

gradual decline in incidence from the sixth to eighth decades.[13]

The Rockwood classification is by far the most widely used classification system for AC separations (**Fig. 8**). In the Rockwood classification, AC separations are divided into 6 types.[14] Type 1 separation represents partial tearing of the AC capsular ligaments. Type 2 separation is rupture of the AC capsular ligaments with intact or incomplete tear of the coracoclavicular ligament. Type 3 separations represent complete rupture of both the AC capsular and coracoclavicular ligaments. Type 4 to 6 AC separations all represent type 3 injuries with an additional soft tissue injury. In type 4 injuries, the distal clavicle is displaced posteriorly through a tear in the trapezius muscle and becomes entrapped. In type 5 injuries, there is significant stripping of the muscle attachments to the distal clavicle, allowing the distal clavicle to become markedly elevated. In type 6 injuries, the distal clavicle is displaced inferiorly and becomes

entrapped below the coracoid process. In general, type 1 and 2 injuries are treated conservatively, type 4 to 6 injuries are treated operatively, and type 3 injuries may be treated conservatively or operatively depending on clinical factors and patient/surgeon preference.

Radiographs are usually adequate for diagnosing and characterizing AC separations. There is quite a bit of variability in the normal AC joint space, which can range from 3 to 6 mm. The coracoclavicular distance is somewhat less variable with a normal distance of approximately 13 mm. Imaging of the contralateral shoulder may be helpful in differentiating AC malalignment from normal anatomic variation in cases of borderline AC widening; however, contralateral films are rarely required. It is imperative that radiographs are performed upright, because an injured AC joint can be partially or completely reduced on a supine radiograph leading to missed diagnosis or underestimating the severity of the AC separation (**Fig. 9**).

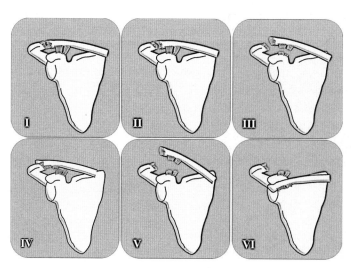

Fig. 8. Rockwood classification for acromioclavicular separations.

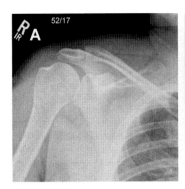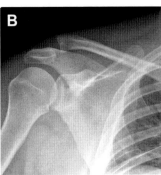

Fig. 9. Missed type III AC separation on supine radiograph. (*A*) Supine AP radiograph demonstrates normal alignment of the AC joint with normal coracoclavicular distance. (*B*) Follow-up upright AP radiograph of the shoulder shows superior displacement of the distal clavicle with widening of both the AC joint and coracoclavicular distance.

The use of a 5-pound weight dangling from the wrist of the injured upper extremity is sometimes used to accentuate the malalignment of the AC joint on radiographs to help with diagnosis. However, the force of gravity on upright imaging provides adequate distraction for grading of AC injuries.

Assessment of AC separations required both upright AP radiograph of the shoulder and an axillary view. The degree of distal clavicle displacement is determined on the AP radiograph. In type 1 injuries, there is minimal or no widening of the AC joint. In type 2 injuries, there is definite widening and/or vertical offset of the AC joint with a normal coracoclavicular distance. In type 3 separations, there is definite widening of the AC joint and coracoclavicular distance. In type 4 separations, the distal clavicle is displaced posteriorly, which may only be appreciated on an axillary view of the shoulder. In type 5 separations, the distal clavicle is markedly displaced superiorly with a coracoclavicular distance more than twice the normal distance (>2.5 cm). In type 6 separations, the distal clavicle is displaced inferiorly below the coracoid process.

In general, MR imaging and CT are not indicated in assessment of AC separations. MR imaging can be useful in confirming entrapment of the distal clavicle within the trapezius muscle in patients with suspected type 4 AC separation on radiographs. MR imaging may also be beneficial in identifying associated injuries as part of preoperative planning for an AC separation requiring surgical treatment, as significant concomitant intraarticular shoulder pathology is identified in between 18% and 39% of patients presenting with high-grade (type III and above) AC separation.[15,16]

Shoulder Dislocation

A "shoulder dislocation" is specifically in reference to dislocation of the glenohumeral joint. Shoulder dislocations are about as common than AC joint separations. The annual incidence of shoulder dislocation has been reported anywhere from 17 to 55 cases per 100,000 people.[1,17,18] Shoulder dislocations have a unimodal distribution in both men and women with peak incidence of male shoulder dislocations in young adults and peak incidence of female shoulder dislocations in elderly patients.[1] Shoulder dislocations are characterized by direction of dislocation, being described as occurring in the anterior, posterior, or inferior direction (**Fig. 10**). Approximately 96% of shoulder dislocations are anterior, 3% are posterior, and less than 1% of dislocations inferior.[17,18] Very rarely, a fracture-dislocation of the humeral head can occur where the humeral head is displaced into the chest cavity, which has been termed an "intrathoracic" dislocation.[19]

A dislocated shoulder requires urgent reduction, so accurate and timely diagnosis is imperative. Anterior dislocations are usually readily apparent on an AP shoulder radiograph depicting the humeral head displaced inferior and medial to its normal articulation with the glenoid. Inferior dislocations are also easily identified on AP shoulder radiographs with the humeral head displaced inferiorly forcing the shoulder into hyperabduction and locking the arm in a raised position termed "luxatio erecta" (see **Fig. 10**B). Unlike anterior and inferior dislocations, posterior dislocations can be very subtle on AP shoulder radiographs. In posterior dislocations, the humeral head is displaced superolateral to its normal articulation with the glenoid; however, this displacement is much less pronounced than the inferomedial displacement seen in anterior dislocations and can be easily missed on AP shoulder radiographs (see **Fig. 10**C, D). A scapula-Y view provides a lateral view of the glenohumeral articulation and can aid in the diagnosis of glenohumeral malalignment. Positioning for the scapula-Y view may be difficult, making it challenging to appreciate subtle malpositioning of the glenohumeral joint that is particularly prevalent in posterior dislocations. A modified axillary view

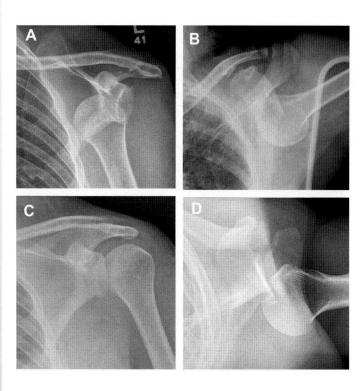

Fig. 10. Glenohumeral shoulder dislocation types. (*A*) Anterior dislocation: the humeral head is displaced inferomedial to its normal location assuming a subcoracoid location. (*B*) Inferior dislocation: the humeral head is displaced inferiorly, forcing the arm into an abduction position termed "luxatio erecta." (*C*) Posterior dislocation: the humeral head is displaced superolateral to its normal position; however, the humeral head displacement is much less pronounced than the displacement seen in other dislocations. (*D*) Axillary view of the patient in image (*C*) shows the posterior dislocation to much better effect.

provides the best image for identifying glenohumeral dislocation. A modified axillary view can be obtained by placing the injured shoulder in 30° of abduction and having the patient lean approximately 10° toward the injured side with the imaging cassette placed either above or below the shoulder. This positioning is much better tolerated in the acute trauma setting than a conventional axillary view that requires 70° to 90° of arm abduction.[20] Although not specific, limited mobility is almost a universal feature of shoulder dislocation. Little change in position between external and internal rotation radiographs of the shoulder should raise suspicion of an occult shoulder dislocation in the setting of trauma. A single AP view with the shoulder in internal rotation in an otherwise normal-appearing examination should also raise concern for a possible posterior shoulder dislocation.

Many patients who have sustained a shoulder dislocation present with reduction of the glenohumeral joint before imaging being obtained. Transient dislocation of the shoulder can be identified by the typical bony injury pattern involving the humeral head and rim of the glenoid. In anterior dislocation, impaction commonly occurs along the posterolateral aspect of the superior humeral head resulting in depression of the humeral head, called a Hill-Sachs lesion. The Hill-Sachs lesion is most commonly appreciated as flattening of the posterosuperior humeral head on an internally rotated AP radiograph of the shoulder (Fig. 11A). A Stryker notch view is a specialized view specifically designed for identification of Hill-Sachs lesions. In a Stryker notch view, the shoulder is placed in abduction and external rotation and a radiograph is obtained with 10° of cephalad angulation.

Impaction also occurs along the anteroinferior rim of the glenoid, which can result in a fracture of the glenoid rim called a Bankart lesion, although a Bankart fracture is less commonly seen than a Hill-Sachs lesion. Bankart fractures are often subtle on AP radiographs of the shoulder but can be appreciated as loss of the thin articular line along the inferior aspect of the glenoid with vertical sclerotic line representing the displaced bone fragment overlying the glenoid neck (Fig. 11B). An axillary view or West Point view is best for identifying Bankart fractures. The West Point view is a modified axillary view where the x-ray beam is directed 25° anterior and 25° medial to obtain an image perpendicular to the glenoid without overlapping of the glenoid by the coracoid or acromion.

Posterior shoulder dislocations result in similar impaction of the humeral head and fracture of glenoid rim as seen in anterior dislocation but in different locations. In posterior dislocations, impaction of the humeral head occurs along the anterior humeral head just medial to the lesser

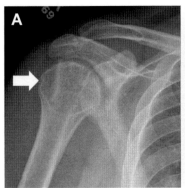 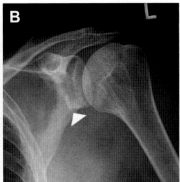 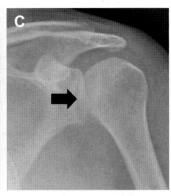

Fig. 11. Fracture patterns of shoulder dislocation. (*A*) Hill-Sachs impaction fracture of the posterosuperior humeral head (*white arrow*). Hill-Sachs lesions often appear as an area of relative lucency with sclerotic margin along the posterior humeral head. (*B*) Bankart fractures are usually seen as a vertical sclerotic line along the inferior aspect of the glenoid neck (*white arrowhead*). (*C*) Reverse Hill-Sachs impaction fracture of the anterior humeral head (*black arrow*). Reverse Hill-Sachs lesions typically appear as vertical lucency along the medial humeral head, which has been termed the "trough sign."

tuberosity and is called a "reverse Hill-Sachs" lesion. This area of impaction can appear as a vertically oriented lucency along the medial humeral head on AP radiographs, which has been termed the "trough sign" (**Fig. 11**C). A reverse Hill-Sachs is best appreciated on an axillary view; the Stryker notch view is not useful in identifying a reverse Hill-Sachs. Posterior dislocations also can cause fractures of the posterior glenoid rim, called a reverse Bankart lesion. A reverse Bankart will appear as loss of the inferior glenoid articular line with medial vertical sclerotic line along the glenoid neck, similar to a regular Bankart lesion. A reverse Bankart is best seen on an axillary view; a West Point view may show a reverse Bankart but does not offer any advantage over an axillary view.

Advanced imaging with MR imaging or CT is often performed after reduction in patients with shoulder dislocation. In the absence of a Bankart fracture, MR imaging is typically the preferred modality for assessment because of the associated soft tissue injuries frequently seen in shoulder dislocation.[21] In the acute setting, a joint effusion is typically present, which causes adequate joint distention, obviating MR arthrography to assess the intraarticular soft tissues.[21] In patients with repeated dislocations or glenoid fracture, CT is often performed to assess degree of glenoid bone loss and planning for fracture fixation.

Scapula Fracture

Scapula fractures are rare, comprising less than 1% of all fractures.[9] Most scapula fractures are the result of a direct blow to the shoulder, usually due to high-energy trauma or fall. Approximately

30% of scapula fractures are intraarticular, involving the glenoid articular surface.[22] The remaining 70% of fractures are extraarticular, involving the scapula body, acromion, and/or coracoid. Scapula fractures follow a unimodal distribution in both men and women. Scapula fractures in men occur most commonly in young adults due to high-energy trauma, whereas scapula fractures in women most commonly occur as fragility fractures in elderly patients.[9] Close inspection of the clavicle should be performed whenever a scapula fracture is identified, because 25% of scapula fractures will have an associated clavicle fracture or AC joint injury.[23] Similar to clavicle fractures, the decision regarding which scapula fractures should undergo surgical fixation is complex and involves many factors including portion of scapula involved, degree of displacement, patient functional status, and associated injuries.[23–25] In general, fractures involving the articular surface of the glenoid, the acromion, or the coracoid process are more likely to require surgical management. Because of this, classification systems have been popularized for guiding surgical management of fractures involving these 3 regions.

The Ideberg classification is a classification for scapula fractures involving the glenoid articular surface (**Fig. 12**).[22] In the Ideberg classification, glenoid fractures are grouped into 6 types. Type 1a fractures are fractures of the anterior glenoid rim and are associated with anterior shoulder dislocation in approximately two-thirds of cases.[22] Type 1b fractures are fractures of the posterior glenoid rim and are associated with posterior dislocations. Type 2 fractures are glenoid fractures that extend through the inferolateral scapula

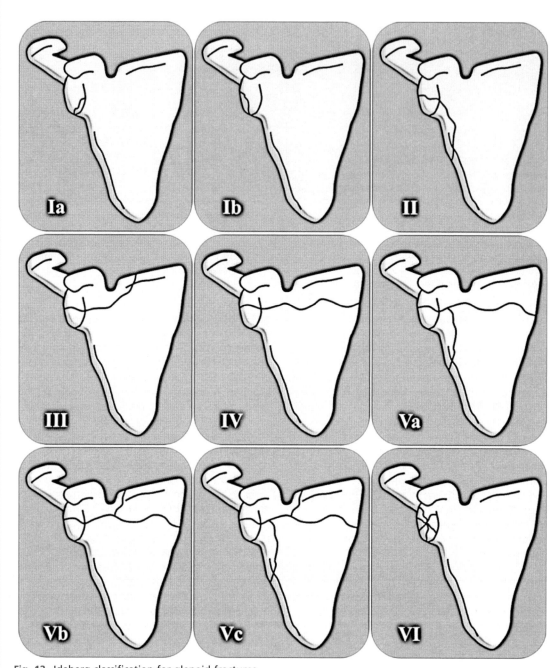

Fig. 12. Ideberg classification for glenoid fractures.

border. Type 3 fractures are glenoid fractures that extend through the superior scapula border, and type 4 fractures extend through the medial scapula border. Type 5 fractures are glenoid fractures that involve more than one scapula border. Type 5a fractures involve the superior and medial borders, type 5b fractures involve the inferolateral and medial borders, and type 5c fractures involve all 3 borders. Type 6 fractures are fractures in which there is significant comminution of the glenoid articular surface.

The Kuhn classification is a system devised to guide surgical management of acromion fractures (**Fig. 13**).[26] Type 1 fractures can be either a nondisplaced complete fracture through the acromion or a fracture that does not result in potential instability of the acromion (eg, an avulsion fracture). Type 2 fractures are displaced complete fractures that do not narrow the subacromial space. Type 3 fractures are displaced complete fractures that narrow the subacromial space. Type 3 fractures can be a fracture where either the acromion is

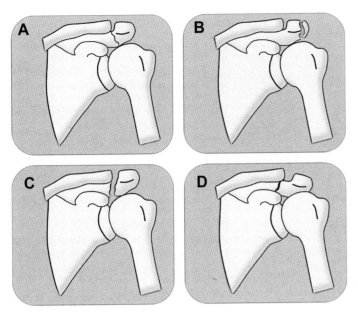

Fig. 13. Kuhn classification for acromion fractures. Type I fractures are fractures that are either nondisplaced (*A*) or do not result in potential instability of the acromion (eg, avulsion fractures) (*B*). Type II fractures are displaced fractures that do not result in narrowing of the subacromial space (*C*). Type III fractures are displaced fractures that do narrow the subacromial space (*D*), which places the rotator cuff at risk for impingement.

displaced inferiorly narrowing the subacromial space or the humeral head migrates superiorly to narrow the subacromial space. Because type 1 and 2 fractures do not narrow the subacromial space, they do not pose a risk for rotator cuff impingement and are usually managed conservatively. Type 3 fractures do place the rotator cuff at risk for impingement; therefore, type 3 fractures often are treated with surgical fixation.

Coracoid process fractures can be classified using the Ogawa system (**Fig. 14**).[27] The Ogawa classification divides coracoid process fractures based on location relative to the insertion of the coracoclavicular ligament. Type 1 fractures occur through the base of the coracoid process proximal to the coracoclavicular ligament insertion. Type 1 fractures can result in scapuloclavicular instability and are often treated with surgical fixation. Type 2 fractures occur distal to the coracoclavicular ligament insertion and represent avulsion fractures of the conjoined tendon of the coracobrachialis and short head of the biceps brachii. Type 2 fractures do not result in scapuloclavicular instability and so are treated conservatively.

The complex osteology of the scapula combined with the overlying soft tissues and osseous structures of the chest makes diagnosis of scapula fractures challenging on radiographs. A standard radiograph series of the scapula is composed of AP and lateral radiographs of the scapula. In the AP radiograph, the shoulder is abducted 90° and the x-ray tube angle is 5° to 10° laterally to obtain an image perpendicular to the scapula. The lateral radiograph is obtained at 90° to the AP view with

the shoulder in slight adduction and flexion to move the humerus away from the scapula body. In practice, a scapula series is primarily used for follow-up of known scapula fractures or for preoperative planning. The most commonly used radiograph series for identifying scapula fractures is a routine shoulder series. An axillary view can be extremely helpful in identifying fractures of the acromion and coracoid processes, which may not be apparent on any other projection (**Figs. 15 and 16**). Many nondisplaced or minimally

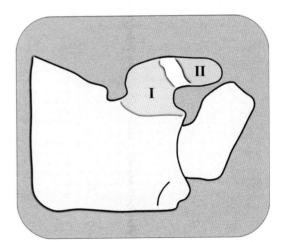

Fig. 14. Ogawa classification for coracoid process fractures. Type I fractures are through the base of the coracoid, proximal to the coracoclavicular ligament insertion. Type II fractures are through the tip of the coracoid, distal to the coracoclavicular ligament insertion.

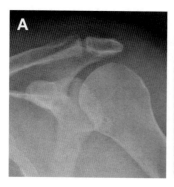
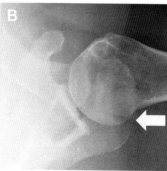

Fig. 15. Type I acromion fracture. (*A*) The nondisplaced acromion fracture is not visible on the standard AP radiograph of the shoulder. (*B*) Axillary view of the shoulder demonstrating the nondisplaced fracture line through the midacromion (*arrow*). Axillary view can be essential for diagnosing nondisplaced acromion fractures.

displaced fractures are not visible on radiographs. A low threshold should be maintained for obtaining CT in the setting of suspected scapula fracture. In the absence of a suspected pathologic fracture, there is no role for MR imaging in the assessment of scapula fractures.[21]

Scapulothoracic Dissociation

Scapulothoracic dissociation is a very rare traumatic injury in which there is extensive osseous and/or soft tissue disruption of the shoulder girdle resulting in disarticulation of the scapula from the chest wall.[28] Most scapulothoracic dissociations are a result of high-energy trauma, with approximately 80% of cases occurring in the setting of a motor vehicle or motorcycle collision.[29] The injury is caused by a strong distracting force across the shoulder girdle, either from a direct blow or rapid deceleration while the injured extremity remains gripped to the handlebar or steering wheel.[28]

Scapulothoracic dissociation can be a challenging diagnosis to make, both clinically and on imaging, because there are no set criteria of clinical examination or imaging findings that define the injury. However, all scapulothoracic dissociations share 2 imaging findings: (1) disruption of clavicular bridge between the shoulder and thorax in the form of sternoclavicular dislocation, clavicle fracture, or AC separation and (2) extensive soft tissue injury of the shoulder girdle allowing lateral migration of the scapula (Fig. 17). Scapulothoracic dissociation can be easily overlooked in the initial clinical assessment, because these patients will often present obtunded or have other distracting injuries, including injuries to the ipsilateral upper extremity.[30,31] It is important to alert clinicians when scapulothoracic dissociation is suspected on imaging, because scapulothoracic dissociation carries a high association with both brachial plexus and major vascular injuries.[32]

The possibility of scapulothoracic dissociation should be considered whenever a clavicle fracture or dislocation of the sternoclavicular or acromioclavicular joint is identified. Appreciable lateral displacement of the scapula is seen in almost all cases of scapulothoracic dissociation.[32] Lateral displacement of the scapula can best be appreciated on an appropriately aligned chest radiograph, where the contralateral scapula is used to define normal alignment. Increased soft tissue density overlying the injured shoulder girdle is commonly seen on radiographs due to extensive edema and hemorrhage frequently occurring with this injury. Scapulothoracic dissociation is assessed on radiographs by measuring a line from midline to the medial border of each scapula. An absolute difference of greater than 1 cm or ratio of greater than 1.29 between the injured and uninjured side

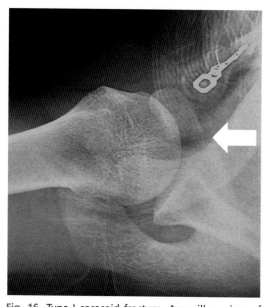

Fig. 16. Type I coracoid fracture. An axillary view of the shoulder shows a mildly displaced fracture through the base of the coracoid, proximal to the coracoclavicular ligament origin (*arrow*). Like acromion fractures, coracoid fractures may only be visible on an axillary radiograph.

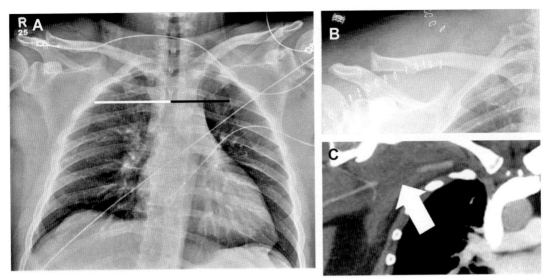

Fig. 17. Scapulothoracic dissociation. (*A*) AP radiograph of the chest showing increased distance of the right medial scapula border from midline (*white line*) compared with the left (*black line*) with a distance ratio of 1.3, consistent with scapulothoracic dissociation. (*B*) AP radiograph of the clavicle shows widening of the AC joint and coracoclavicular distance, consistent with a type 3 AC separation. (*C*) Coned coronal postcontrast CT image of the chest demonstrates transection of the axillary artery (*arrow*) with surrounding axillary hematoma.

is consistent with scapulothoracic dissociation (see **Fig. 17**A).[32–34] The use of this technique, although, depends on an appropriately positioned radiograph and uninjured contralateral shoulder girdle. Rotation of the chest or bilateral shoulder injuries can make assessment of scapulothoracic dissociation on radiographs unreliable.

CT or MR imaging can aid in the diagnosis of scapulothoracic dissociation by identifying muscle disruption and/or deep soft tissue edema and hemorrhage (see **Fig 17**C). CT angiography is indicated in all patients with confirmed or suspected scapulothoracic dissociation because almost all patients will present with evidence of some degree of vascular compromise, and as much as 10% of patients will have a limb threatening vascular injury.[30,32,34] Noncontrast brachial plexus MR imaging and/or CT myelography is indicated if the patient has an associated neurologic impairment. Both MR imaging and CT myelography are acceptable methods for assessing preganglionic nerve root avulsion, which is a common injury pattern in distraction injuries of the shoulder resulting in nerve injury.[28,35] However, MR imaging is preferred to CT in the evaluation of postganglionic nerve root injuries and more distal injuries to the brachial plexus.[21,35]

SUMMARY

Traumatic shoulder girdle injuries are a common injury encountered in the emergency center.

Many radiographic views have been described for evaluating traumatic shoulder girdle injuries. It is vital that the appropriate radiographic positioning is performed when evaluating for suspected injury of the shoulder girdle, because shoulder girdle injuries can be easily missed on imaging. Upright radiographs should also be performed whenever possible to avoid misdiagnosis or underdiagnosis of injury to the shoulder. Advanced imaging using CT or MR imaging is usually not required to assess shoulder girdle injuries. However, a low threshold should be held for performing advanced imaging when there is suspected scapula injury, shoulder instability, or injury to the medial clavicle.

REFERENCES

1. Enger M, Skjaker SA, Melhuus K, et al. Shoulder injuries from birth to old age: A 1-year prospective study of 3031 shoulder injuries in an urban population. Injury 2018;49(7):1324–9.
2. Gun B, Dean R, Go B, et al. Non-modifiable risk factors associated with sternoclavicular joint dislocations in the U.S. military. Mil Med 2018;183(5–6): e188–93.
3. Boesmueller S, Wech M, Tiefenboeck TM, et al. Incidence, characteristics, and long-term follow-up of sternoclavicular injuries: An epidemiologic analysis of 92 cases. J Trauma Acute Care Surg 2016; 80(2):289–95.

4. Glass ER, Thompson JD, Cole PA, et al. Treatment of sternoclavicular joint dislocations: a systematic review of 251 dislocations in 24 case series. J Trauma 2011;70(5):1294–8.

5. Tepolt F, Carry PM, Heyn PC, et al. Posterior sternoclavicular joint injuries in the adolescent population: a meta-analysis. BMC Musculoskelet Disord 2017; 18(1):82.

6. Wirth MA, Rockwood CA. Acute and chronic traumatic injuries of the sternoclavicular joint. J Am Acad Orthop Surg 1996;4:268–78.

7. Lee JT, Nasreddine AY, Black EM, et al. Posterior sternoclavicular joint injuries in skeletally immature patients. J Pediatr Orthop 2014;34(4):369–75.

8. Beckmann N, Crawford L. Posterior sternoclavicular Salter-Harris fracture-dislocation in a patient with unossified medial clavicle epiphysis. Skeletal Radiol 2016;45(8):1123–7.

9. Court-Brown CM, Caesar B. Epidemiology of adult fractures: A review. Injury 2006;37(8):691–7.

10. Herteleer M, Winckelmans T, Hoekstra H, et al. Epidemiology of clavicle fractures in a level 1 trauma center in Belgium. Eur J Trauma Emerg Surg 2017; 44(5):717–26.

11. Kihlström C, Möller M, Lönn K, et al. Clavicle fractures: epidemiology, classification and treatment of 2 422 fractures in the Swedish Fracture Register; an observational study. Am J Sports Med 2014; 42(10):2517–24.

12. Takase K. The coracoclavicular ligaments: an anatomic study. Surg Radiol Anat 2010;32(7):683–8.

13. Clayton RA, Court-Brown CM. The epidemiology of musculoskeletal tendinous and ligamentous injuries. Injury 2008;39(12):1338–44.

14. Rockwood CA Jr. Fractures and dislocations of the shoulder. In: Rockwood CA Jr, Green DP, editors. Fractures in adults. Philadelphia: Lippincott; 1984. p. 860–910.

15. Tischer T, Salzmann GM, El-Azab H, et al. Incidence of associated injuries with acute acromioclavicular joint dislocations types III through V. Am J Sports Med 2009;37(1):136–9.

16. Markel J, Schwarting T, Malcherczyk D, et al. Concomitant glenohumeral pathologies in high-grade acromioclavicular separation (type III - V). BMC Musculoskelet Disord 2017;18(1):439.

17. Krøner K, Lind T, Jensen J. The epidemiology of shoulder dislocations. Arch Orthop Trauma Surg 1989;108(5):288–90.

18. Shields DW, Jefferies JG, Brooksbank AJ, et al. Epidemiology of glenohumeral dislocation and subsequent instability in an urban population. J Shoulder Elbow Surg 2018;27(2):189–95.

19. Sola Junior WC, Santos PS. Intrathoracic fracture-dislocation of the humerus - case report and literature review. Rev Bras Ortop 2017;52(2):215–9.

20. Senna LF, Pires E, Albuquerque R. Modified axillary radiograph of the shoulder: a new position. Rev Bras Ortop 2016;52(1):115–8.

21. Amini B, Beckmann NM, Beaman FD, et al. ACR appropriateness criteria® shoulder pain-traumatic. J Am Coll Radiol 2018;15(5S):S171–88.

22. Ideberg R, Grevsten S, Larsson S. Epidemiology of scapular fractures. Incidence and classification of 338 fractures. Acta Orthop Scand 1995;66(5):395–7.

23. Lantry JM, Roberts CS, Giannoudis PV. Operative treatment of scapular fractures: a systematic review. Injury 2008;39(3):271–83.

24. Anavian J, Gauger EM, Schroder LK, et al. Surgical and functional outcomes after operative management of complex and displaced intra-articular glenoid fractures. J Bone Joint Surg Am 2012;94(7): 645–53.

25. Königshausen M, Coulibaly MO, Nicolas V, et al. Results of non-operative treatment of fractures of the glenoid fossa. Bone Joint J. 2016;98-B(8):1074–9.

26. Kuhn JE, Blasier RB, Carpenter JE. Fractures of the acromion process: a proposed classification system. J Orthop Trauma 1994;8(1):6–13.

27. Ogawa K, Yoshida A, Takahashi M, et al. Fractures of the coracoid process. J Bone Joint Surg Br 1997;79(1):17–9.

28. Choo AM, Schottel PC, Burgess AR. Scapulothoracic dissociation: evaluation and management. J Am Acad Orthop Surg 2017;25(5):339–47.

29. Damschen DD, Cogbill TH, Siegel MJ. Scapulothoracic dissociation caused by blunt trauma. J Trauma 1997;42(3):537–40.

30. Lee L, Miller TT, Schultz E, et al. Scapulothoracic dissociation. Am J Orthop (Belle Mead NJ) 1998; 27(10):699–702.

31. Flanagin BA, Leslie MP. Scapulothoracic dissociation. Orthop Clin North Am 2013;44(1):1–7.

32. Zelle BA, Pape HC, Gerich TG, et al. Functional outcome following scapulothoracic dissociation. J Bone Joint Surg Am 2004;86(1):2–8.

33. Lange RH, Noel SH. Traumatic lateral scapular displacement: An expanded spectrum of associated neurovascular injury. J Orthop Trauma 1993; 7(4):361–6.

34. Sampson LN, Britton JC, Eldrup-Jorgensen J, et al. The neurovascular outcome of scapulothoracic dissociation. J Vasc Surg 1993;17(6):1083–8.

35. Beckmann NM, West OC, Nunez Jr. D, et al. ACR Appropriateness Criteria Suspected Spine Trauma. American College of Radiology. Revised 2018. Available at: https://acsearch.acr.org/docs/69359/Narrative. Accessed January 14, 2019.

Imaging Acetabular Fractures

David Dreizin, MD[a],*, Christina A. LeBedis, MD[b], Jason W. Nascone, MD[c]

KEYWORDS

- Acetabular fractures • Transverse fractures • Column fractures • Wall fractures
- Computed tomography • Surface rendering • Cinematic rendering

KEY POINTS

- Judet and Letournel described 10 fracture types: 5 elemental (simple) and 5 associated (complex). The Judet-Letournel classification system is challenging to learn by rote memorization.
- Systematic stepwise approaches to classification often divide acetabular fracture into 3 families: transverse, column, and wall. Each fracture family is distinguishing based on the orientation of the dominant fracture line on supra-acetabular computed tomography (CT) images.
- A pattern seen almost exclusively in elderly patients is the geriatric protrusion fracture, a variant of anterior column and anterior wall fracture. The quadrilateral plate is comminuted, hinged posteriorly, and medially rotated. The dome may be impacted.
- CT improves characterization of articular incongruities, nondisplaced fractures, intra-articular fragments, impaction injuries, quadrilateral plate involvement, and femoral head subluxations.
- Imaging criteria of instability include the CT subchondral arc for the weight-bearing dome, and percentage involvement of the posterior wall.

INTRODUCTION

Acetabular fractures are encountered by radiologists in a variety of practice settings. They occur overwhelmingly in the adult population,[1–3] with a bimodal age distribution; fractures in younger patients result from high-energy trauma, such as traffic accidents.[4] As the population has aged, there has been a disproportionate increase in the incidence of acetabular fractures in elderly patients after low-energy trauma. These patients often initially present to community emergency departments before transfer to trauma referral centers, where orthopedic expertise in acetabular trauma is concentrated.[2,5–8] Imaging is routinely used to plan open reduction and internal fixation (ORIF). Surgeries are lengthy and carry the risk of complications, and benefits must always be measured against risks.[9] Various imaging criteria have evolved to identify the subset of patients for whom ORIF may be unnecessary or of limited benefit. The Judet-Letournel classification system helps determine the most appropriate surgical approach[10,11] but is nonintuitive and challenging to learn by rote memorization.[12,13] Systematic classification algorithms that incorporate multiplanar reformatted (MPR) and three-dimensional (3D) images can substantially improve the accuracy,

Disclosures: The authors have no relevant financial activities or conflicts of interest to disclose.
[a] Department of Diagnostic Radiology and Nuclear Medicine, R Adams Cowley Shock Trauma Center, University of Maryland School of Medicine, 22 South Greene Street, Baltimore, MD 21201, USA; [b] Department of Radiology, Boston University Medical Center, 715 Albany Street, Boston, MA 02118, USA; [c] Department of Orthopaedics, University of Maryland School of Medicine, R Adams Cowley Shock Trauma Center, 22 South Greene Street, Baltimore, MD 21201, USA
* Corresponding author.
E-mail address: daviddreizin@gmail.com

Radiol Clin N Am 57 (2019) 823–841
https://doi.org/10.1016/j.rcl.2019.02.004
0033-8389/19/© 2019 Elsevier Inc. All rights reserved.

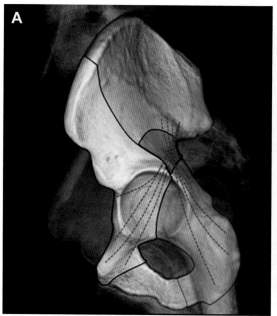
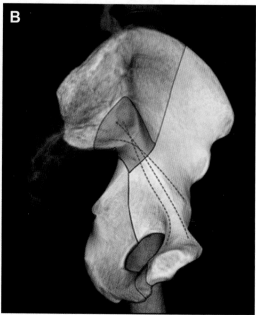

Fig. 1. Lateral (*A*) and medial (*B*) surface-rendered CT images of the acetabulum and innominate bone showing columnar anatomy. Dashed lines approximate trabeculae of the 2 columns (*yellow,* anterior; *blue,* posterior), which converge in the supra-acetabular region to form the sciatic buttress (*red*).

agreement, and speed of classification.[12–16] Postoperatively, computed tomography (CT) is increasingly used to assess the quality of reduction and evaluate for postsurgical and posttraumatic complications. This article is a primer for radiologists seeking to provide added value to orthopedists in decision making and surgical management of patients with acetabular fractures. Concepts covered include basic anatomy and biomechanics, systematic classification, surgical approaches and fixation principles, imaging predictors of poor outcome, and imaging of common complications.

ACETABULAR ANATOMY AND BIOMECHANICS

The acetabulum includes not only the acetabular cup but also the structures of the innominate bone that support it and are used as sites of reduction and placement of orthopedic hardware.[10] Judet and Letournel[10] were the first to conceptualize the weight-bearing component of the acetabular fossa as a keystone between 2 structural columns (anterior and posterior) formed by the innominate bone (the ischium, ilium, and pubis). This explicitly surgical concept informs all aspects of classification and management.[13]

The columns are not discretely defined anatomic structures, instead representing aggregates of trabecular bone along stress vectors, as governed by Wolff's law (remodeling of bone through deposition and resorption in response to physical stresses).[17] When the acetabulum is viewed en face from its lateral aspect, the columns are oriented in the shape of the Greek letter lambda (Λ).[13,18] The trabeculae of the posterior (or ilioischial [II]) column extend from the ischial spine down the ischial tuberosity,[17] forming the short limb of the lambda. The anterior column (the long limb), is formed by bony trabeculae along the iliac crest, pelvic brim, and pubic rami.[7,13,18,19] The columns coalesce in the supra-acetabular region and course posteriorly to form the thick and compact sciatic buttress, which transmits load from the axial skeleton via the sacroiliac (SI) joint[7,10,18] (**Fig. 1**). The acetabular cup is a laterally located, inferiorly tilted, and anteverted hemispheric depression lined by an inverted U-shaped acetabular cartilage.[7,20] The walls of the acetabular cup extend from the columns, converging with the roof to form the weight-bearing dome (WBD).

Under normal conditions, both columns and walls play a role in weight transference. Peak pressures are seen at the WBD in a standing position. The posterior wall takes a more prominent role in resisting stress when rising from a sitting position or descending stairs.[9,21–23] Physiologic compression of the cartilage along any vector dissipates forces more peripherally and results in a relatively even distribution of pressure within the joint.[21,22]

IMAGING MODALITIES

Anteroposterior (AP) radiographs of the pelvis are part of the secondary advanced trauma life support (ATLS) survey and may reveal posterior femoral head dislocations that require urgent reduction to correct vascular compromise.[4,10,24] Complete acetabular series (radiographic AP and Judet views) can play an important role for operating surgeons. The uninjured side is a useful radiographic representation of the patient's normal anatomy. In addition, these images are consistent with the fluoroscopic images and plain radiographs obtained intraoperatively. However, plain radiographs have many drawbacks, including difficulty positioning patients because of pain and multiple injuries, and poor image quality. Portable technique is associated with superimposition of oblique fracture fragments and overlapping soft tissues, bowel gas, or external devices.[5,18,25–30] With thin sections, near-isotropic MPRs, and bone convolution kernels, CT improves characterization of articular incongruities, nondisplaced fractures, intra-articular fragments, impaction injuries, quadrilateral plate involvement, and femoral head subluxations.[13,16,20,24–27,31] Intravenous contrast-enhanced abdominopelvic or whole-body CT is widely used after high-energy trauma, allowing assessment of concomitant soft tissue and vascular injury.[26,32,33] With modern scanners and reconstruction algorithms, pelvic CT dose is comparable with radiographic series.[34]

Volume-rendered and surface-rendered images equivalent to optimally positioned radiographic views are unobstructed by overlying structures.[25,27] High-quality MPRs and 3D images help make sense of complex comminuted fractures,[31] resulting in improved classification agreement and accuracy,[5,12] and a change in management in up to 30% of patients.[5,35] Virtual disarticulation using region-of-interest masking allows direct visualization of the acetabular fossa from its lateral aspect,[6,27,36] whereas half-space images that remove the contralateral hemipelvis increase the range of viewing angles of the iliac fossa and quadrilateral plate.[37] Real-time 3D image manipulation allows characterization of the degree of fragment rotation and areas of greatest displacement.[25] At this time, 3D images generated using traditional ray tracing techniques can obscure nondisplaced fractures from volume-averaging effects[3,5,18]; however, new developments such as cinematic rendering, which generates photorealistic images by simulating billions of light rays using a Monte Carlo–based algorithm, may improve detection of nondisplaced and minimally displaced fractures[38] (**Fig. 2**).

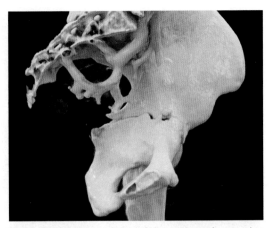

Fig. 2. Medial view of the left innominate bone using cinematic rendering in a 40-year-old woman after motor vehicle collision (MVC). The fine detail of a minimally displaced left transverse acetabular fracture is shown to advantage.

IMAGING LANDMARKS
Anteroposterior View and Computed Tomography Correlates

Judet described classification based on examination of radiographic cardinal lines on an AP view of the pelvis. The lines are created by x-ray beams passing structures in tangent[17] and are approximate representations of the individual columns and walls. The AP view is supplemented by information from 2 orthogonal oblique Judet views: the iliac oblique (IO) and obturator oblique (OO) views, each taken with the patient tilted right or left side up at 45° of offset from the coronal plane.[16,20,26,27] Each landmark has been subsequently correlated to anatomy on two-dimensional and 3D CT images using pelvic models labeled with radiographic markers.[17,18] CT bypasses the need to assess radiographic lines because the walls and columns are viewed in their entirety with much greater detail. Familiarity with Judet views, Judet lines, and their CT correlates remains necessary because surgeons rely on them during intraoperative fluoroscopy and plan surgeries accordingly.[26,27]

The Judet lines include the radiologic roof, the posterior lip, the acetabulo-obturator line, the II line, and the iliopectineal (IP) line[17,25] (**Fig. 3**). On CT, anterior column fragments include the anterior two-thirds of the WBD, the anterior wall, superior pubic ramus, pelvic brim, and variable portions of the iliac wing.[7,10,13,18,20,26] The IP line corresponds perfectly with the pelvic brim along its distal three-quarters, which is always disrupted in anterior column fractures.[17,20,26]

Posterior column fragments contain the ischial spine, the posterior WBD and wall, the ischial

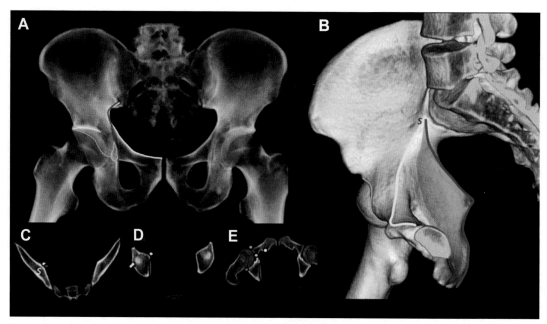

Fig. 3. Bone template volume-rendered (*A*), half-space surface-rendered 3D image of the medial innominate bone (*B*), and axial CT images at the level of the sciatic buttress (denoted by *S*) (*C*), acetabular roof (*D*), and acetabular fossa (*E*). Yellow, IP line denoting acetabular rim; red, II line, formed by the posterior four-fifths of the quadrilateral plate and ischial tuberosity; green, rim of the anterior wall (delimited by the acetabulo-obturator line in *A*); dark blue, rim of the posterior wall; light blue line in (*A*) and arrow in (*D*), subchondral bone of the acetabular roof; orange, pelvic teardrop formed by the medial margin of the cotyloid fossa and lateral margin of the obturator canal.

tuberosity, and most of the quadrilateral plate. The fracture line extends inferiorly from the retroacetabular region at the greater sciatic notch through the ischiopubic junction.[7,10,13,20] On CT, the II and IP lines diverge from a common origin above the greater sciatic notch.[17] The II line is formed by an x-ray beam in tangent to the posterior four-fifths of the quadrilateral plate.[10,17] Inferiorly, the II line follows the medial ischial border. The II line is always disrupted in posterior column fractures. Some anterior wall fractures that involve the quadrilateral surface also result in disruption of the II line and initially can be mistaken for posterior column fracture on plain radiographs.

At the radiologic roof, the beam is in tangent to only a small 2-mm to 3-mm region of the WBD. The roof extends medially to the top of the cotyloid fossa.[17] The posterior lip represents the edge of the posterior wall. The acetabulo-obturator line (from the superior border of the obturator foramen to the lateral margin of the roof) marks the shallow and horizontal anterior wall.[17]

Judet Views and Computed Tomography Correlates

Each view best visualizes 3 key landmarks. On the IO view, which has a posterior oblique orientation

with respect to the injured side, these are the iliac wing, margin of the posterior column, and margin of the anterior wall.[13,16,27] On the OO view, these are the obturator ring viewed en face, the iliac wing in profile, and the rim of the posterior wall.[13,27]

JUDET-LETOURNEL CLASSIFICATION

The Judet-Letournel classification remains a cornerstone of treatment planning. Judet and Letournel[10] described 10 fracture types. There are 5 elemental (simple) fractures in which a single dominant fracture line divides the acetabulum into 2 fragments, and 5 associated (complex) fractures, which are combinations of 2 elemental fracture types with 2 dominant fracture lines.[10,16] Elemental fractures include anterior and posterior column, anterior and posterior wall, and transverse fractures. Associated fractures include associated both column (ABC), transverse with posterior wall (TPW), T-type, posterior column posterior wall (PCPW), and anterior column hemitransverse (ACHT) fractures.[16] By descending order of prevalence, posterior wall fractures (23.6%), ABC fractures (21.7%), transverse and posterior wall fractures (17.4%), T-type fractures (9.3%), and elemental transverse fractures (8.3%) together account for 80% to 90% of acetabular fractures.[4,16]

Biomechanical Principles

Almost all acetabular fractures result from forces that drive the femoral head into the acetabular fossa.[26] Fracture patterns are determined by femoral head position and direction of the force vector, magnitude of transmitted force, and bone quality.[7,10,17,26] Posterior wall fractures are produced by direct trauma to a flexed knee with the hip in flexion. The classic mechanism is dashboard impact during a motor vehicle collision. With sufficient external rotation, the femoral head impacts the acetabulum more medially, resulting in a posterior column fracture.[10] Transverse fractures are caused by lateral blows to the greater trochanter. The degree of abduction determines the craniocaudal location of the fracture. More severe forces cause T-type fractures. TPW fractures result if the hip is internally rotated. Anterior column and wall fractures result from a blow to the posterolateral aspect of the greater trochanter with the hip externally rotated, which is a common mechanism in elderly falls.[10] There has been a 2.4-fold increase in incidence of acetabular fractures among patients older than 60 years in the past 3 decades,[39,40] and fractures involving the front part of the acetabulum (anterior column, anterior wall, and ACHT fractures) are becoming more common.[8] A pattern seen almost exclusively in elderly patients is the geriatric protrusion fracture, a variant of anterior column and anterior wall fracture. The head is driven into the acetabulum anteromedially, resulting in comminution, quadrilateral plate and femoral head medialization, and dome impaction.[8,40,41]

Fracture Typing and Stepwise Classification

Brandser and Marsh[16] used a systematic stepwise approach to classification with the Judet-Letournel system based on the concept of 3 fracture families: transverse, column, and wall. Many similar variations have subsequently been described that largely maintain fidelity with Brandser and Marsh's system.[12–16,20,25,27,30,37,42] Tools including a smartphone app[12] and 3D-printed acetabular fracture models[43,44] can further enhance understanding and streamline classification. The transverse family includes elemental transverse, TPW, and T-type fractures[13,16] (Fig. 4). The column family includes elemental anterior or posterior, ABC, PCPW, and ACHT fractures (Fig. 5). Typical wall family fractures are simply isolated fractures of the anterior and posterior wall (Fig. 6).

Axial images of the supra-acetabular region greatly simplify classification and are a useful starting point.[13,27] Each fracture family is distinguished based on the orientation of the dominant fracture line.[13] Transverse fractures are sagittally oriented, column fractures are coronally oriented, and wall fractures extending to the dome have a lateral oblique orientation[13,16] (Fig. 7). After examining the sciatic buttress on axial images (Fig. 8), 3D images seem adequate for further stepwise classification.[12] Subsequent decision points allow classification by inspection of the iliac wing, retroacetabular surface, obturator ring, and walls.[13,16,27]

Column Family Fractures

Unifying features of column family fractures are the coronal orientation of the dominant supra-acetabular fracture line and involvement of the obturator ring.[13,16] In elemental anterior and posterior column fractures, the fragment is dissociated from the sciatic buttress and no longer contributes to load transmission. Elemental anterior column fractures involve the iliac wing but not the retroacetabular surface. Elemental posterior column fractures involve the retroacetabular surface but not the iliac wing. ABC fractures are the only fracture type in which the entire articular surface is dissociated from the sciatic buttress.[30,42] Scrolling caudally through axial images, there is no continuity between the buttress and any part of the dense subchondral bone of the WBD[13,16] (see ABC fracture in Figs. 5C and 8). A CT spur sign representing the distal shard of the sciatic buttress may be present if the articular acetabulum is medialized.[13,16,20] A posterior column fracture that also involves the posterior wall is a PCPW fracture, and this is the only associated fracture that only involves the posterior half of the acetabulum.[27] The combination of a coronally oriented column fracture and lateral oblique wall fracture imparts a complex appearance on the supra-acetabular image.[25]

Transverse Family Fractures

The unifying feature of transverse family fractures is the sagittal orientation of the dominant fracture.[13,16] Elemental transverse fractures extend through the walls but do not result in dissociated wall fragments that require separate fixation.[27] TPW fractures are distinguished from elemental transverse fractures by the presence of both a sagittal fracture line and lateral oblique fracture line on supra-acetabular axial images.[20] However, not all posterior wall fractures extend to the dome, and assessment at the level of the acetabular fossa is necessary. Elemental transverse fractures show a single dissociated ischiopubic fragment,

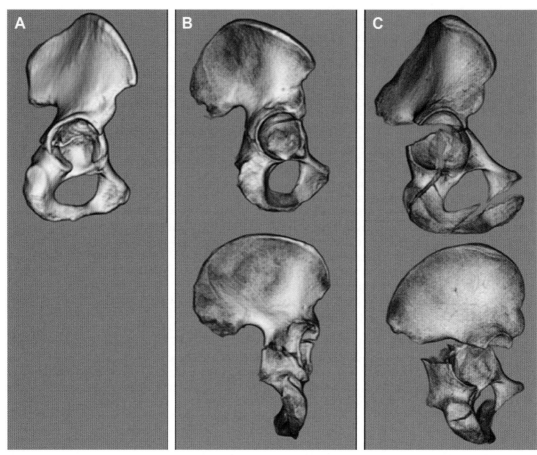

Fig. 4. Transverse family fractures include elemental transverse (*A*), TPW (*B*), and T type (*C*). (*A*) A 35-year-old man after MVC with juxtatectal elemental transverse fracture. (*B*) A 45-year-old man after MVC with transtectal TPW fracture; (*C*) A 22-year-old man after MVC with transtectal T-type fracture and marked medial displacement of the ischiopubic fragments.

and the obturator ring is intact.[16,27] In T-type fractures, the obturator ring is disrupted by a coronally oriented vertical stem extending through the quadrilateral plate, inferior margin of the cotyloid fossa, and variable locations of the inferior obturator ring, most commonly the ischiopubic region.

The inferior tilt and anteversion of the acetabulum explains the use of the term transverse for an oblique fracture that runs superomedially to inferolaterally in the anatomic plane. The term refers to the orientation of the dominant fracture line when the acetabulum is viewed en face (in the acetabular plane), with the notch facing inferiorly.[37] The sagittal fracture line shifts laterally with caudal progression of axial images, with the inferior fragment always located medially.[20,42] Transverse family fractures are divided into 3 categories (infratectal, juxtatectal, and transtectal) based on the relationship of the fracture line with the upper margin of the cotyloid fossa.[18] The distinction is best made with coronal CT images.

Approximately 20% of transverse fractures are transtectal.[10] Transtectal fractures extend through the WBD, allowing the inferior fragment and femoral head to translate medially as a unit (see T-type fracture, **Fig. 4**C). The likelihood of femoral head damage and posttraumatic arthritis is greatly increased, and operative control is very difficult.[20] Unlike ABC fractures, there is still some continuity between the sciatic buttress and the cranialmost portion of the WBD subchondral bone.

Wall Family Fractures

Isolated wall fractures extending to the roof are obliquely oriented on supra-acetabular axial images.[20] A dissociated fragment will also be present on 3D images and axial images through the midfossa. Simple wall fractures do not violate the columns; the retroacetabular surface, obturator ring, and iliac wing are intact. The precise anatomic boundaries of dissociated anterior

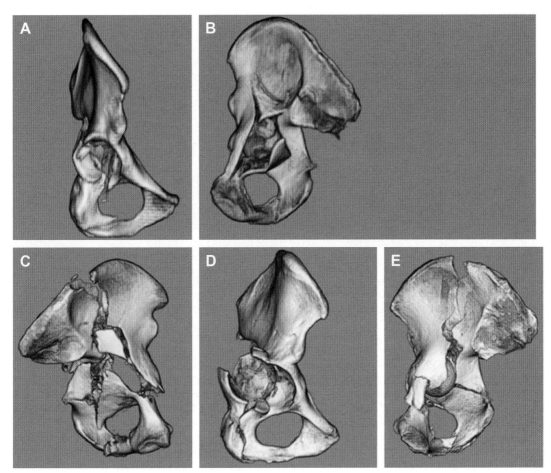

Fig. 5. Column family fractures include elemental posterior (*A*), elemental anterior (*B*), ABC fractures (*C*), PCPW fractures (*D*), and ACHT fractures (*E*). (*A*) A 35-year-old male unrestrained passenger in an MVC with a posterior column fracture. (*B*) A 69-year-old man after a mechanical fall while walking with an anterior column protrusion fracture. (*C*) A 53-year-old man after a fall from a 15-m (50-foot) bridge with a comminuted ABC fracture. Note the complete dissociation of both columns and WBD from the sciatic buttress. (*D*) A 44-year-old man following MVC with a comminuted PCPW fracture. (*E*) A 63-year-old man following a fall with an ACHT protrusion fracture. Anterior column, anterior wall, and ACHT fractures are frequently components of a geriatric protrusion fracture pattern involving dome impaction and quadrilateral plate comminution following low-energy trauma.

wall fragments are a source of confusion and poor interobserver agreement[5] because of ambiguity in differentiating low anterior column from anterior wall fractures.[13,16] Up to 65% of unclassifiable fractures involve the anterior column and quadrilateral plate.[30,45] Anterior wall fractures are trapezoidal and do not cross above the anterior inferior iliac spine (AIIS). The fragment involves a portion of the anterior roof and articular facet. The fracture line traverses the root of the superior pubic ramus distally and involves a portion of the quadrilateral plate and pelvic brim.[20,46] Unlike anterior column fractures, these fractures do not traverse the obturator foramen[37] (see anterior wall fracture, **Fig. 6**B).

Geriatric Protrusion Fractures

In geriatric protrusion fractures, the quadrilateral plate is comminuted, hinged posteriorly, and medially rotated (see anterior wall, **Fig. 6**B; anterior column, **Fig. 5**B; and ACHT fractures, **Fig. 4**E). The anterior column or wall component is usually markedly medially displaced along with the femoral head. The femoral head impacts the osteoporotic dome, resulting in a medial hollow, with 2 adjacent curves on coronal images resembling the wings of a gull (the gull-wing sign)[26,47] (impaction fractures, **Fig. 9**). In ACHT fractures, a coronally oriented fracture bearing the anterior column component propagates superiorly above the acetabulum into the ilium and crosses the

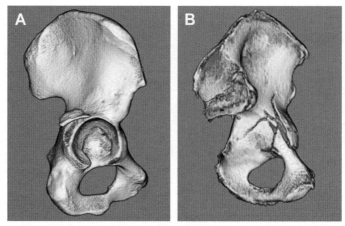

Fig. 6. Wall family fractures are elemental fractures of the posterior (*A*) and anterior (*B*) walls of the acetabulum. Anterior wall fractures are often components of a geriatric protrusion pattern fracture pattern and are usually trapezoidal in shape, involving the pelvic brim and quadrilateral plate. The superior extent is below the anterior inferior iliac spine (AIIS), differentiating these fractures from elemental anterior column fractures. (*A*) A 29-year-old pedestrian struck by a vehicle with a high posterior wall fragment. (*B*) An 83-year-old pedestrian struck by a vehicle with a trapezoidal anterior wall fragment below the AIIS. The fracture involves the pelvic brim and extends to the quadrilateral plate.

obturator ring inferiorly at the superior pubic ramus. A sagittally oriented fracture line is seen posteriorly resembling the posterior half of an elemental transverse fracture.[18] The periarticular and comminuted nature of geriatric protrusion fractures makes repair very difficult, and outcome is usually poor.[26]

Other Atypical Fractures

As with all classification systems, the Judet-Letournel system is oversimplified, projecting discrete categories onto a continuous spectrum of injury.[7] Atypical fractures are commonly comminuted with secondary or incomplete fracture lines.[30] Comminuted T-type fractures may resemble ABC fractures.[25] T-type, ACHT, and ABC fractures may have a separate posterior wall component, which can change the surgical approach.[11,30] Extended posterior wall fractures may propagate into the sciatic notch, quadrilateral plate, and supra-acetabular region,[25] and a variant T type with posterior column pattern may also occur.[20]

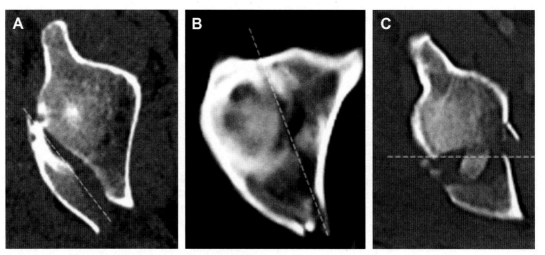

Fig. 7. Orientation of (*A*) wall, (*B*) transverse, and (*C*) column fractures on axial supra-acetabular CT images. Wall fractures are obliquely oriented and laterally located. Transverse fractures propagate in an AP (sagittal or near-sagittal) direction, and column fractures are coronally oriented.

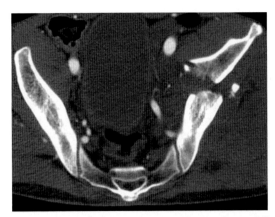

Fig. 8. Axial CT image of 53-year-old man after a fall from a 15-m (50-foot) bridge with a comminuted ABC fracture (surface-rendered image previously shown in Fig. 5C). The sciatic buttress is fractured and there is no continuity between the buttress and the weight-bearing portions of the acetabulum.

IMAGING IN THE CHOICE OF SURGICAL APPROACH AND FIXATION TECHNIQUES

Basic familiarity with surgical principles is important to understand how CT findings influence the surgical approach and hardware used. Surgeons frequently achieve articular reduction by realignment of the extra-articular cortical surfaces.[48] Direct visualization or palpation of the fractured front or back halves of the acetabulum gives the surgeon an indirect cortical read of the articular reduction. Cortical reads are used together with

fluoroscopy to reduce the joint.[1,49] At times, direct intra-articular exposure is required, which may be performed via arthrotomy or by using the fracture as a window to the joint. The choice of anterior versus posterior surgical exposure for reduction and fixation is simple for fractures involving only the front or back parts of the acetabulum but is less straightforward when both are involved.[10,19,49] In these cases, imaging features help determine the optimal approach. More than 90% of acetabular fractures can be treated with a single anterior or posterior exposure.[19,50] However, the approach for fractures involving both columns (transverse, TPW, T-type, and ABC fractures) is not consistent and depends on the surgical pattern, specifically the degree of rotation and displacement of anterior and posterior fragments (best appreciated on surface-rendered images) and obliquity of fracture lines.[19] The general rule of thumb is that the approach should address the aspect of the pelvis with the most displacement. Transverse family fractures are usually addressed from a posterior approach. Fractures with a predominantly anterior column component (anterior column, ABC, and ACHT fractures) are most commonly addressed via an anterior approach. Combined anterior and posterior approaches are unavoidable for some complex fractures with displacement of both front and back parts of the acetabulum, such as transtectal transverse or T-type fractures, ACHT fractures with significant posterior column

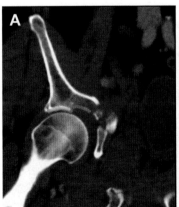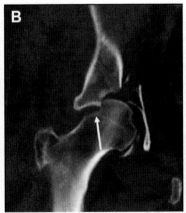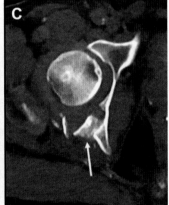

Fig. 9. Impaction fractures involving the dome (A), femoral head (arrow, B), and posterior wall (arrow, C) all confer a poor prognosis. In (A), dome impaction gives a characteristic gull-wing appearance formed by the intact dome, and medial hollow at the site of impaction (blue outline). (A) A 77-year-old man who fell 2.5 m (8 feet) off a ladder, with an ACHT pattern geriatric protrusion fracture. The patient underwent acute total hip arthroplasty (THA). The course was complicated by lower extremity deep venous thrombosis. (B) A 73-year-old woman after MVC with anterior column protrusion fracture and femoral head impaction (arrow), who expired from multiple severe injuries. (C) A 60-year-old man after MVC with posterior wall marginal impaction (arrow). He underwent meticulous reconstruction of the posterior wall using femoral head as a template via Kocher-Langenbeck (KL) approach.

involvement, and ABC fractures.[19,50,51] Single approaches are preferred whenever possible because of lower operative time, blood loss, and overall surgical insult.[1,48,51] Surgical modifications that increase access and visibility; specialized bone-holding instruments such as clamps, hooks, and forceps that allow reduction of minor displacements of remote fragments; and the use of percutaneous or conventional screws placed along reproducible osseous corridors have made it possible to achieve fixation of most fractures involving both columns with a single approach. The component remote to the surgical field should be reducible and not markedly displaced if a single approach is planned.[6,19,27,48,49,52–55] The ability to reduce fragments remote to the exposure requires a complex series of reduction maneuvers and increases with the surgeon's experience level.

Surgical Exposures

The most common exposures are the Kocher-Langenbeck (KL) approach posteriorly and the ilioinguinal or modified Stoppa approaches anteriorly (**Fig. 10**). Posterior wall fragments requiring fixation, which are seen in approximately half of acetabular fractures, preclude a single approach with an anterior exposure, and a KL approach is typically used.[4,51] The KL approach exposes the retroacetabular surface and posterior wall for direct visualization and plate placement as well as the sciatic notches for clamp insertion and digital palpation of the quadrilateral surface. Exposure involves splitting the gluteus maximus along its fibers, and medial reflection of the short external rotators: the piriformis, gemelli, and obturator internus.[48,51] It is the most common surgical exposure, used in nearly half of patients.[4,49] Several modifications allow direct visualization of a greater portion of the cranial and anterior aspects of the supra-acetabular surface. These modifications are helpful for large posterior wall fragments extending into the dome, and for corridor screw placement for fractures that involve both columns.[49] The most common modification is a trochanteric flip osteotomy (TFO). The trochanteric osteotomy fragment is retracted anteriorly with the gluteus minimus, gluteus medius, and vastus lateralis muscles.[48] A TFO also facilitates posterior femoral head dislocation for joint inspection and removal of intra-articular fragments through a capsulotomy or disrupted capsule and may limit heterotopic ossification by reducing the force of retraction.[48] The Gibson modification involves a more lateral incision that allows posterior retraction of the gluteus maximus, and unencumbered anterior retraction of the gluteus medius, greatly improving access to more anterior and cranial portions of the supra-acetabular region.[48]

The ilioinguinal approach is used to access the entire anterior column from the SI joint to the pubis.[48,49] Three windows (lateral, middle, and medial) are developed. The lateral window (lateral to the iliopsoas), created by releasing the attachments of the abdominal wall and iliacus muscle, exposes the iliac fossa down to the pelvic brim.[48] The medial window (between the iliac vessels and spermatic cord or round ligament) is accessed by division of the aponeurosis of the external abdominal oblique muscle and transversalis abdominis (anterior and posterior inguinal walls) and exposes the superior pubic ramus.[48,49] The middle window (between the iliopsoas and iliac vessels), developed by dissecting the IP fascia in the femoral canal, gives access to the true pelvis and indirect access to the quadrilateral plate.[48,49] Placement of hardware along the quadrilateral surface is difficult because access is incomplete.[48] Use of the modified Stoppa exposure, in which an expanded medial window is created using a Pfannenstiel incision and division of the rectus sheath, provides much better access of the medial

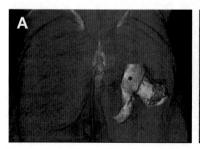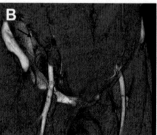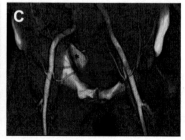

Fig. 10. Simulations of the 3 most common surgical exposures to acetabular fractures created using 3D CT images and region of interest masking. (*A*) KL approach with virtual trochanteric osteotomy, exposing the posterior column retroacetabular surface (*asterisk*) with improved access to the supra-acetabular region and joint capsule. (*B*) Ilioinguinal approach, exposing the anterior column from the SI joint (*arrow*) to the pubis. (*C*) Modified Stoppa approach with improved access to the quadrilateral plate (*asterisk*).

quadrilateral plate and posterior column surfaces via the true pelvis from an angle of 45° (see **Fig. 10C**). Dissection of the inguinal canal is not performed using a modified Stoppa approach alone but may be combined with a traditional ilioinguinal approach to increase exposure.[48,56]

The extended iliofemoral (EIF) approach is an extensile exposure of the entire lateral surface of the acetabulum for wide access to both columns.[19] The EIF approach is used rarely because of high rates of complications related to extensive muscle dissection, including abductor weakness, deep hematoma, devascularization of bone fragments, muscle necrosis, and fulminant infection.[1,8,19,49,57] EIF is reserved for severely disorganized fractures involving both columns not amenable to a combined approach, and for fractures treated subacutely (after 3 weeks) when callus formation and scar retraction limit fragment mobilization.[48]

Principles of Fixation

Buttress plating

Acetabular fragments always displace away from the joint, and realignment is achieved using buttress plating. Tightening of screws placed through a contoured malleable plate and secured into stable intact bone pushes the plate against displaced fragments, returning them to normal alignment.[49] At least 2 screws are used on each side of the fracture where possible for torsional stability. Buttress plates along the retroacetabular surface secured to the posterior sciatic buttress and ischium are used for posterior column and wall fractures. Undercontouring and eccentric placement of screws tension the plate, which results in compressive forces that help reduce anterior parts of the fracture.[46] Pelvic brim plates secured to the anterior aspect of the sciatic buttress and pubic body are used for anterior column fractures. An infrapectineal plate with a free distal end, oriented orthogonally to a pelvic brim plate, secured to the intact buttress typically via a modified Stoppa approach, can help reduce and stabilize a medially displaced quadrilateral plate in some geriatric protrusion fractures.[40,49,53,58,59] Comminution of posterior wall fragments is more common in the elderly than in younger adults, and mediolaterally oriented spring plates affixed to the stable medial wall afford additional buttress support of comminuted fragments. Hooks at the lateral ends press against bone fragments, aiding stabilization[8,46,60] (hardware, **Fig. 11**).

Screw corridors

Screw corridors are regions of the innominate bone with sufficient bone for screw placement under fluoroscopy. Partially threaded cannulated percutaneous screws placed using a guidewire and conventional lag screw techniques are typically used to supplement ORIF and secure non or minimally displaced portions of complex acetabular fractures remote to the exposure. In all cases, corridor screws must be oriented perpendicular to the axis of the fracture line to achieve adequate compression. The feasibility of a single approach to both columns therefore depends in part on the orientation and obliquity of dominant fracture lines.[48,54]

The anterior column corridor runs from the posterolateral supra-acetabular aspect of the ilium down to the pubic bone. Antegrade screws placed into the supra-acetabular surface are particularly useful for fractures involving both columns that require a posterior approach because of a posterior wall fragment.[53,55] Posterior column corridor screws are typically conventional screws placed through a pelvic brim plate used to secure the posterior fragment of a fracture involving both columns approached through a single anterior exposure (see **Fig. 11E, F**). Two screws are typically placed toward the ischial spine and tuberosity for tortional stability. Screws along the iliac corridor from the AIIS to the posterior sciatic buttress are used to stabilize high anterior column fragments. Percutaneous axial posterior column screws directed superiorly through the ischial tuberosity may be used for high posterior column fractures.[8,27,39,53–55]

Primary total hip arthroplasty

In elderly patients with poor bone stock and severe disorganization of the joint, the goal may be to provide sufficient stability to support a total hip arthroplasty (THA).[41] As many as 12% of elderly patients receive THA as their initial treatment, primarily because of the higher incidence of dome, wall, and femoral head impactions.[61] Acute THA involves first gaining stability of the 2 columns using standard techniques of ORIF and percutaneous screws. The columns do not require anatomic reduction because the press-fit acetabular implant replaces the articular surface.[39,41] Multi-holed acetabular components and reinforcement rings or cages allow placement of screws directed in ideal planes into the columns, perpendicular to fracture lines; in this way the acetabular component functions as an internal fixation device[8,41] (see **Fig. 11F**). Excision of the femoral head provides direct exposure of the joint, and the resected femoral head can be used as bone graft to reinforce the reconstruction.[8,41] Cerclage cables encircling the columns and quadrilateral plate promote stable cup fixation.[8,41,62] Postoperatively,

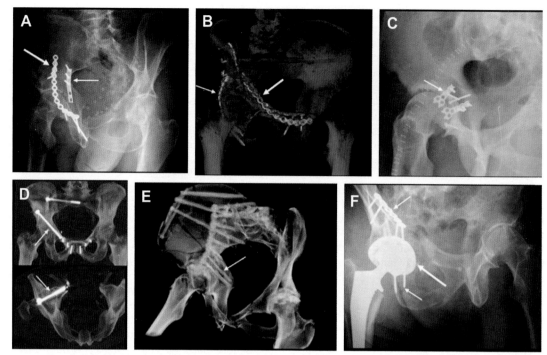

Fig. 11. Common acetabular hardware and screw corridors. (*A*) Anterior column protrusion fracture in 69-year-old man shown in **Fig. 5**B fixed with a pelvic brim plate (*thick arrow*) and orthogonal infrapectineal buttress plate (*thin arrow*). (*B*) Posterior column plate with eccentrically directed screws into the sciatic buttress and ischial tuberosity (*thin arrow*) and pelvic brim plate (*thick arrow*) placed via staged modified Stoppa and KL approaches in a 22-year-old man with a T-type transtectal acetabular fracture (previously shown in **Fig. 4**C). Marked medialization of front and back parts precluded repair using a single approach. (*C*) Comminuted posterior wall fracture in a 26-year-old man following MVC fixed with interfragmentary screws and spring-hook plates. (*D*) A 41-year-old man with transverse fracture following MVC, transfixed with an antegrade anterior column screw (*arrows*). (*E*) A 57-year-old woman with severely comminuted ABC fracture. Minimally displaced posterior column fragment transfixed remotely with posterior column screws (*arrow*) placed through a pelvic brim plate. (*F*) Acute THA (*thick arrow*) in a 77-year-old man with ACHT geriatric protrusion fracture and dome impaction (shown in **Fig. 9**A). The patient underwent acute THA (*thick arrow*) following fixation of anterior and posterior components with a pelvic brim plate and posterior column corridor screws (*thin arrows*).

the degree of subsidence on imaging may indicate loosening. Slight (1–3 mm) central and superior subsidence is expected while bone becomes consolidated; however, spontaneous loosening is more likely with subsidence of more than 3 to 5 mm[8]

Postoperative imaging with plain radiography or CT is performed to assess for quality of reduction and to ensure there is no articular perforation of interfragmentary screws, cortical penetration by corridor screws, or extension of spring-hook plates into the labrum.[46,54] CT is increasingly used postoperatively because presence of hardware does not obscure assessment of fracture reduction.[25,63] When plain radiographs are used, oblique Judet views are vital. Postoperative appearances can be confusing without knowledge of surgical exposures and fixation techniques to provide context for efficient and clinically relevant reporting.

IMAGING CRITERIA FAVORING CONSERVATIVE MANAGEMENT

Articular incongruities of the weight-bearing portions of the acetabulum, subluxation and mobility of the femoral head, and intra-articular osteochondral fragments stress and abrade the cartilage. All of these phenomena are considered under the loose umbrella term of instability. Instability and incongruity lead to unacceptable rates of posttraumatic arthritis and are therefore an indication for operative management. Bed rest and long-term traction are of historical interest only. Patients who are not candidates for operative management are mobilized despite articular incongruity. When operative management is indicated, traction is used in the preoperative period to maintain the head in a located nonsubluxed position.

In the short term, instability connotes inability to bear weight, preventing early mobilization.

Mortality is up to 4 times higher in patients treated with bed rest compared with early mobilization. Prolonged periods of recumbency cause thromboembolic phenomena, deconditioning with loss of ambulatory function, pressure sores, and septic complications.[41] In the long term, instability causes cartilage damage in a vicious cycle that results in osteoarthritis.[23,50,61] Surgery is difficult and risky, particularly in elderly and debilitated patients, and nonoperative management should be considered when feasible. Patients without WBD involvement, sufficiently intact posterior walls, and absence of intra-articular osteochondral fragments represent a small but important subset of patients that have a good prognosis with nonoperative management.[22] Special considerations apply to elderly patients with secondary congruence after ABC fractures. In all other patients, the acetabulum should be stable with normal joint contact stress in the presence of physiologic loads. Over time, concrete CT-based criteria conferring stability at the WBD and posterior wall have replaced vague concepts of the "personality" of the fracture.[28,64]

Roof Arc Angles and the Subchondral Computed Tomography Arc

The status of the WBD has been termed the greatest prognostic indicator in acetabular fractures.[65] Distribution of load must extend over a sufficient area of the WBD to prevent cartilage matrix deterioration.[22,65] Furthermore, when the more cranial extent of the articular surface is intact, the femoral head is more likely to maintain its relationship with the acetabulum. More cranial patterns result in subluxation of the femoral head and often warrant intervention. In cadaver specimens, excision of the acetabular roof within an arc of 45° produces marked deformation from increased pressure concentrations,[65] whereas excision outside of this cutoff produces only small increases in deformation.[65] Most acetabular fractures involve the acetabular roof at a measurement of less than 45°. However, when fractures are outside of this weight-bearing area, prognosis is excellent with nonoperative management if there is no other indication for ORIF.[1,22,27] Quantitative measurements may be necessary to determine whether the WBD is involved.[65] Matta and colleagues[65] described a method of measuring medial, anterior, and posterior roof arcs on AP, IO, and OO views respectively. On each of the 3 views, 2 lines are drawn from the center of the acetabulum-, 1 extending vertically and a second extending to the fracture. The orthogonal roof arcs form a hemisphere.[65,66] If the roof arc angle (the angle subtended by the 2 lines) is less

than 45° on any view, the WBD is involved. Assessment of WBD involvement is greatly improved with CT. The superior 10 mm of the acetabulum is equivalent to a roof arc of 45°[22] (**Fig. 12**). With knowledge of the section thickness, axial images are counted down from the most superior slice depicting the dense articular roof. If the fracture is visualized within this 10-mm interval (the CT subchondral arc), the WBD is involved and nonoperative management is contraindicated. Fractures that typically occur below the CT subchondral arc are infratectal transverse and low anterior column fractures.[2,22]

The Posterior Wall

Both the WBD and posterior wall must be stable in the presence of physiologic loads.[3,27] Measurements of CT subchondral arcs do not apply to fractures of the posterior wall, which occur beyond the plane of measurement.[9] Marked alterations in the mechanics of load transmission across the hip result after posterior wall fractures.[23] Creation of

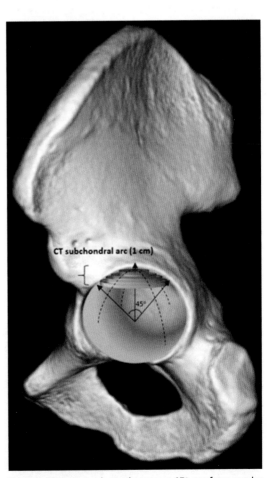

Fig. 12. Correspondence between 45° roof arc angles and the 1-cm CT subchondral arc. Fractures within this region involve the WBD.

fractures in the posterior wall of cadaver specimens results in decreased peripheral contact and increase in maximal contact force in the WBD.[23] Cadaver studies have shown that posterior wall fractures with more than 20% involvement of the wall are always stable, whereas those with more than 50% involvement are always unstable.[9,67,68] Counterintuitively, fractures involving a more superior portion of the acetabulum may be more stable than same-size fractures located more inferiorly.[28] Assessment of percentage posterior wall involvement should be made using the axial section with the largest fragment, typically at the central fossa.[28] If the amount of posterior wall involvement is between 20% and 50%, and all other imaging criteria suggest nonoperative management, dynamic stress testing with the patient under anesthesia can be an important problem-solving tool.[9,27] Approximately 7% of patients without definitive CT evidence of instability are unstable on fluoroscopic examination.[9] Late subluxations are possible despite initial stability in patients treated nonoperatively, and follow-up imaging with serial radiographs may be necessary.[28] Late instability is a devastating complication and difficult to salvage in young patients, which drives a low threshold for fixation. The current surgical trend is to proceed with fixation of most posterior wall fragments unless truly nondisplaced or stress negative under fluoroscopic evaluation.

Femoral Head Congruity

For nonsurgical management to be considered, all parts of the weight-bearing acetabular surface must maintain a congruent relationship with the femoral head out of traction, with parallel equidistant alignment at all points.[27] Loss of head-roof congruence often results from posterior femoral head subluxation and is a major predictor of hip survival[61]; 60% of hips showing this feature develop arthritis.[3,11] A posterior femoral head

subluxation of as little as 0.5 mm compared with the contralateral side on CT can result in cartilage wear and joint degeneration.[28] Because the patient is lying supine in the CT scanner, this is akin to a stress view.[28] If subluxation is visible on the CT scan, instability is already established, nonoperative management is not feasible, and posterior wall or CT subchondral arc measurements become extraneous.[3]

Absence of Intra-articular Fragments

Intra-articular fragments are seen in 25% to 35% of acetabular fractures[24,31,69] and are a source of severe hip pain and decreased range of motion, preventing early mobilization.[31] Fragments may be dragged into and trapped within the joint after reduction of dislocation[24] (**Fig. 13**). Presence of intra-articular bone fragments does not necessarily indicate open reduction, unless fragments are trapped in the weight-bearing area,[28,70] but should always be noted.

Absence of Dome, Marginal, and Femoral Head Impaction

Forceful impact of the femoral head against the acetabulum causes plastic deformation of metaphyseal trabecular bone and flattening of the acetabular fossa in the affected area.[7,16,49] Posterior wall impaction is best visualized on axial CT images, whereas dome impaction is best characterized with coronal images[27] (see **Fig. 9**). Restoration of joint congruity requires the use of elevators or an osteotome to raise the impacted fragment using the femoral head as a template,[71] either through a capsulotomy for posterior wall impaction or by working through the fracture or a surgically created defect under fluoroscopic guidance in the case of dome impaction.[46,49] The intervening metaphyseal defect may need to be filled with synthetic bone substitute or autograft before fixation with interfragmentary

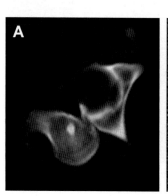
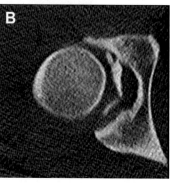

Fig. 13. A 26-year-old man following MVC with comminuted posterior wall fracture and posterior hip dislocation (*A*). Intra-articular fragments dragged into the joint during emergent reduction (*B*).

screws.[71] If dome, posterior wall, or femoral head impaction is present, nonoperative management is not a viable option. After repair, impaction has a high risk of collapse and good outcomes are elusive.[71]

Secondary Congruence

Fractures that are treated nonoperatively are deemed stable based on the criteria presented earlier. ABC fractures are one notable exception in which roof arc angles do not apply.[9] Because both columns completely dissociate from the sciatic buttress, the entire acetabular surface displaces medially along with the femoral head. With secondary congruence, both columns remain in alignment with each other and maintain congruence with the femoral head.[9,11,26] Letournel and Judet[11] described complete secondary congruence in greater than 80% of both column fractures. The concept of complete congruence has changed with the improved ability to detect steps and gaps with CT and the realization that small (1 mm) incongruities can be deleterious.[50] Biomechanical studies have shown that stress concentrations increase in the dome of the acetabulum with secondary congruence.[39,72] Malunion of the medialized acetabulum also results in abnormal biomechanics. Despite this, in elderly patients for whom surgical risk outweighs the potential benefit of an anatomic result, secondary congruence may be sufficient to restore a pain-free mobile hip with nonsurgical management using therapy-guided toe-touch weight bearing.[11,39,73] Serial radiographs obtained at intervals such as 2, 6, and 12 weeks are appropriate to evaluate for late displacement.[39]

Special Considerations in Geriatric Protrusion Fractures

Anatomic reduction is very hard to achieve after these fractures, and outcomes are often unfavorable, with rapid progression of posttraumatic osteoarthritis, particularly when medial dome impaction is present.[39,41] Anatomic reduction is achieved in less than 50% of patients more than 60 years old.[41,50] Again, the risks of surgery in elderly patients may outweigh any benefit, and nonoperative management may be favored for minimally displaced fractures because of poor bone quality, multiple comorbidities, and inability to tolerate the stress of major surgery.[8,41] Comminution greatly increases the likelihood of late displacement.[41] If there is central protrusion of the femoral head greater than 10 mm, nonoperative management is unlikely to be successful.[8]

IMAGING OF COMPLICATIONS
Osteoarthritis

Osteoarthritis is the primary complication following acetabular fracture, with an incidence of 27% to 38%.[1,4] ORIF halves the incidence of osteoarthritis.[2] The likelihood of requiring delayed THA within 2 years is high if age is greater than 40 years, reduction is nonanatomic, there is roof and posterior wall involvement, articular impaction is present, the femoral head is injured, or initial fracture displacement is more than 20 mm.[74] Postoperative imaging has prognostic value. If residual articular incongruities are less than 2 mm, the incidence of osteoarthritis is 13.2% compared with 43.5% with incongruities greater than 2 mm.[4] CT detects more articular incongruities than plain radiographs immediately after surgery and following healing, and deformities are consistently greater on CT.[29] CT is increasingly the preferred imaging modality postoperatively; however, it is unclear what benefit this may have in terms of improving clinical outcome.[6,25,27] CT findings that require revision surgery, including articular instrumentation, unacceptable reduction, and residual osteochondral fragments, are seen in approximately 2.5% of patients.[24,27,75]

Coarse categorical systems are used to grade radiographic evidence of osteoarthritis. Matta[50] introduced the following criteria: grade I (excellent) corresponds with normal appearance of the hip; grade II (good) with mild changes, including small osteophytes, less than 1-mm joint space narrowing, and minimal sclerosis; grade III (fair) with moderate osteophytes, less than 50% joint space narrowing, and moderate sclerosis; and grade IV (poor) describes advanced changes, large osteophytes, severe (>50%) joint space narrowing, and severe collapse or wear of the head.[50] Radiographic results have been shown to correlate well with functional outcomes.[65]

Heterotopic Ossification

Heterotopic ossification (HO) develops after long periods and may require resection months to years after ORIF. The abductors and short external rotators are usually affected.[76] Severe HO (Brooker class III, <1 cm between opposing bone surfaces; or class IV, ankylosis), causing contractures and stiffness, is seen in approximately 6% of patients overall but increases to 23.6% with extensile approaches.[4] When the abductor muscles are contused, the KL approach can also result in severe HO.[4] Additional risk factors include morbid obesity, traumatic brain injury, and prolonged mechanical ventilation.[77,78] CT provides better detail for grading HO than plain radiography (**Fig. 14A**).

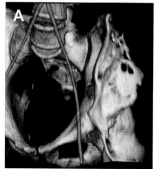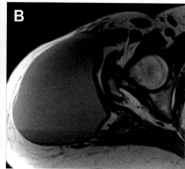

Fig. 14. (*A*) A 3D surface-rendered image of a 22-year-old man with multitrauma, including severe traumatic brain injury and anterior column acetabular fracture following motorcycle collision, who developed bridging (Brooker grade IV) heterotopic ossification over several years. (*B*) T1-weighted axial image in a 46-year-old woman following MVC, with right anterior wall acetabular fracture and Morel-Lavallee lesion showing intermediate signal intensity and layering debris. She underwent incision and drainage given the high risk of infection.

A hip that may appear completely ankylosed on radiographs may show discontinuity on CT.[76,77]

Avascular Necrosis of the Femoral Head

Avascular necrosis after posterior dislocation of the femoral head causes poor outcomes regardless of the method of treatment but is rare, occurring in 3% to 4% of patients.[10,11,50] Immediate reduction may decrease the risk of osteonecrosis.[3,79]

Sciatic Nerve Injury

Sciatic nerve damage is associated with displaced posterior column and wall fractures. Twenty percent of patients with posterior wall or column fractures, and 40% of patients with posterior dislocation of the femoral head, have sciatic nerve injury.[3,4,80] The peroneal division is most at risk, and sciatic nerve palsies typically result in foot drop.[3] Mild palsies generally improve, whereas severe palsies have unfavorable outcomes.[7,81]

Other Complications

Thromboembolic and local wound infections both occur with an incidence of approximately 4%.[4] Closed soft tissue degloving injuries (Morel-Lavallee lesions) shear the subcutaneous tissue from underlying fascia, typically over the greater trochanter, resulting in an infection-prone potential space.[3,7] Magnetic resonance imaging may better characterize Morel-Lavallee lesions, which are culture positive in a third of cases, requiring debridement and negative pressure dressing[3,7,82,83] (**Fig. 14**B). To prevent intra-articular spread, acetabular fracture repair must be delayed until infections resolve. Intra-articular infection is usually seen in the setting of posterior KL approaches.[50]

Septic arthritis destroys the articular surface of the joint, and salvage is difficult.[3] Infection, HO, and neurologic injury have potentially catastrophic effects on outcomes.[3] Nonunion is a rare complication, but fractures may take a long time to unite and changes of healing should normally be expected to last an average of 14 weeks, and up to 5 months in some patients.

SUMMARY

Acetabular fractures are encountered by radiologists in a wide spectrum of practice settings. The radiologist's value in the acute and long-term management of acetabular fractures is augmented by familiarity with systematic CT-based algorithms that streamline and simplify Judet-Letournel fracture typing, together with an appreciation of the role of imaging in initial triage, operative decision making, postoperative assessment, prognostication, and evaluation of complications. The steep increase in incidence of acetabular fractures in the elderly over the past several decades places special emphasis on familiarity with geriatric fracture patterns.

REFERENCES

1. Briffa N, Pearce R, Hill A, et al. Outcomes of acetabular fracture fixation with ten years' follow-up. J Bone Joint Surg Br 2011;93(2):229–36.
2. Laird A, Keating J. Acetabular fractures: a 16-year prospective epidemiological study. J Bone Joint Surg Br 2005;87(7):969–73.
3. Tornetta P. Displaced acetabular fractures: indications for operative and nonoperative management. J Am Acad Orthop Surg 2001;9(1):18–28.
4. Giannoudis P, Grotz M, Papakostidis C, et al. Operative treatment of displaced fractures of the

acetabulum: a meta-analysis. J Bone Joint Surg Br 2005;87(1):2–9.

5. Ohashi K, El-Khoury GY, Abu-Zahra KW, et al. Inter-observer agreement for Letournel acetabular fracture classification with multidetector CT: are standard Judet radiographs necessary? Radiology 2006;241(2):386–91.

6. Mears DC. A sobering message to acetabular fracture surgeons: commentary on an article by Diederik O. Verbeek, MD, et al. "Predictors for long-term hip survivorship following acetabular fracture surgery. importance of gap compared with step displacement". J Bone Joint Surg Am 2018; 100(11):e81.

7. Coughlin TA, Shivji FS, Quah C, et al. Acetabular fractures, anatomy and implications for treatment. Orthopaedics and Trauma 2018;32(2):116–20.

8. Mears DC. Surgical treatment of acetabular fractures in elderly patients with osteoporotic bone. J Am Acad Orthop Surg 1999;7(2):128–41.

9. Tornetta P III. Non-operative management of acetabular fractures: the use of dynamic stress views. J Bone Joint Surg Br 1999;81(1):67–70.

10. Judet R, Judet J, Letournel E. Fractures of the acetabulum: classification and surgical approaches for open reduction: preliminary report. J Bone Joint Surg Am 1964;46(8):1615–75.

11. Letournel E, Judet R. Fractures of the acetabulum. Springer-Verlag Berlin Heidelberg; 1993.

12. Riouallon G, Sebaaly A, Upex P, et al. A new, easy, fast, and reliable method to correctly classify acetabular fractures according to the Letournel system. JB JS Open Access 2018;3(1):e0032.

13. Saterbak AM, Marsh J, Turbett T, et al. Acetabular fractures classification of Letournel and Judet–a systematic approach. Iowa Orthop J 1995;15:184.

14. Ly TV, Stover MD, Sims SH, et al. The use of an algorithm for classifying acetabular fractures: a role for resident education? Clin Orthop Relat Res 2011; 469(8):2371–6.

15. Jouffroy P, Sebaaly A, Aubert T, et al. Improved acetabular fracture diagnosis after training in a CT-based method. Orthop Traumatol Surg Res 2017; 103(3):325–9.

16. Brandser E, Marsh J. Acetabular fractures: easier classification with a systematic approach. AJR Am J Roentgenol 1998;171(5):1217–28.

17. Saks B. Normal acetabular anatomy for acetabular fracture assessment: CT and plain film correlation. Radiology 1986;159(1):139–45.

18. Martinez CR, Di Pasquale TG, Helfet DL, et al. Evaluation of acetabular fractures with two-and three-dimensional CT. Radiographics 1992;12(2): 227–42.

19. Gusic N, Sabalic S, Pavic A, et al. Rationale for more consistent choice of surgical approaches for acetabular fractures. Injury 2015;46:S78–86.

20. Lawrence DA, Menn K, Baumgaertner M, et al. Acetabular fractures: anatomic and clinical considerations. Am J Roentgenol 2013;201(3):W425–36.

21. Hodge W, Carlson K, Fijan R, et al. Contact pressures from an instrumented hip endoprosthesis. J Bone Joint Surg Am 1989;71(9):1378–86.

22. Olson SA, Matta JM. The computerized tomography subchondral arc: a new method of assessing acetabular articular continuity after fracture (a preliminary report). J Orthop Trauma 1993;7(5): 402–13.

23. Olson SA, Bay BK, Chapman MW, et al. Biomechanical consequences of fracture and repair of the posterior wall of the acetabulum. J Bone Joint Surg Am 1995;77(8):1184–92.

24. Pascarella R, Maresca A, Reggiani LM, et al. Intra-articular fragments in acetabular fracture–dislocation. Orthopedics 2009;32(6). Available at: https://doi.org/10.3928/01477447-20090511-15.

25. Geijer M, El-Khoury GY. Imaging of the acetabulum in the era of multidetector computed tomography. Emerg Radiol 2007;14(5):271.

26. Chotai N, Arshad H, Bates P. Radiographic anatomy and imaging of the acetabulum. Orthopaedics and Trauma 2018;32(2):102–9.

27. Mauffrey C, Stacey S, York PJ, et al. Radiographic evaluation of acetabular fractures: review and update on methodology. J Am Acad Orthop Surg 2018;26(3):83–93.

28. Calkins MS, Zych G, Latta L, et al. Computed tomography evaluation of stability in posterior fracture dislocation of the hip. Clin Orthop Relat Res 1988; 227:152–63.

29. Borrelli J Jr, Ricci WM, Steger-May K, et al. Postoperative radiographic assessment of acetabular fractures: a comparison of plain radiographs and CT scans. J Orthop Trauma 2005;19(5):299–304.

30. Herman A, Tenenbaum S, Ougortsin V, et al. There is no column: a new classification for acetabular fractures. J Bone Joint Surg Am 2018;100(2):e8.

31. Griffiths HJ, Standertskjöld-Nordenstam CG, Burke J, et al. Computed tomography in the management of acetabular fractures. Skeletal Radiol 1984;11(1):22–31.

32. Dreizin D, Munera F. Blunt polytrauma: evaluation with 64-section whole-body CT angiography. Radiographics 2012;32(3):609–31.

33. Baghdanian AH, Armetta AS, Baghdanian AA, et al. CT of major vascular injury in blunt abdominopelvic trauma. Radiographics 2016;36(3):872–90.

34. Favinger JL, Zamora DA, Kanal KM, et al. Imaging of acetabular fractures: a phantom study comparing radiation dose by radiography and computed tomography. Semin Roentgenol 2018.

35. Fishman EK, Kuszyk B. 3D imaging: musculoskeletal applications. Crit Rev Diagn Imaging 2001;42(1): 59–100.

36. Burk D Jr, Mears D, Kennedy W, et al. Three-dimensional computed tomography of acetabular fractures. Radiology 1985;155(1):183–6.

37. Scheinfeld MH, Dym AA, Spektor M, et al. Acetabular fractures: what radiologists should know and how 3D CT can aid classification. Radiographics 2015;35(2):555–77.

38. Dreizin D, Nam AJ, Hirsch J, et al. New and emerging patient-centered CT imaging and image-guided treatment paradigms for maxillofacial trauma. Emerg Radiol 2018. https://doi.org/10.1007/s10140-018-1616-9.

39. Antell NB, Switzer JA, Schmidt AH. Management of acetabular fractures in the elderly. J Am Acad Orthop Surg 2017;25(8):577–85.

40. Ferguson T, Patel R, Bhandari M, et al. Fractures of the acetabulum in patients aged 60 years and older: an epidemiological and radiological study. J Bone Joint Surg Br 2010;92(2):250–7.

41. Cornell CN. Management of acetabular fractures in the elderly patient. HSS J 2005;1(1):25–30.

42. Durkee NJ, Jacobson J, Jamadar D, et al. Classification of common acetabular fractures: radiographic and CT appearances. Am J Roentgenol 2006;187(4):915–25.

43. Awan OA, Sheth M, Sullivan I, et al. Efficacy of 3D printed models on resident learning and understanding of common acetabular fracturers. Acad Radiol 2019;26(1):130–5.

44. Lim PK, Stephenson GS, Keown TW, et al. Use of 3D printed models in resident education for the classification of acetabulum fractures. J Surg Educ 2018; 75(6):1679–84.

45. Hutt J, Ortega-Briones A, Daurka J, et al. The ongoing relevance of acetabular fracture classification. Bone Joint J 2015;97(8):1139–43.

46. Ferguson T, Forward D. AO Surgery reference-acetabular fractures 2018. Available at: https://www2.aofoundation.org/wps/portal/surgery?showPage=diagnosis&bone=Pelvis&segment=Acetabulum. Accessed June 8, 2018.

47. Anglen JO, Burd TA, Hendricks KJ, et al. The "Gull Sign": a harbinger of failure for internal fixation of geriatric acetabular fractures. J Orthop Trauma 2003;17(9):625–34.

48. Cutrera NJ, Pinkas D, Toro JB. Surgical approaches to the acetabulum and modifications in technique. J Am Acad Orthop Surg 2015;23(10):592–603.

49. Rawal J, Arshad H, Bates P. Surgical stabilization of acetabular injuries: approaches and methods. Orthopaedics and Trauma 2018;32(2):121–30.

50. Matta JM. Fractures of the acetabulum: accuracy of reduction and clinical results in patients managed operatively within three weeks after the injury. J Bone Joint Surg Am 1996;78(11):1632–45.

51. Jimenez ML, Vrahas MS. Surgical approaches to the acetabulum. Orthop Clin North Am 1997;28(3):419–34.

52. Bozzio AE, Johnson CR, Mauffrey C. Short-term results of percutaneous treatment of acetabular fractures: functional outcomes, radiographic assessment and complications. Int Orthop 2016; 40(8):1703–8.

53. Hammad A, El-Khadrawe T. Accuracy of reduction and early clinical outcome in acetabular fractures treated by the standard ilio-inguinal versus the Stoppa/iliac approaches. Injury 2015;46(2):320–6.

54. Starr AJ, Reinert CM, Jones AL. Percutaneous fixation of the columns of the acetabulum: a new technique. J Orthop Trauma 1998;12(1):51–8.

55. Bates P, Gary J, Singh G, et al. Percutaneous treatment of pelvic and acetabular fractures in obese patients. Orthop Clin North Am 2011;42(1):55–67.

56. Karunakar MA, Le TT, Bosse MJ. The modified ilioinguinal approach. J Orthop Trauma 2004;18(6):379–83.

57. Helfet DL, Borrelli JJ, DiPasquale T, et al. Stabilization of acetabular fractures in elderly patients. J Bone Joint Surg Am 1992;74(5):753–65.

58. Archdeacon MT, Kazemi N, Collinge C, et al. Treatment of protrusio fractures of the acetabulum in patients 70 years and older. J Orthop Trauma 2013; 27(5):256–61.

59. Laflamme G, Hebert-Davies J, Rouleau D, et al. Internal fixation of osteopenic acetabular fractures involving the quadrilateral plate. Injury 2011;42(10):1130–4.

60. Goulet JA, Rouleau JP, Mason DJ, et al. Comminuted fractures of the posterior wall of the acetabulum. A biomechanical evaluation of fixation methods. J Bone Joint Surg Am 1994;76(10):1457–63.

61. Manson TT, Reider L, O'Toole RV, et al. Variation in treatment of displaced geriatric acetabular fractures among 15 Level-I trauma centers. J Orthop Trauma 2016;30(9):457–62.

62. Mouhsine E, Garofalo R, Borens O, et al. Cable fixation and early total hip arthroplasty in the treatment of acetabular fractures in elderly patients1. J Arthroplasty 2004;19(3):344–8.

63. Ohashi K, El-Khoury GY, Bennett DL, et al. Orthopedic hardware complications diagnosed with multidetector row CT. Radiology 2005;237(2):570–7.

64. Tile M, Pennal GF. Pelvic disruption: principles of management. Clin Orthop Relat Res 1980;(151):56–64.

65. Matta JM, Anderson LM, Epstein HC, et al. Fractures of the acetabulum. A retrospective analysis. Clin Orthop Relat Res 1986;(205):230–40.

66. Matta JM, Merritt PO. Displaced acetabular fractures. Clin Orthop Relat Res 1988;(230):83–97.

67. Keith JJ, Brashear JH, Guilford W. Stability of posterior fracture-dislocations of the hip. Quantitative

assessment using computed tomography. J Bone Joint Surg Am 1988;70(5):711–4.

68. Vailas JC, Hurwitz S, Wiesel SW. Posterior acetabular fracture-dislocations: fragment size, joint capsule, and stability. J Trauma 1989;29(11): 1494–6.

69. Rubenstein J, Kellam J, McGonigal D. Acetabular fracture assessment with computerized tomography. J Can Assoc Radiol 1982;33(3):139–41.

70. Rosenthal RE, Coker WL. Posterior fracture-dislocation of the hip: an epidemiologic review. J Trauma 1979;19(8):572–81.

71. Meena U, Tripathy S, Sen R, et al. Predictors of postoperative outcome for acetabular fractures. Orthop Traumatol Surg Res 2013;99(8):929–35.

72. Levine RG, Renard R, Behrens FF, et al. Biomechanical consequences of secondary congruence after both-column acetabular fracture. J Orthop Trauma 2002;16(2):87–91.

73. Gänsslen A, Hildebrand F, Krettek C. Conservative treatment of acetabular both column fractures: does the concept of secondary congruence work. Acta Chir Orthop Traumatol Cech 2012;79(5):411–5.

74. Tannast M, Najibi S, Matta JM. Two to twenty-year survivorship of the hip in 810 patients with operatively treated acetabular fractures. J Bone Joint Surg Am 2012;94(17):1559–67.

75. Archdeacon MT, Dailey SK. Efficacy of routine postoperative CT scan after open reduction and internal fixation of the acetabulum. J Orthop Trauma 2015; 29(8):354–8.

76. Wu X-B, Yang M-H, Zhu S-W, et al. Surgical resection of severe heterotopic ossification after open reduction and internal fixation of acetabular fractures: a case series of 18 patients. Injury 2014; 45(10):1604–10.

77. Mears DC, Velyvis JH, Chang C-P. Displaced acetabular fractures managed operatively: indicators of outcome. Clin Orthop Relat Res 2003;407: 173–86.

78. Firoozabadi R, O'Mara TJ, Swenson A, et al. Risk factors for the development of heterotopic ossification after acetabular fracture fixation. Clin Orthop Relat Res 2014;472(11):3383–8.

79. Tornetta P, Mostafavi HR. Hip dislocation: current treatment regimens. J Am Acad Orthop Surg 1997; 5(1):27–36.

80. Middlebrooks ES, Sims SH, Kellam JF, et al. Incidence of sciatic nerve injury in operatively treated acetabular fractures without somatosensory evoked potential monitoring. J Orthop Trauma 1997;11(5): 327–9.

81. Fassler PR, Swiontkowski MF, Kilroy AW, et al. Injury of the sciatic nerve associated with acetabular fracture. J Bone Joint Surg Am 1993;75(8):1157–66.

82. Hak DJ, Olson SA, Matta JM. Diagnosis and management of closed internal degloving injuries associated with pelvic and acetabular fractures: the Morel-Lavallee lesion. J Trauma Acute Care Surg 1997;42(6):1046–51.

83. Nickerson TP, Zielinski MD, Jenkins DH, et al. The Mayo Clinic experience with Morel-Lavallée lesions: establishment of a practice management guideline. J Trauma Acute Care Surg 2014;76(2): 493–7.

Frequently Missed Fractures in Pediatric Trauma
A Pictorial Review of Plain Film Radiography

Michael P. George, MD, MFA*, Sarah Bixby, MD

KEYWORDS

• Pediatric • Radiology • Fracture • Missed • Emergency • Radiography

KEY POINTS

- Missed fractures are common in pediatric patients because of the subtlety of findings, significant normal variation in the developing skeleton, and unique site-specific fracture patterns found only in children.
- Bones in children are distinguished by increased elasticity and porosity, the relative strength of the periosteum, and the vulnerability of the physis compared with bones in adults.
- Unique fracture types of the pediatric skeleton include torus or "buckle" fractures, plastic bowing and greenstick fractures, and physeal injury.
- Pediatric fractures are subtle. Understanding the mechanism and common patterns of site-specific injuries facilitates detection.

INTRODUCTION

Missed fractures are common in pediatric trauma patients. Fractures in children differ substantially from those in adults, because injuries may be subtle or even radiographically occult. Additionally, there is substantial variation in the contour of developing bones and the growth plate, such that normal findings may sometimes mimic injury. When left undiagnosed, untreated fractures can have serious cosmetic and functional consequences in children.[1] They are also the most common cause of medicolegal complications for pediatric trauma physicians, emergency room physicians, and radiologists.[2,3]

Understanding the mechanism and radiographic appearance of pediatric skeletal trauma facilitates detection of these injuries, which results in better outcomes for patients. This article examines the unique features of pediatric bone contributing to missed fractures, the incidence of missed

fractures, common injury types of the pediatric skeleton, and frequently missed site-specific fracture patterns, highlighting problem-solving techniques for challenging cases.

UNIQUE FACTORS OF PEDIATRIC BONE

It is an axiom of pediatric medicine that "children are not just small adults." This is also true of the immature skeleton. In adults, when a force is applied to a mature bone, the force propagates through the bone because of its rigidity, until the point of fracture, which manifests as a cortical discontinuity. Children have proportionately more cartilage and collagen than the adult skeleton and their bones are thus less rigid.[4] The increased elasticity and porosity of immature bone leads to a higher likelihood of fracture,[5] although the fracture is less likely to propagate. Furthermore, the outer periosteal sleeve of a child's bone is proportionally tougher than the inner fibrous cortex. As such

Disclosure: The authors have no financial interest, commercial interest, or potential conflict of interest with respect to this article and its publication.
Department of Radiology, Boston Children's Hospital, 300 Longwood Avenue, Boston MA 02115, USA
* Corresponding author.
E-mail address: Michael.george@childrens.harvard.edu

Radiol Clin N Am 57 (2019) 843–855
https://doi.org/10.1016/j.rcl.2019.02.009
0033-8389/19/© 2019 Elsevier Inc. All rights reserved.

pediatric fractures may demonstrate cortical deformity rather than discontinuity (the torus or "buckle" fracture).

The physis adds an element of complexity to the pediatric skeleton. This highly vascular structure is the site of longitudinal and transverse growth of long bones and manifests radiographically as a straight or undulating lucent band. Histologically, the physis is composed of resting, proliferating, and hypertrophying chondrocytes that undergo provisional calcification before being incorporated into the ossified metaphysis.[6] The physis is surrounded peripherally by the tough fibrous ring of Lacroix, which connects the epiphyseal and metaphyseal periosteum.[7] Because the periosteum at the level of metaphysis is weaker than the ring of Lacroix and epiphyseal periosteum,[8] fractures through the growth plate tend to deviate through the metaphysis (Salter-Harris II injury). Overall, physeal cartilage is the weakest structure in a child's skeleton.[9]

INCIDENCE OF MISSED FRACTURES IN PEDIATRIC TRAUMA

Musculoskeletal injuries comprise most occult injuries in the setting of trauma.[10] A review of the orthopedic and surgical trauma literature suggests that missed fractures are common, with retrospective studies demonstrating an incidence of between 2% and 9%,[11,12] and prospective studies showing higher rates of injury (11%–27%).[1,13] Unfortunately, most of these studies do not distinguish occult from missed fractures; and those studies that focus on missed fractures are retrospective in nature, comparing preliminary interpretations by radiology residents or nonradiologists with the gold standard of the finalized report. In such studies, the most frequently missed pediatric fractures are those of the fingers, distal radius, elbow, and proximal fibula.[14,15] Further prospective studies are needed to adequately characterize the true incidence and distribution of missed fractures in pediatric trauma.

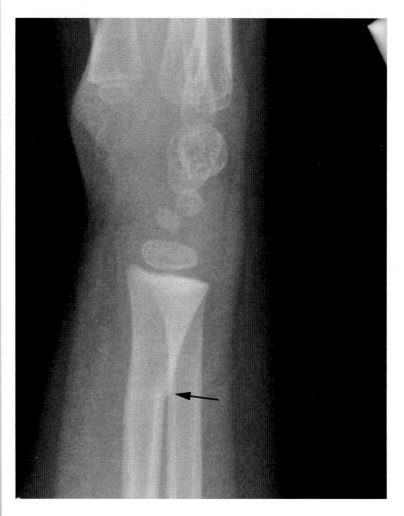

Fig. 1. A 4-year-old girl with buckle fracture of the distal radius (*arrow*) after fall.

UNIQUE FRACTURE TYPES OF THE PEDIATRIC SKELETON
Torus Fractures

Torus or "buckle" fractures are common in the pediatric population. These fractures most frequently involve the distal radius and ulna,[4] although they are frequently missed in the small bones of the hands and feet. The mechanism of the buckle fracture is an axial load, most often on an outstretched hand. There is focal convexity on the compression side of the bone and the tension side of the bone remains intact (Fig. 1).[16]

One notable variant of the classic torus fracture is the angled buckle, in which a primary axial and additional secondary force is applied to the bone. In this setting, the cortex does not bulge convexly, but angles sharply inward in the direction of the secondary force (Fig. 2).[17] These fractures occur most frequently through the metaphysis of the proximal radius, distal tibial, and distal humerus.

Both classic and angled buckle fractures are stable, treated conservatively with immobilization, and typically heal without complication.[18]

Plastic and Greenstick Fractures

Plastic or "bowing" fractures also result from excessive axial loading. In these fractures, the elasticity of immature bone permits increased curvature over the full length of the shaft, without cortical discontinuity or offset (Fig. 3).[19] These fractures most commonly occur in the radius, ulna, and clavicle.[20] Subtle plastic fracture may sometimes mimic physiologic bowing, but are easily distinguished with comparison views.[21] Although considered stable injuries, some authors advocate reduction of plastic fractures when the degree of angulation exceeds 20°, or if the bowing is cosmetically unacceptable.[22]

At some point, axial loading exceeds the elasticity of the immature bone, which fractures along the tensile side of the shaft, leaving the compressive side intact (Fig. 4). This a greenstick fracture. Unlike plastic fractures, greenstick injuries are unstable, and frequently displace even after splinting.[23]

Physeal Fractures

Salter-Harris I and II injuries are the most frequently missed growth plate fractures because of their subtlety. Salter-Harris I injuries result from shearing

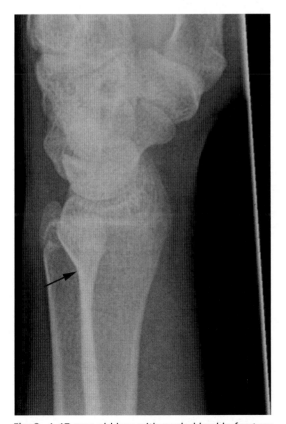

Fig. 2. A 17-year-old boy with angled buckle fracture of the distal left radius after a fall (arrow).

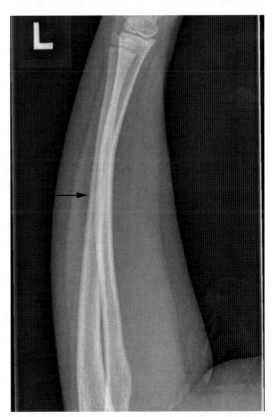

Fig. 3. An 11-year-old boy with bowing fractures of left radius and ulna (arrow) after fall.

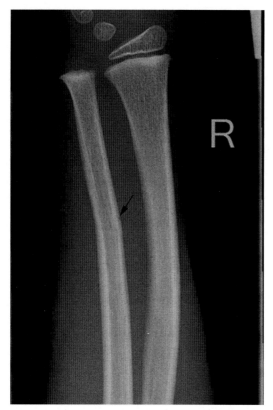

Fig. 4. A 5-year-old boy with greenstick fracture of the distal ulnar shaft (*arrow*) after fall.

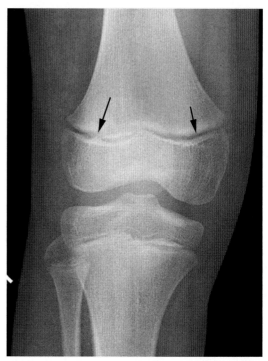

Fig. 5. Anteroposterior (AP) radiograph of the knee in an 8-year-old girl with a Salter I fracture of the distal femur demonstrates widening of the distal femoral physis (*arrows*).

forces applied to the physis, with the fracture plane passing exclusively through the growth plate.[24] Although offset of the metaphysis and epiphysis is easily recognizable, physeal widening may be the only sign of injury in some cases of Salter-Harris I fracture (**Fig. 5**). Comparison views are confirmatory when physeal widening is suspected,[21] because growth plate closure is typically symmetric. By contrast, Salter-Harris II injuries result from shear and angular forces, and deviate through the metaphysis (**Fig. 6**). The metaphyseal component may be subtle. A helpful sign in this setting is a bone fragment along the most distal aspect of the metaphysis (Thurston-Holland fragment) indicating metaphyseal involvement.[25] Finally, it is worth mentioning that physeal injury is often overlooked in older children, in whom the growth plate may nearly be fused. In this setting, the only suggestion of injury may be asymmetric sclerosis along the developing physeal scar.[26]

SPECIFIC PEDIATRIC FRACTURES PATTERNS THAT ARE FREQUENTLY MISSED
Shoulder and Clavicle

Coracoid process fractures are uncommon, but easily missed injuries resulting from a direct impact to the coracoid process secondary ossification center, typically during a contact sport (50%).[27,28] Fracture typically takes place at the base of the coracoid process,[29] in which the secondary ossification center is avulsed from the physis by the blow (Salter-Harris I injury). This manifests radiographically as widening of the coracoid growth plate (**Fig. 7**), best appreciated on the axillary view.[29] There is no standard management of coracoid process fractures.[30]

Little leaguer shoulder is an overuse injury of the proximal humeral physis that typically manifests in baseball pitchers aged 11 to 16 years.[31] Repeated overhead throwing motions damage the vessels within the metaphysis, altering the pattern of new bone mineralization at the provisional zone of calcification. This manifests radiographically as a widened and sclerotic physis (**Fig. 8**). Prompt diagnosis is critical, because bone bridges may develop without appropriate cessation of activity.[30]

So-called sternoclavicular (SC) dislocation is typically a Salter-Harris fracture at the level of the proximal clavicular physis. These injuries require significant compressive force to the sternum or clavicle, typically in the setting of motor vehicle collision.[32] The proximal clavicular physis, which does not close until 23 to 25 years, is the weakest

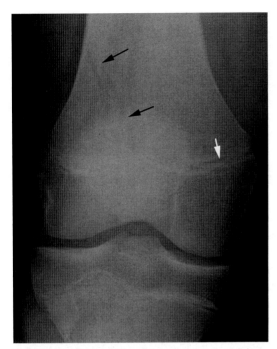

Fig. 6. AP radiograph in a 15-year-old boy with knee pain after trauma demonstrates an oblique fracture through the distal femoral metaphysis (*black arrows*) and widening of the medial physis (*white arrow*) consistent with a Salter II fracture.

component of the SC unit and fracture typically occurs through the physis.[26] Radiographic signs of clavicular physeal injury (or true SC dislocation) are subtle, and are suggested by asymmetric clavicular height (**Fig. 9**). Specifically, on a frontal radiograph, the difference in the craniocaudal positions of the medial clavicles should be less than 50% of the width of the clavicular heads.[26] If abnormal, cross-sectional imaging is recommended to distinguish Salter-Harris injury from SC

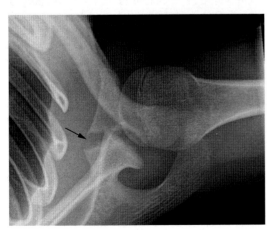

Fig. 7. A 14-year-old boy with coracoid process fracture (*arrow*).

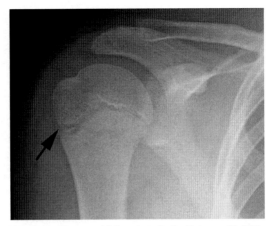

Fig. 8. A 13-year-old boy baseball pitcher with little leaguer shoulder. The proximal humeral physis is widened and irregular (*arrow*).

dislocation and assess for mediastinal complications, which are frequent.

Elbow

Supracondylar fractures are the most common elbow fracture in children. During a fall on an outstretched hand, exaggerated hyperextension displaces the ulnar olecranon into the dorsal humeral metaphyseal plate,[33] and the olecranon acts as the fulcrum of supracondylar fracture. Radiographically, the fracture manifests as transversely oriented supracondylar radiolucency (**Fig. 10**). Associated dorsal displacement disrupts the anterior humeral line, which normally passes through the posterior third of the capitellum,[34] although this finding is less sensitive in children younger than 4 years old.[35] Fractures are often subtle and a joint effusion may be the only radiographic sign of injury,[36] with elevation of posterior fat pad (**Fig. 11**). Because the anterior humeral line and fat pad are detected on the lateral radiograph, patient positioning is crucial. A good rule of thumb is that on a properly positioned lateral radiograph, a supracondylar "teardrop" should be formed by the anterior concavity of the coronoid fossa and the posterior concavity of the olecranon fossa.[36]

Radial neck fractures were considered rare, but a recent study by Emery and colleagues[37] suggests that these may be the second most common fractures of the pediatric elbow. Radial neck fractures are most commonly buckle injuries that result from hyperextension in the setting of an additional valgus force. These deformities are often subtle (**Fig. 12**) and comparison views may be necessary. They are frequently associated with olecranon fractures, which are the most common occult elbow fracture in children (**Fig. 13**).[37]

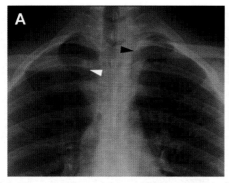 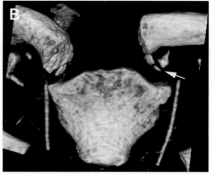

Fig. 9. (*A*) A 17-year-old boy with concern for sternoclavicular dislocation after trauma. The left clavicular head (*black arrowhead*) is asymmetric and projects higher than the right (*white arrowhead*). (*B*) Three-dimensional reconstruction from a computed tomography scan demonstrating a Salter II fracture through the proximal left clavicle on same patient, with the epiphysis and small metaphyseal fragment (*arrow*) maintaining alignment with sternoclavicular joint with superior displacement of the left clavicle.

Lateral condyle fractures are historically described as the second most common elbow fracture in children. These fractures result from a varus force on an extended elbow.[30] These fractures are easily missed, because they often primarily involve cartilaginous injury to the intercondylar region or capitellum, with only a slender bony fragment along the lateral condyle (Fig. 14). These injuries are often occult on the anteroposterior view, and an external oblique view may be necessary for confirmation.[33]

Medial epicondyle avulsions are considered the third most common pediatric elbow fracture, and typically occur in older children. The mechanism is typically a fall on an outstretched hand, combining hyperextension with valgus stress.[33] They may also occur in the setting of posterior elbow dislocation. The degree of avulsion varies from subtle widening of the medial epicondylar physis to intraarticular displacement, in which the displaced medial epicondyle mimics a trochlear ossification center (Fig. 15). For this reason, whenever "trochlear" ossification is noted, an orthotopic position of the medial epicondyle should be confirmed. It is

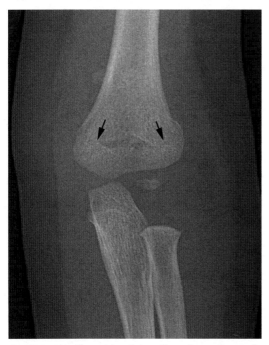 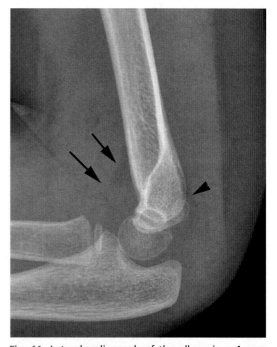

Fig. 10. AP radiograph of the elbow in a 20-month-old boy after a fall demonstrates a nondisplaced supracondylar fracture (*arrows*).

Fig. 11. Lateral radiograph of the elbow in a 4-year-old girl after fall demonstrates elevation of the anterior fat pad (*arrows*) and posterior fat pad (*arrowhead*) indicating joint effusion.

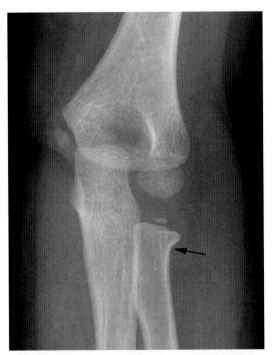

Fig. 12. Oblique radiograph of the elbow in a 4-year-old girl with pain 2 weeks after a fall demonstrates a nondisplaced radial neck (*arrow*) with subtle periosteal new bone formation).

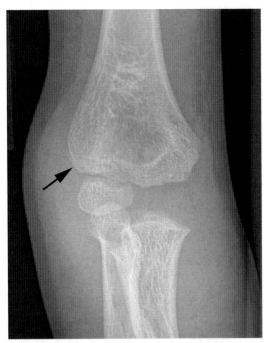

Fig. 14. AP radiograph in a 7-year-old boy with a lateral condylar fracture (*arrow*) of the elbow.

also worth noting that, unlike supracondylar and lateral condylar fractures, injuries of the medial epicondyle can occur without a joint effusion.[36]

Epiphyseal separation of the distal humerus is a rare but frequently missed (56%) Salter-Harris I fracture in young children and infants.[37] In infants, the cause is typically obstetric, but in younger children the injury raises concern for nonaccidental trauma. Radiographs most frequently demonstrate medial (93%) and posterior displacement of nonossified distal humeral epiphysis, radius, and ulna (**Fig. 16**). Confirmatory ultrasound is performed in difficult cases.

Wrist

Scaphoid bone impaction fractures are frequently missed buckle fractures that result from axial loading of the wrist during hyperextension. In children, scaphoid bone fractures often demonstrate shortening or contour deformity of the scaphoid (**Fig. 17**), sometimes with a thin dense band representing superimposition of trabecula. Loss of the navicular fat pad is another subtle sign of injury.[21] Given the substantial variation in the normal appearance of the scaphoid, comparison views are often helpful.

Hip and Pelvis

Slipped capital femoral epiphysis (SCFE) is the most common abnormality of the hip in adolescence.[38] It most commonly results from repetitive microtrauma to the developing femoral neck, often during growth spurts, with predisposing

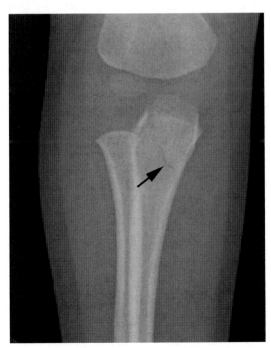

Fig. 13. AP radiograph of the elbow in a 32 month old with a nondisplaced olecranon fracture (*arrow*).

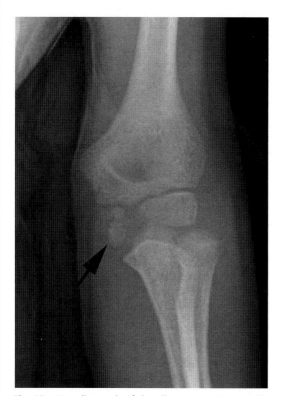

Fig. 15. AP radiograph of the elbow in an 11-year-old boy with a medial epicondylar avulsion fracture demonstrates the displaced epicondyle within the joint space (*arrow*) mimicking a trochlear ossification center. Lateral radial head subluxation is also noted.

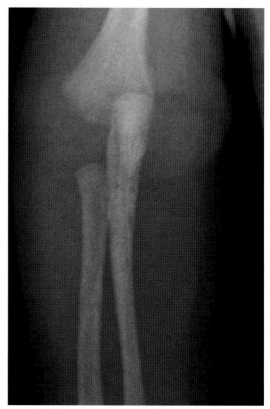

Fig. 16. AP radiograph of the elbow in an 11-day-old girl refusing to move the right arm demonstrates medial displacement of the proximal ulna and radius with respect to the distal humerus. Epiphyseal separation at the distal humerus was confirmed with ultrasound.

factors including hypothyroidism, hypopituitarism, hyperparathyroidism, obesity, and renal osteodystrophy.[39] SCFE is a Salter-Harris I fracture of the femoral neck. Muscular insertions below the great trochanter cause the femoral metaphysis to migrate anteriorly, laterally, and superiorly, causing the appearance of "epiphyseal" slippage. This is detected on AP radiographs by disruption of Klein's line and epiphyseal foreshortening. Performing a frog-lateral view increases the sensitivity of radiographs, although this risks worsening the slip in unstable (nonambulatory) SCFE (**Fig. 18**).[40]

SCFE is rarely missed in the setting of significant metaphyseal offset. However, it is more challenging to detect the preslip phase of SCFE, in which the epiphysis and metaphysis align. It is important to emphasize that early detection can have a profound impact on the patient's prognosis. Findings of preslip SCFE include physeal widening and demineralization.[39] Early or subtle SCFE can also be easily missed, because up to 60% of cases may present with a preserved Klein's line. The sensitivity of the AP radiograph is increased by comparing the width of the

epiphyses lateral to Klein's line, with a greater than 2 mm discrepancy suggestive of SCFE.[41]

Pelvic avulsion fractures are common injuries in adolescents and young adults, and reflect the relative vulnerability of the pelvic apophyses in the setting of forceful myotendinous contraction.[42] Acutely avulsed fragments are sharply demarcated, displaced along the path of their myotendinous unit, and with time become more sclerotic and ill-defined.[43] Nondisplaced avulsions are easily missed because the apophyses normally demonstrate a lucent physis. As such, any asymmetry of the pelvic apophyses should be treated with suspicion. Subacute or chronic avulsions can stimulate an aggressive periosteal reaction, mimicking osteomyelitis or malignancy.[44]

Knee

Tibial tubercle avulsion fractures occur secondary to forceful traction of the quadriceps during extension, frequently during jumping sports. They are most

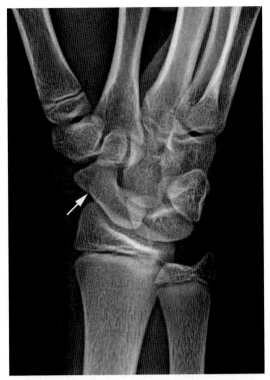

Fig. 17. Oblique radiograph of the wrist in a 9 year old with wrist pain after fall demonstrates mild buckling of the radial cortex of the scaphoid bone (*arrow*) at the site of a distal pole scaphoid fracture.

common in teenage boys, often with preexisting traction osteochondritis (Osgood-Schlatter) of the tibial tuberosity. Radiographically, avulsion fractures of the tibial tubercle may demonstrate discontinuity of the tuberosity tip, physeal widening, or intra-articular fracture. Isolated foci of mineralization adjacent to the tubercle are common normal variants, and typically do not reflect either avulsion fracture or Osgood-Schlatter.[45]

Patellar sleeve fractures also stem from contraction of the quadriceps, but typically during flexion.[45] In this fracture the intact patellar tendon avulses the cartilaginous inferior pole of the patella, potentially with a small bone fragment.[46] Patella alta and a joint effusion may be present. Because the insult of patellar sleeve fractures is primarily cartilaginous, plain film radiography tends to underestimate the extent of injury.

Tibial spine fractures result from forced hyperextension of the knee with avulsion at the insertion of the anterior cruciate ligament.[47] These fractures are difficult to detect on the AP view because of superimposition of bone, and are best seen on the tunnel or oblique views.[43] In the acute phase the superior border of the fragment is sharp and well corticated at the ligamentous attachment, whereas the inferior border lacks cortication (**Fig. 19**). These injuries are considered "anterior cruciate ligament equivalents," with operative management depending on the degree of displacement and size of the fragment.

Tibia

Classic toddler's fractures are common spiral fractures of the tibial diaphysis that often extend into the distal metaphysis. They result from torsional forces during early walking, but often present with pain referable to the ankle. These hairline fractures are usually nondisplaced and subtle cases are notoriously difficult to detect (**Fig. 20**).[21] Furthermore, in children who cannot bear weight, lower extremity fracture is often present even

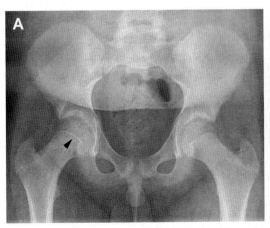
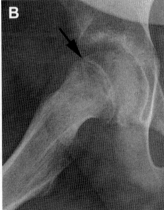

Fig. 18. (*A*) A 13-year-old boy with right slipped capital femoral epiphysis. AP radiograph of the pelvis demonstrates widening and irregularity of the proximal right femoral physis (*arrowhead*). (*B*) A 13-year-old boy with right slipped capital femoral epiphysis. Frog leg lateral radiograph of the right hip demonstrates mild posteromedial displacement of the femoral head with respect to the neck (*arrow*).

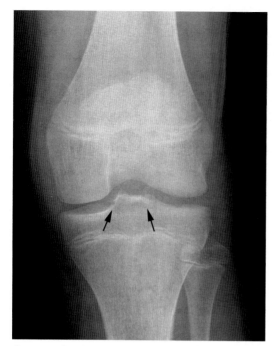

Fig. 19. AP radiograph in a 13-year-old boy after left knee injury demonstrates a minimally displaced tibial spine fracture (*arrows*). Incidental note is also made of a Segond fracture.

with "normal" radiographs.[48] Given the insensitivity of plain film radiography for this common injury, follow-up radiographs in 10 to 14 days (vs MR imaging) may be beneficial if the clinical suspicion is high.

Variant (type II) toddler's fractures have been recently described by Swischuk and colleagues.[49] These are also seen during early ambulation, and result from impaction and hyperextension forces at the level of the developing tibial tuberosity. Radiographically, they present with anterior or lateral buckling, transverse hairline fracture, and increasing concavity of the tuberosity (**Fig. 21**). The tibial plateau may be tilted anteriorly and inferiorly.[21]

Trampoline fractures are similar injuries of the tibial metaphysis, although they occur in older children (2–5 years). These fractures result when a trampoline is shared between partners of unequal weight. The mat recoils upward, meeting the descending child and loading the tibia with impaction and hyperextension forces.[50] The tibial metaphysis fractures transversely and the plateau tilts anteriorly and inferiorly. Like toddler's fractures, these injuries are often subtle or occult (75%) on plain film radiography.[51]

Foot and Ankle

The cuboid toddler's fracture is a frequently missed fracture[52,53] that results from vertical loading of a

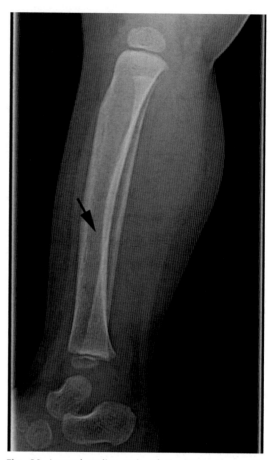

Fig. 20. Lateral radiograph of the tibia in an 18-month-old boy with limp demonstrates subtle nondisplaced toddler's fracture of the tibia (*arrow*).

hyperflexed forefoot, often during a fall from a bunk bed. The cuboid is impacted between the calcaneus and lateral metatarsals.[54] Acutely, radiographs demonstrate bandlike density of the cuboid because of superimposition of the trabecula, possibly with cortical deformation (**Fig. 22**). In the subacute and chronic phase, sclerosis predominates. Because there is substantial variation in the normal contour of the cuboid, comparison views may be helpful.

Metatarsal bunk bed fractures also involve an axial load, typically affecting the first metatarsal.[55] The typical radiographic appearance is of a buckle fracture with angulation (but no outward convexity) of the cortex (**Fig. 23**).

SUMMARY

Pediatric musculoskeletal trauma is easily missed on plain film radiography. Compared with the adult skeleton, immature bone is more porous and flexible, and the developing physes and apophyses are particularly prone to injury. Knowledge of

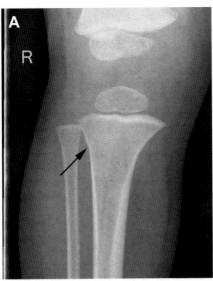
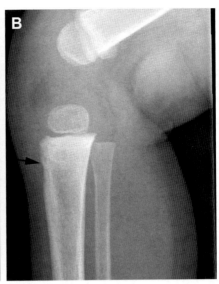

Fig. 21. (*A*) AP radiograph of the right knee in a 24 month old with limp demonstrates a subtle buckle fracture (*arrow*) at the proximal tibia near the tibial tubercle. (*B*) Lateral radiograph of the right knee in a 24 month old with limp demonstrates a subtle buckle fracture (*arrow*) at the proximal tibial tubercle.

unique fracture types and site-specific injury patterns is crucial to detecting subtle injury, and correct and early diagnosis can have a significant cosmetic and functional impact. Given the high degree of normal variation in the developing skeleton, comparison views of the (asymptomatic) contralateral limb, and/or short-term radiographic follow-up are reasonable strategies for managing equivocal cases. MR imaging may be considered in children who do not require sedation, if a confirmed diagnosis would lead to a change in management. Prompt diagnosis and management

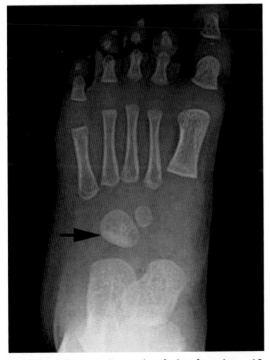

Fig. 22. Oblique radiograph of the foot in a 16-month-old boy with limp demonstrates sclerosis within the proximal cuboid (*arrow*) in keeping with a healing toddler's fracture.

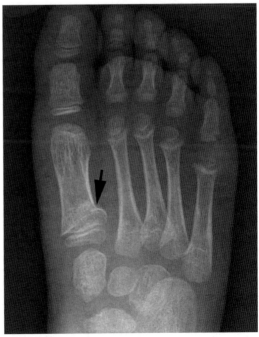

Fig. 23. AP radiograph of the foot in a 7-year-old boy with pain demonstrates a "bunk bed" fracture at the base of the first metatarsal (*arrow*).

has important implications for fracture healing, symptom relief, return to play/normal activities, and avoiding potential deformity. Understanding the classic imaging findings in subtle, common pediatric fractures helps ensure that these injuries are not missed.

REFERENCES

1. Heinrich SD, Gallagher D, Harris M, et al. Undiagnosed fractures in severely injury children and young adults. J Bone Joint Surg Am 1994;76-A: 561–72.
2. Segal LS, Shrader MW. Missed fractures in paediatric trauma patients. Acta Orthop Belg 2013;79: 608–15.
3. Berlin L. Malpractice and radiologists: an 11.5 year perspective. AJR Am J Roentgenol 1986;147:1291–8.
4. Little JT, Klionsky NB, Chaturvedi A, et al. Pediatric distal forearm and wrist injury: an imaging review. Radiographics 2013;34(2):472–90.
5. Frost HM, Schonau E. The "muscle-bone unit" in children and adolescents: a 2000 overview. J Pediatr Endocrinol Metab 2000;13(6):571–90.
6. Wattenbarger JM, Gruber HE, Phieffer LS. Physeal fractures: part I: histologic features of bone, cartilage, and bar formation in a small animal model. J Pediatr Orthop 2002;22(6):703–9.
7. Rathjen KE, Birch JG. Physeal injuries and growth disturbances. In: Beaty JH, Kasser JR, editors. Rockwood and Wilkins' fractures in children. 7th edition. Philadelphia: Lippincott Williams & Wilkins; 2010. p. 91–119.
8. Dwek JR. The periosteum: what is it, where is it, and what mimics it in its absence? Skeletal Radiol 2010; 39(4):319–23.
9. Jaimes C, Jimenez M, Shabshin N, et al. Taking the stress out of evaluating stress injuries in children. Radiographics 2012;32:537–55.
10. Soundappan SV, Holland AJ, Cass DT. Role of an extended tertiary survey in detecting missed injuries in children. J Trauma 2004;57:114–8.
11. Brooks A, Holroyd B, Riley B. Missed injury in major trauma patients. Injury 2004;35:407–10.
12. Enderson BL, Reath DB, Meadors J, et al. The tertiary trauma survey: a prospective study of missed injury. J Trauma 1990;30:666–9.
13. Sobus KM, Alexander MA, Harcke HT. Undetected musculoskeletal trauma in children with traumatic brain injury or spinal cord injury. Arch Phys Med Rehabil 1993;74:902–4.
14. Davis IC. Location of commonly missed fractures in a level 1 trauma center. RSNA 2012 conference paper.
15. Mounts J, Clingenpeel J, McGuire E, et al. Most frequently missed fractures in the emergency department. Clin Pediatr (Phila) 2011;50(3):183–6.
16. Slongo TF, Audigé L, AO Pediatric Classification Group. Fracture and dislocation classification compendium for children: the AO pediatric comprehensive classification of long bone fractures (PCCF). J Orthop Trauma 2007;21(suppl 10):S135–60.
17. Hernandez JA, Swischuk LE, Yngve DA, et al. The angled buckle fracture in pediatrics: a frequently missed fracture. Emerg Radiol 1996;(10):71–2.
18. Bae DS, Howard AW. Distal radius fractures: what is the evidence? J Pediatr Orthop 2012;32(suppl 2): S128–30.
19. Malik M, Demos TC, Lomansney LM, et al. Bowing fracture with literature review. Orthopedics 2016; 39(1):e204–8.
20. Siwschuk LE. Emergency imaging of the acutely ill or injured child. 4th edition. Lippincott Williams & Wilkings. p. 306–10.
21. Swischuk LE, Hernandez JA. Frequently missed fractures in children (value of comparative views). Emerg Radiol 2004;11:22–8.
22. Vorlat P, De Boeck H. Bowing fractures of the forearm in children: a long-term followup. Clin Orthop Relat Res 2003;413(413):233–7.
23. Randsorg PH, Siversten EA. Classification of distal radius fractures in children: good inter- and intra-observer reliability, which improves with clinical experience. BMC Musculoskelet Disord 2012;13:6.
24. Rogers LF, Poznanski AK. Imaging of epiphyseal injuries. Radiology 1994;191(2):297–308.
25. Cope R. Radiologic history exhibit. Charles Thurstan Holland, 1863-1941. Radiographics 1995;15(2):481–8.
26. Jadhav SP, Swischuk LE. Commonly missed subtle skeletal abnormalities in children: a pictorial review. Emerg Radiol 2008;15:291–8.
27. May MM, Bishop JY. Shoulder injuries in young athletes. Pediatr Radiol 2013;43(suppl 1):S135–40.
28. DiPaola M, Marchetto P. Coracoid process fracture with acromioclavicular joint separation in an American football player: a case report and literature review. Am J Orthop 2009;38:37–9 [discussion: 40].
29. Davis KW. Imaging pediatric sports injuries: upper extremity. Radiol Clin North Am 2010;48(6):1199–211.
30. Delgado J, Jaramillo D, Chauvin NA. Imaging of the injured pediatric athlete: upper extremity. Radiographics 2016;26:1672–2678.
31. Carson WG Jr, Gasser SI. Little leaguer's shoulder: a report of 23 cases. Am J Sports Med 1998;26(4): 575–80.
32. McCulloch P, Henley BM, Linnau KF. Radiographic clues for high-energy trauma: three cases of sterno clavicular dislocation. AJR Am J Roentgenol 2001; 176:1534.
33. Dwek JR, Chung CB. A systematic method for evaluation of pediatric sports injuries of the elbow. Pediatr Radiol 2013;43(suppl 1):S120–8.
34. Rogers LF, Mabave S Jr, White H, et al. Plastic bowing, torus, and greenstick supracondylar fractures of the

humerus: radiographic clues to obscure fractures of the elbow in children. Radiology 1978;128:145–50.

35. Greenspan A. Orthopedic imaging, a practical approach. Lippincott Williams & Wilkins; 2004. ISBN:0781750067.

36. John SD, Wherry K, Swischuk LE, et al. Improving detection of pediatric elbow fractures by understanding their mechanics. Radiographics 1996; 16(6):1443–60.

37. Emery KH, Zingula SN, Anton CG, et al. Pediatric elbow fractures: a new angle on an old topic. Pediatr Radiol 2016;46(1):61–6.

38. Crawford AH. Current concepts review: slipped capital femoral epiphysis. J Bone Joint Surg Am 1988; 70:1422–7.

39. Boles CA, El-khoury GY. Slipped capital femoral epiphysis. Radiographics 1997;17(4):809–23.

40. Hesper T, Zilkens C, Bittersohl B, et al. Imaging modalities in patients with slipped capital femoral epiphysis. J Child Orthop 2017;11:99–106.

41. Green DW, Mogekwu N, Scher DM, et al. A modification of Klein's line to improve sensitivity of the anterior-posterior radiograph in slipped capital femoral epiphysis. J Pediatr Orthop 2009;29(5):449–53.

42. Sanders TG, Zlatkin MB. Avulsion injuries of the pelvis. Semin Musculoskelet Radiol 2008;12(1):42–53.

43. Stevens MA, El-Khoury GY, Kathol MH, et al. Imaging features of avulsion injuries. Radiographics 1999;19:655–72.

44. Brandser EA, El-Koury GY, Kathol MH. Adolescent hamstring avulsions that simulate tumors. Emerg Radiol 1995;2:273–8.

45. Dupuis CS, Westra SJ, Makris J, et al. Injuries and conditions of the extensor mechanism of the pediatric knee. Radiographics 2009;29:877–86.

46. Green NE, Swiontkowski MF, editors. Skeletal trauma in children. 3rd edition. Philadelphia: Saunders; 2002.

47. Gottsegen CJ, Eyer BA, White EA, et al. Avulsion fractures of the knee: imaging findings and clinical significance. Radiographics 2008;28(6):1755–70.

48. Naranja RJ, Gregg JR, Dormans JP, et al. Pediatric Fracture without radiographic abnormality. Clin Orthop Relat Res 1997;342:141–6.

49. Swischuk LE, John SD, Tschoepe EJ. Upper tibial hyperextension fractures in infants: another occult toddler's fracture. Pediatr Radiol 1999;29:6–9.

50. Boyer RS, Jaffe RB, Nixon GW, et al. Trampoline fracture of the proximal tibia in children. AJR Am J Roentgenol 1986;146(1):83–5.

51. Hauth E, Jaeger H, Luckey P, et al. MR imaging for detecting trampoline fractures in children. BMC Pediatr 2017;17:27.

52. Simonian PT, Vaheyj W, Rosenbaum DM, et al. Fracture of the cuboid in children: a source of leg symptoms. J Bone Joint Surg Am 1995;77:104–6.

53. Englaro EE, Gelfand MJ, Paltiel HJ. Bone scintigraphy in preschool children with lower extremity pain of unknown origin. J Nucl Med 1992;33:351–4.

54. John SD, Moorthy CS, Swischuk LE. Expanding the concept of the toddler's fracture. Radiographics 1997;17:367–76.

55. Johnson GF. Pediatric Lisfranc injury: "bunk-bed" fracture. AJR Am J Roentgenol 1981;137:1041–4.